THE
TENNIS PARTNER

Abraham Verghese

HARPER ⬤ PERENNIAL

NEW YORK • LONDON • TORONTO • SYDNEY • NEW DELHI • AUCKLAND

HARPER ● PERENNIAL

A hardcover edition of this book was published in 1998 by HarperCollins Publishers.

P.S.™ is a trademark of HarperCollins Publishers.

HarperCollins books may be purchased for educational, business, or sales promotional use. For information please write: Special Markets Department, HarperCollins Publishers, 10 East 53rd Street, New York, NY 10022.

FIRST HARPER PERENNIAL EDITION PUBLISHED 1999.
REISSUED IN 2009 AND 2011.

Designed by Elina D. Nudelman

The Library of Congress has catalogued the hardcover edition as follows:
    Verghese, A. (Abraham)
    The tennis partner : a doctor's story of friendship and loss / Abraham Verghese.
        p. cm
    ISBN 978-0-06-017405-7
    1. Verghese, A. (Abraham), 1955– . 2. Physicians—Texas—El Paso—Biography. I. Title.
    R154.5.V53A3   1988
    610'.92—dc12   98-6749

ISBN 978-0-06-211639-0 (pbk.)

11   12   13   14   15   OV/RRD   10   9   8   7   6   5   4   3   2   1

For my sons, Steven, Jacob, and Tristan,
and especially for Sylvia

O

In memory of David Smith, M.D., 1959–1994,
James Searcy, 1936–1995,
and Adolph Sanchez, 1950–1996

Prologue

He had started rounds at five-thirty in the morning, working his way from one room to the next, writing progress notes as he went. He was at the bedside of his last patient when his beeper went off.

When he saw the number displayed, his throat constricted. A crimson flush spread up his neck, to his cheeks. The elderly woman with Crohn's disease and a short-bowel syndrome, who quite liked this blond, boyish doctor, looked up at him with concern. A minute ago he had been listening to her heart; now she could almost swear she heard his.

He staggered out into the corridor, and stood there, leaning on the chart rack. He took a step in the direction of the stairwell. Then stopped. Then took another step that way. Then turned back.

The flush on his face retreated, taking every drop of color from his skin until it matched the whiteness of the walls. His world and his vision narrowed and he was unaware of the nurse who walked by him.

He did not notice that his patient had come out of the bed, pushing her IVAC pump before her, the yellow, white, and clear bags dangling from their hooks. She stood staring at him through the doorway.

With great difficulty he wheeled the charts back to the nurses' station and took up his pen in a peculiar four-fingered, childlike grip. His hand trembling, he brought the progress note he was writing to a close. To anyone but a nurse, his handwriting would have been completely illegible.

He did not answer the page from the phones nearby. Instead, he took the elevator down from the fifth floor to the lobby and walked directly to Dr. Lou Binder's office.

Binder was waiting for the phone to ring. When he saw the intern in his doorway, he stood up. Before the intern could so much as open his mouth, Binder said, "Let's go to the lab."

But the intern could not move. He held Binder's gaze for a second, then his face crumpled, his shoulders sagged, and he slumped into a chair in front of Binder's desk.

"What have you done?" Lou asked, softly.

The intern sobbed, but no words came out.

○

An hour later, the two of them were at the El Paso International Airport, boarding a plane. Dr. Binder had not allowed him to go home for clothes. He had given one of his own jackets to the intern to put over his scrubs. The intern called his girlfriend from a pay phone but again the sobs robbed him of words. "I'm sorry" was all he could manage.

On the plane, a flight attendant had to remind him twice to put on his seat belt. He stared out the window as the plane took off, then made a steep, banking left turn allowing him to see the hospital clearly, and a few blocks beyond it, the Rio Grande, and Juárez, Mexico. The pilot leveled the plane, pointing it east for the one-and-a-half-hour flight to Dallas. Soon, El Paso receded from view, and with it his hopes and dreams. He had tried so hard, he told himself. Then he slapped himself in the face. Binder turned at the sound but was not surprised. "Not hard enough," the intern said aloud, to no one but himself.

○

In Dallas, Binder walked him over to the gate for the flight to Atlanta, and handed him his ticket. "The Talbott-Marsh clinic is your only chance."

The flight attendant collecting boarding passes could tell this was a significant leave-taking. She had a good sense about people, knew how to read the signs, having had years of practice. She was about to say something lighthearted about his scrubs, but decided not to when she looked in the man's face.

Binder watched the intern walk down the jet way. He remained at the window until the plane pulled away from the gate.

O

In Atlanta, four men awaited him. They introduced themselves: two were surgeons, one was an orthopedist, and one was an anesthesiologist. One of the surgeons was his father's age; the rest looked to be in their thirties or early forties. In the car, one of them said, "You won't believe me, but you'll look back and think of this day as the first day of your real life."

O

When they arrived at the cluster of buildings in suburban Atlanta that constituted the clinic, he was taken in to meet Dr. Talbott.

Doug Talbott, a big man with thick, silvery hair, came around his desk with an alacrity that belied his seventy years. His handshake was firm, and he took the young man's hand in both of his and led him to one of two armchairs that faced each other next to a fireplace. His smile, under a brigadier's mustache, was warm and unaffected.

They sat without speaking, the older man's fingers resting thoughtfully on the side of his face. Despite the scar over his eyebrow and a sunken cheek from what looked like an old orbital fracture, his face was kindly. After a long while, his voice emerged from the depths of his chest, soothing and with no trace of a Southern drawl, pausing after every sentence, letting each thought hang there before he brought out the next one.

"You have a terrible disease. You need lifelong treatment."

The intern sat, mesmerized, numb, conscious only of the sound of his own breathing.

"I am told I was a world-famous cardiologist," Talbott continued, his gnarled hands moving like delicate wands to punctuate his words. "But I don't know how. I was an alcoholic. When I couldn't swallow alcohol anymore because of the vomiting, the hiatal hernia, I switched to meprobamate, which was not considered addictive. Then Demerol, which was not considered addictive, then Talwin, which was not considered addictive, then Equinil, which was not considered addictive . . ." He smiled as he recited this, a tale he had told thousands of times, as if the naïveté of his generation of physicians still amazed him.

Talbott had been institutionalized several times, at one point spending a year and a half with psychiatrists who dismissed his alcohol use as a "cover-up for something deeper that you need to lie down on the couch and tell us about." After many relapses, after many rounds with AA, after his oldest son, disgusted with him, beat him over a kitchen table, his wife finally committed him to an asylum for the criminally insane.

"When the inmates found out I was a doctor," he said, his eyes twinkling, as if the funny part was coming, "they beat the hell out of me. Broke my face. Cracked my ribs. I remember lying on the floor in my own blood, spitting out fragments of my teeth."

He smiled, and the intern could see the glint of a gold tooth peeking out from behind the mustache. The smile evaporated, leaving in its place an expression of pain that the younger man recognized as the equal of his.

"It was at that moment, lying on the floor, I swore to myself that if I ever got out of that place alive, I would find treatment that was specific for doctors. I would make that my life's mission.

"Sobriety," he said, shaking his head gently, "is the easiest part of recovery. We are only peripherally involved with sobriety here. You can get sobriety in El Paso detox, or the county jail. What you *will* get here is true recovery. This will come from your recognizing that you have a disease, like diabetes. And just like a diabetic taking insulin and monitoring blood sugars, every day for the rest of your life, you will need to monitor and treat your disease.

"Unfortunately, society doesn't understand that you have a disease, a disorder in your forebrain, a genetic defect that makes you so susceptible. *You*—despite being a doctor—don't understand that you have a disease. Instead you see yourself as reprehensible, morally flawed." He leaned forward, as if imparting a secret. "And now, now that they caught you, you feel intense *shame*."

That word seemed to pierce the thin veneer of the intern's composure and, his facial muscles drawing up, he began to whimper. Shame was what he had tried to keep bottled in all day, shame had made it difficult to breathe on the plane, made it impossible to eat, and now shame overtook him completely and he boo-hooed like a baby.

The older man leaned back in his chair, his hands forming a steeple in front of his face. He made no effort to intervene. But he observed the young man, felt his grief, watched him weep just as he had watched four thousand or so other doctors over the years weep tears of shame.

He could see their faces clearly. Some were now dead from their disease. He could picture, as if it were a road map, the events that had led them to this state. When they were young college students, they had worked incredibly hard to get into medical school, forgoing the parties, the quick pleasures, in pursuit of the doctor dream. When they were accepted into medical school, and then later, when they graduated and survived the ordeal of internship, they had come to feel special. They had learned to be self-sufficient, and even to think of themselves as invulnerable, as if they had struck a bargain with the Creator in return for caring for the ill. The very qualities that led them to be doctors—compulsiveness, conscientiousness, control over emotions, delayed gratification, fantasies of the future—predisposed them to use drugs. When they did, to the very end, the physician-patient denied his or her patienthood. And when it all came crashing down, what they felt was monstrous, crippling shame.

"Don't confuse shame with guilt," he said eventually. "Shame says, 'I *am* the mistake,' while guilt says, 'I *made* a mistake.' You made a mistake, but you are not a mistake."

The young man composed himself as best he could. Despite what he was hearing, he could still think only of what he had lost, of how he had blown it, of how he was once again in a rehabilitation program. He had been on probation as a student, carefully monitored as an intern, given numerous chances, and now he felt in the pit of his stomach that he had blown the doctor dream, erased his ability to ever get a medical license in any state. What did it matter if he were sober or not—if he couldn't be a doctor, what was the point of any of this?

"I know you've been to recovery programs many times before, probably to some good ones, but none that specialized in doctors with addiction. As a physician, you have unique issues that we will address here. Don't get me wrong—the twelve steps are at the core of recovery, wherever you are. But as a doctor, what makes you unique is that your denial is exquisite, a hundredfold more entrenched than non-physicians. Even now as you sit there, you are in massive denial. In the back of your mind, you think that your biggest misfortune was to get caught."

The intern had his head down. He did not try to deny this.

"We'll talk more in the morning," Dr. Talbott said, standing up. "You're lucky to have arrived on the night of our weekly Caduceus Club. We started our first Caduceus Club here in Georgia twenty years ago." He glowed with pride. "We now have seventy-three Caduceus Clubs all over the United States and Canada."

○

They strolled across the grounds to a large building, the Anchor Hospital. Off to one side were some tennis courts, but if the intern, whose life and livelihood had for so long revolved around tennis, saw the courts, he gave no sign. The two men entered the building through a side door. The intern who had been to so many AA and NA meetings was unprepared for what he saw. Chairs had been pushed to the edges of a large dining hall to form a giant circle, and about a hundred physicians were seated, filling the room with a steady drone, as if this were a medical convention. Everyone was dressed casually, and he saw only one other person dressed in scrubs. His fear and shame rose again as his peers turned to glance at the newcomer with Dr. Talbott. But then, when he realized that every one of them was here for the same reason he was, he felt, for the first time that day, an easing of the weight in his chest. Some of the doctors smiled at him.

"If you think your problems are unique, you get over that in a heartbeat here," his older companion whispered to him, putting an arm on his shoulder. "Terminally unique. Every one of us thought we were terminally unique. We thought that M.D. stood for M. Deity." He sat down and guided the intern to a chair on his right.

"Shall we begin?" Dr. Talbott said, and the room quieted. Dr. Talbott nodded to a man sitting on his left.

"Hi, I'm Steve; I'm a neurosurgeon and an alcoholic," the man began. He was an intense, dark-haired man, with spidery hands and quick, birdlike movements of his head.

"HI, STEVE!" a chorus of voices said.

"I'm leaving here tomorrow after a four-month stay," he said, beaming. Others looked happy for him. "I feel good, grateful . . .

This is my second stay at Talbott-Marsh. I'm looking forward to being with my wife and kids. Lots of issues there, many things she has to forgive me for . . . I'm not going back into practice just yet. Still a few licensing issues that are being sorted out . . . But I'm not worried about that . . ."

"When you look back, Steve," Talbott asked, "what were the factors that made you relapse?"

"I stopped communicating," he said quickly. "Hid my feelings, started looking for faults in other people—my wife, my partners, anyone to blame for what I felt. I got on my 'pity pot,' started with the 'stinking thinking,'" he said, using his fingers to make quotation marks in the air, his words tripping over each other. "I was a dry drunk for months before I actually relapsed. I forgot that I had a disease. I thought I could actually take a drink and nothing would happen, no one would know. But I'm on a contract now with my medical society that involves daily Antabuse, urine checks, sponsor visits . . ." He had run out of steam. He added brightly, "One day at a time."

The baton was passed to the left.

"Hi, I'm Judy; I'm an ER physician and a cocaine addict."

"Hi, I'm Todd; I'm a nephrologist and a crack addict."

"Hi, I'm Bob; I'm a radiologist and an alcoholic."

Around the room, the litany continued: alcohol, amphetamines, crack, Valium, Lomotil, Xanax. Codeine in many forms. Every specialty in medicine seemed to be represented, particularly anesthesia. Fentanyl and sufentanil (both very potent narcotics) seemed to be the favorite of the anesthesiologists and surgeons.

It was now the turn of the other man in a scrub suit. He had linebacker shoulders, brown, curly hair, and handsome, movie-star features. The man had sat there with his arms folded, leaning back in his chair, wary of the proceedings. Now he uncrossed his arms.

"I just got in today. From California. I'm a vascular surgeon. I guess I'm here to find out if there is a problem. I'm here for . . . evaluation," he said, looking at Dr. Talbott.

"Tell us what happened, Kurt," Dr. Talbott said.

"I operated early this morning . . . As I was leaving the operating room, the administrator confronted me, along with the head of anesthesia. They said some fentanyl was missing." He shrugged. "I told them I had nothing to do with it—"

The other doctors were shifting in their chairs. The momentum of the meeting had been retarded.

"And the reason they suspected you?"

"Allegations at another hospital I go to that I had removed fentanyl. I was under observation, I guess, though no one told me." The silence in the room seemed to weigh on him. "No one has had any complaints about my work, I take good care of my patients—"

"Are you here of your own volition?"

"Well, yeah, I guess. If I didn't agree to come out here for an evaluation, they were going to report me to the medical society. Which meant automatic suspension of my license. Takes away my livelihood. So . . . I said I'd come. I didn't get a chance to pack, or to—"

"Tell us, Kurt, how is your marriage?" Talbott interrupted.

"My wife left me two months ago."

"And I understand you have been having a major problem with your finances?"

"I have a lot of debt, if that's what you mean. My partnership dissolved, so I had to set up my own office. But I'm getting back on track. I cover four different hospitals. No one has ever complained about my work—"

"The *work* is the last thing to suffer," an intense older man across the room burst in, unable to keep quiet any longer. He wore half-moon glasses over which he peered at the newcomer. He had a thick Southern accent. "The order in which you dee-stroy your life," he said, holding out his hand and pulling down fingers, "is first family, then you screw your partners, then you screw up your finances, then your health goes. Hell, your job performance is the last thing to go."

The burly Californian stirred in his chair. He was embarrassed. If this had been a staff meeting at his own hospital, he would have told this hick to go to hell.

"I should know, son," the man went on, whipping off his glasses, his tone softening, but not much. "I was confronted only when I passed out in the OR and fell face forward into the abdomen I had just opened. In the two years preceding that, I'd lost everything: my family, my friends, my money. I protected my job till the very end, and even when they sent me here, I still didn't think I really had a problem, came here to be ee-valuated . . ."

The surgeon from California was still. He had thought he could finesse his way through this evaluation, get back home in a few days, but it was starting to look more difficult.

"Okay," Dr. Talbott said. "Welcome, Kurt."

Kurt's stay—if he wanted a license to practice medicine—would be more than just a few days.

The bouncing ball was coming closer to the young intern from El Paso. He could feel his face getting hot, his mouth getting dry.

All eyes were now on him.

○

Later that night, in the on-site apartment he was assigned to share with three others, he went to the bathroom to wash up. He saw his face in the mirror above the sink, and he recoiled from it, the sight causing him to sit down on the edge of the tub. The image he had seen was of the person who had betrayed him yet again, a person he loathed.

Despite the stories he had heard that evening, despite the empathy of his new housemates, who had lent him clothes and toiletries, he was, if anything, more fearful. He had a sense of dread, of tremendous apprehension, and it had come to a head when he looked at his reflection.

More than any place he had been through before, he knew that the Talbott-Marsh clinic—if he wanted to practice medicine again—would force him to face that person in the mirror, would make him take down the bricks and mortar he had used to entomb his deepest, darkest secret. Out it would come, bellowing, ferocious and savage after years of confinement, and he would be forced to stand in front of it, puny and defenseless to face its wrath.

He raised his head slowly, lifted his chin, until once again his face appeared in the mirror. He ducked, and with an anguished grunt, he slumped to the floor, screwing his eyes shut and covering his face, believing, like a child, that if he closed his eyes and didn't look at the monster, it would go away.

Part I

Never ask a better player to hit with you . . .

—*Pancho Segura*

1

There are two Thanksgivings in El Paso. The one in November is observed much as it is in the rest of America: turkey, dressing, corn, sweet potatoes, and pumpkin pie, then motor shutdown, a retreat to the couch and TV. Six hundred thousand *Paseños* watch the Cowboys play in Texas Stadium six hundred miles east.

The other Thanksgiving is celebrated on the last Sunday in April. It commemorates the day Don Juan de Oñate's party of one hundred and thirty families, two hundred and seventy single men, eleven Franciscan friars, eighty-three wagons, and seven thousand cattle discovered *El Paso del Norte*, the Pass to the North. Previous Spanish explorers had taken the routes along the Conchos River to the Rio Grande, but Oñate's colonists had marched from Santa Barbara in New Spain (Mexico) straight up and across the treacherous desert north of Chihuahua city. By the time the advance party of eight horsemen scuffed through brush and cottonwood and finally saw the Rio Grande, they were cotton-mouthed, crazy with thirst. Two horses plunged in and were swept away. Two others drank enough to rupture their stomachs. What Oñate had discovered after the fifty-day desert crossing—the last five days with no water at all—was a magnificent valley formed by the Rio Grande as it emerged from the southernmost spurs of the Rockies.

Here, on April 20, 1598, Oñate stopped and held a Mass of thanksgiving. He claimed the new territory—New Mexico—in the name of Philip II of Spain a full two decades before the Pilgrims landed at Plymouth Rock. "I take all jurisdiction, civil as well as criminal, high as well as low, from the edge of the mountains to the stones and sand in the rivers, and the leaves of the trees . . ." This opening into the new territory—*el paso*—would be the caravan route, the lifeline of New Mexico, the jewel in the Camino Real.

○

Just as there are two Thanksgivings, there are two El Pasos. One is visible from the highway, an El Paso that a trucker traversing America on Interstate 10 from Jacksonville to Los Angeles might see and find nothing to distinguish it from any other American city but for the way it and the Franklin Mountains spring out of the parched and desolate land. He might catch glimpses of the Rio Grande bordering the freeway and beyond that see houses in Juárez, Mexico, sitting on a rise.

It might seem to such an observer as if a desert wind had gleaned pieces of Sacramento, Hackensack, Des Moines, and Dallas and deposited them here where they have rooted and now sprout Blockbusters, Kmarts, Targets, U-Hauls, and every other franchise flavor, their fluorescent signs beckoning like listless whores from both sides of the freeway. And to the trucker's eyes, what little desert he can see past the strip malls and billboards is occupied by bull-dozers and cement mixers that are paving over cactus and creosote with the same abandon they had shown Phoenix only twenty years before. From the cab of the truck, the town's founding father would appear to be Sam Walton, and the Wal-Mart edifice its epicenter. And then, fifteen or so exits later, the vision is gone—a forgettable mirage perhaps.

○

¿Dónde está la estación del ferrocarril? asked the audio Spanish tape in my car.

"La estación del ferrocarril está a la derecha," I replied, though I had no idea where the train station was.

After three days of unpacking boxes in our new El Paso house, I had risen before dawn, dressed for my first day at work, and then joined a wagon train of early risers, speeding in two columns, head-lights on, down a looping access road to that same freeway. Fortunately, the sign clearly said I-10 EAST, because in the limitless desert, without the sun, there was almost no way to tell. When Vásquez de Coronado and his party explored the Southwest in 1541, they used the sunrise as a guide, firing an arrow at the sun, and then, before they overtook the first arrow, letting fly another one and another, following this aerial trail until they came to the Rio Grande.

I sped past a square building, and off to one side I saw into a lighted window. A white-uniformed, dark-haired man hovered over someone else's knees, snowcaps on shapeless thighs. He stood as if picking logs from a woodpile. That's all I saw as I passed by. I swiveled my neck against the edge of the seat belt. I thought I saw a sign for the Coronado Nursing Center.

Then I was on the freeway, racing through the desert, the Franklin Mountains now on my left, the river on my right, that tableau from the nursing home well behind me.

But my mind insisted on lingering there, filling in the blanks. I could see the attendant folding over and wedging the soiled draw sheet under the bottom of a withered woman as she lay on one side. I could see him flip her over, using her knees as a lever. One tug and the bundled-up sheet was free and joined the growing pile in the laundry bag. She looked at his face, unable to speak, a prisoner in her own stroke-ravaged brain. And on his face was the set look of a man finding the necessary distance needed to finish work that was not particularly gratifying.

○

Alone behind our bedroom windows, alone in our cars, towns give us the necessary illusion that we belong. Until that moment, I had felt camouflaged in this new town, shielded from prying eyes, free in my new job to spin a new persona, to pitch my myth, the African-born-but-of-Indian-parentage-naturalized-American saga and to weave it into all the other dusty histories of The Pass. I loved the role of newcomer to town, relished the contrast between the lands I had left behind and this desert where there were broad spaces even between raindrops. I was still probing new words with my tongue, words like "cholla cactus" and "Mormon tea" that felt as strange as a new filling on a tooth. The novelty of the landscape, as brown and arid as Tennessee was green and fertile, its huge horizons, made it possible for me to feel I was on a spiritual quest. And yet, even as one reinvented a self, the things that made a journey tolerable were close at hand: paved roads, an airport, Midas mufflers, the Village Inn, and any number of places to buy thermal paper for the fax machine.

A newcomer is unencumbered by his past, his mistakes and

secrets unknown. This is the great promise of moving: that if you fold your life into a U-Haul truck and put it on the road, you will be given a clean plate with which to approach the buffet.

I had come barreling across the plains and the desert to settle in El Paso, driven by the same forces that brought Coronado and Oñate from New Spain looking for the City of Gold, the Fountain of Youth, the Seven Cities of Cibola, the Grand Quivira, El Dorado . . .

Their failure meant nothing to me.

But the sight of that nursing-home window had unnerved me, made me feel as if a giant eye had me in its sights.

Look here, the window had said, and I had looked.

2

Cartons full of my books and papers were stacked shoulder high, awaiting filing cabinets and shelves. The carpet was red. The walls were ivory colored, still exhaling the scent of paint. I ran my fingers over the surface. The new latex coat had formed dimples over old nail holes, dimples that in a few places had cracked to form tiny mouths. Once I could see the nail holes, my eyes played connect the dots to see if there was some clue there to the previous occupant. This was my new medical-school office, but on this first day it resisted me, or I it.

Through an entire wall of waist-to-ceiling windows I saw two pregnant women sitting side by side, rooted to a bench in the court-yard, motionless, their bodies having conceded to the new life within. Dark-haired both, and easily last trimester. The tan mask of gravidity on their cheeks and over the bridges of their noses made them look as if they were sisters. One covered her mouth and laughed as the other said something.

A new-issue white coat with the red Texas Tech School of Medicine logo on the breast pocket lay folded on my desk. It was longer than I was used to, reaching to my knees. I distributed my stethoscope, reflex hammer, handbook, tuning fork, flashlight, oph-thalmoscope, and my trusty Olympus among its pockets. The cam-era was the size of a pack of cards, with a built-in flash and autofo-cus. I held it at arm's length, looked into its iris, and snapped.

○

My office was in the Texas Tech Health Sciences Center building, a low-slung, two-story, ultramodern structure that housed classrooms, auditoriums, the medical library, the dean's office, and the offices of all the different clinical departments. My department, internal medicine, was on the ground floor.

Opposite the Tech building was its younger twin, the smaller, more anxious one, which housed the outpatient clinics. Both twins sat behind and in the shadow of the brooding mother, the eight-story Thomason Hospital building. We Texas Tech faculty and our house staff were the doctors for Thomason Hospital, and the hospital, in turn, served as our sole clinical and teaching base. Two mutually dependent institutions, connected by walkways and tunnels.

As I came out of Tech, I could hear a helicopter. I walked around the hospital to its side entrance and saw the snub-nosed insect, buzzing noisily, settling on the painted X in the middle of the parking lot, kicking up great clouds of dust. One of the realtors who had driven me around El Paso had told me he got his medical care at the fancy Hospi-Hiltons clustered on a rise north of the freeway called Pill Hill. But he had made no bones about where he wanted to be airlifted if he smashed up on I-10: Thomason, the best trauma center in West Texas. I hurried indoors, my tie clasped over my nose.

○

As I walked into Enrique's room, he asked his mother, in Spanish, to wait outside. She left without a murmur of protest.

"My mother has no idea," were his first words.

A teenager, would have been my guess, but the chart said he was twenty-two. His pale skin stood out against the jet black hair that he had corralled into a ponytail. He had a hairline so straight and low that it looked as if it had been drawn across his forehead with a ruler. Against a bounty of good looks, the violaceous bunionlike swelling on the tip of his nose seemed like a joke, a party gag he had strapped on. But his eyes said that this was no joke, and that the tip-of-the-nose lesion bothered him more than all the others that dotted his body, more than the elephantiasislike swelling of his legs. The intern's admission note said that six months ago Enrique's skin had blossomed with the purple spots of Kaposi's sarcoma, at which point he had shown up at the Texas Tech clinic, had blood drawn, and was found to have AIDS. He had bolted, failed to keep his follow-up appointment. For six months, I imagined, he had lived in denial, powdering over his most visible lesion. But three days of increasing shortness of breath had brought him back. His skin lesions were so numerous and so vivid now that when I pulled the sheet back, his body looked as if he had walked in front of a spray gun. His chest X ray had a ratty, moth-eaten appearance with indistinct opacities in both lung fields that obscured the heart borders, almost certainly more Kaposi's tumors in the lung.

"How did you explain the skin spots to your mother?"

He shrugged, the movement knocking his oxygen mask to one side. I put it back.

"I hid it. Till today." As far as he was concerned, only the lesion on the tip of his nose existed. "My sister is the only one who knows. She told my mother it was a cancer."

"Does your mother know you are gay?"

Again the shrug, a gentler movement. He stared straight ahead, depressed, fearful. I tried to see him with the eyes of his mother. She would have stroked his brow, seen that his eyebrows were plucked into sharp arcs, a stubble now growing back. She would have noted the clear polish on his nails. She knew he worked as a hairdresser. She knew.

"Maybe it will help you to tell her. You have enough to worry about—"

He shook his head.

"No . . . She has a weak heart. The news would kill her."

How many men in other cities had told me the same thing? And always their mothers' hearts had proved stronger than their sons gave them credit for.

In my previous positions in Iowa and Tennessee, I had taken care of a generation of gay men who had been infected in the early eighties, before that cumbersome word "AIDS" had found its niche on our tongues, before anyone knew for sure how it was spread. The message of safe sex had come too late for so many. But I guessed that Enrique had been infected long after the word about HIV was out.

"Had you heard about HIV before . . . ?"

"Yes . . . I just didn't think . . . the man I was with . . ."

I pictured him, when he was younger and unscathed, seeing the storm ahead but unable to resist pointing the prow of his boat right at it. It was, for me, the metaphor of all sexually transmitted illnesses. We talked about STDs cognitively, preached protection, as if the cognitive mind were in control. But it was some other part of the body that ruled at such moments.

He was breathless and aggravated even by the effort of speaking. I eased him into a sitting position. His lungs sounded better than his X ray had suggested. Over his heart, I heard a coarse, superficial scratchy sound with each beat—a pericardial rub, probably a sign of metastasis to the heart lining. I did not tell him this. In the creases of his groin were hard lumps—more Kaposi's invading the inguinal and iliac nodes and choking off the lymphatic return from his legs, making them swell. Each toenail emerged from the puffiness of a toe like a pig in a blanket.

With his permission, I pulled out my camera and took a picture of his feet. And his trunk. And his nose. It would allow me to make comparisons later, to see how he responded to chemotherapy. I saw four dots tattooed on the back of his hand, between the thumb and index finger, on the webbed area that is called the anatomical snuff-box.

"Oh, that? When I was a teen," he said dismissively, as if that were aeons ago. "It's a *pachuco* thing . . . the sign of the cross. Because of Cristo Rey."

Cristo Rey was a striking monument that sat about five thousand feet above sea level on a peak where the three states of Texas, New Mexico, and Chihuahua came together. It was visible from just about everywhere in El Paso. The figure of Christ, with outstretched arms, standing thirty-three feet tall on a nine-foot base, was an icon for the city. I had heard that on the last Sunday in October pilgrims wound their way up the mountain, stopping at the fourteen stations of the cross.

○

In the hallway, his mother stood with folded arms, squat and as solid as granite. Her face was pockmarked with acne scars. The same dark and intense eyes as her son, but otherwise nothing that would predict his beauty. Enrique had told me that she lived in Juárez and spoke no English. He lived in El Paso with his sister.

"*Momentito, señora,*" I said to her and sought out his nurse in the treatment room to ask her to translate for me. The ward, I noticed, was airy and clean. Sunlight from the big picture windows at both ends flooded the corridors and reflected off the waxed floor and the baby-blue walls.

Rosa was the nurse's name. I explained that I was the infectious diseases consultant called to see her patient. In a county hospital on the East Coast I might have had to wait, and she might have expressed resentment at being pressed into this service. But Rosa put down her pen, closed the cardex, and came with me.

"If I were to say 'SIDA' to the mother, would she know what we're talking about?"

"She knows already," Rosa said, smiling gently at me. "Trust me."

○

I tried out a Spanish phrase of introduction with the mother, one that I had memorized, offering her my name and the fact that I was *un especialista en enfermedades infecciosas*. The words felt like dry ice cubes on my tongue. Rosa pitched in when I faltered. Through her, I explained: A pneumonia . . . we had started antibiotics . . . hopefully, he would get better . . . awaiting tests . . .

The mother nodded with each piece of information, with each half-truth. And if she was curious about the skin lesions, she didn't ask. Nor did she bring up SIDA. I didn't mention the chemotherapy we would probably have to start that very day, his only hope. Then I spoke for myself, bypassing Rosa:

"*¿Tiene alguna pregunta, señora?*"

Her eyes dropped immediately.

"*Pos . . . no. Gracias.*"

No questions at all.

○

"*La* cafeteria *está en el* basement," I replied to an older man in a straw Stetson who had asked directions, hoping that border Spanglish would allow me the liberty of throwing in English when nothing else came to mind. His wife peered through lenses as thick as soda bottles. She wore a print dress that went to her ankles. The two of them appeared out of place and lost.

He thanked me and then added a lengthy postscript in Spanish that I didn't get. I explained that I spoke only a little Spanish. He smiled broadly, showing me a gold upper incisor, sheepish for having taken *me* to be Mexican. I smiled back. Had they been wearing a dhoti and a sari, he and his wife could just as easily have passed for natives in the corridors of Government General Hospital in Madras, South India, where I went to medical school. They shuffled off.

Behind the nurses' station, I found a chair and a section of counter space to appropriate so as to write my note in the chart. There were interns and students milling around, waiting for their attending physician. The academic year had started a month before, and I imagined that I stood out as a new face. Soon I would give a lecture, take morning report, have students sign up for an elective on infectious diseases, and thereby find my place, but for now I experienced the self-consciousness of a newcomer.

The four students with white coats that ended at their hips were Anglos. The interns in the longer white coats were foreign-trained physicians: There was one who was probably from India or Pakistan, another from the Middle East, and another who I guessed was Mexican or South American. And yet "foreignness"—my own and that of others—seemed less noticeable to me in El Paso than it had been in Iowa, or Tennessee. It was more than a question of the prevalent skin tone. One took a different view of foreignness when living on the border, when many of one's patients were wading across the river for care. By county edict, the hospital didn't ask for proof of citizenship. A billing address sufficed. It was common for a patient from Juárez to use the name and identity of a relative in El Paso. When the person whose name had been borrowed showed up as a patient, it caused all kinds of confusion in medical records.

3

A short and dark period from my childhood lingers, linked with the mem-
ory of a gloomy Abyssinian church. My parents, along with several
hundred other Indian college graduates, were recruited to teach in
the new schools Emperor Haile Selassie built all over Ethiopia. Like
the other Indian teachers, my parents were Syrian Christians, their
religion having its roots in the church St. Thomas the Apostle had
set up in South India after the death of Christ.

Every Sunday, after the Ethiopian throngs had packed into
church, worshiped, and left, the Indian community gathered in the
same church. It was a church the emperor had built—a scaled-down
version of St. Peter's in Rome. I recall the gargoyles, the basilica, and
the emperor's future tomb, already constructed in the nave. Despite
or perhaps because of the stained-glass windows, the church was as
dark as a catacomb, and the thick Persian carpets used as prayer
mats and rolled to the side after the morning service gave off a cor-
poreal odor to match.

I remember the boredom of standing through that interminable
service, listening to the nasal singsong of the priests, also recruited
from South India to teach in the theological college. The congrega-
tion pitched in tunelessly at the requisite times, unaccompanied by
any musical instrument. The service was in Syriac, an ancient Coptic
language, never used except in the liturgy and therefore gibberish to
us children.

It was a sad, serious, funereal ritual, and tears were rolling down
the cheeks of the women as they recalled God only knows what.
Smiling or giggling got your ear pulled. And so you stood, breathing
in the incense, eyelids getting heavy as you watched the to-and-fro
of the censer, only to be startled awake by the sacring bell.

After the service, the adults stood around and engaged in the insincere post-church palaver that was perhaps the social highlight of the week. Then we retreated home to that brooding silence with the lingering question always of what would happen next.

o

My memory of that period is tied up with sounds and smells: rain rattling on a corrugated tin roof, the scent of wet eucalyptus, raised voices inside the house that brought my heart to my throat, the telephone shattering against a wall, wood smoke from the fireplace, and, worst of all, silences that settled like a shroud and heightened until they were a constant keening.

But to the outside world, what was presented was a front of normality, a smooth surface where children went to school and adults to work, and maids clanged and cooked in the kitchen, and the gardener sang to himself as he cut the grass with his sickle, squatting and crab-walking across the lawn.

I was nine and clinging to the surface appearance, not fully subscribing to it but frightened of what lay beneath if I let go. And of course, I was convinced that I was in some way responsible for my parents' troubles. Though my parents' squabbling stopped in a year, my emotional barometer had already been established. I was suspicious of normality.

If as a child I could not understand the dynamics of what was happening *inside*, I did not need to go far to escape. I would say anything, lie like a grown-up just to get *outside*. I didn't care about the certain punishment for unfinished homework that awaited me at school. The sting of a ruler was sharp but lasted only a minute, whereas the walls of our house, the furniture, crowded around my head like a vice. The sound of rain pinging against the tin roof drove me mad.

Outdoors, I needed only my tennis racket and a ball. Against the warped side of a shed, I played imaginary opponents, humbling Tilden, Laver, and Pancho Segura with my Slazenger. There were so many erratic ways the ball could come off that shed and I knew every one of them. With my eyes shut, I could predict the trajectory of the ball. That triplet of sounds the ball made as it looped between racket, shed, and ground was utterly mesmerizing, soothing, and I yearned to keep it going without interruption.

Years later, in medical school, when we learned to auscultate the heart, I leaned over a patient's wicker-basket chest and heard a gallop rhythm of heart failure for the first time—*lub-de-uh, lub-de-uh*. My own heart quickened in recognition. When I lifted my stethoscope off the patient, a dark, bilious wave swept over me, carried me to the exact state of mind that I must have had as a child: a precocious anxiety that could only be obliterated by constant activity, by the metronomic tattoo of the ball.

My parents perhaps wondered if I was autistic, but at least that *thunk-a-thup* told them that I was at home, not off somewhere on my bicycle, my other more elaborate escape. During school vacations, I could stay on the saddle from dawn to dusk, the whirring wheels pacifying me, that sound perhaps linked to the hum of the umbilical artery, or the uterine soufflé, or some other maternal murmur.

I fancied myself a spy. I kept tiny notebooks—a kind I can no longer find—and filled them with detailed entries on the half-caste, Italian-Ethiopian madam who ran the bar opposite our house, sketches of the open-toed high-heeled pumps that did something remarkable to her ankles and calves, a drawing of the tribal tattoo that circled her neck like a choker. There was an army general who inadvertently became one of my subjects when I saw his Mercedes parked discreetly at the back of the bar on two separate occasions. I knew where he lived, and even followed him to his office.

I thought of myself as invisible, then. I wonder now how others must have viewed me. I can see it now, as if in a movie: A medium shot from twelve feet high: a brown Indian kid with unruly hair flying around on his blue Hercules, hands rarely on the handles, the bike an extension of his body. He sails into the frame and eyes everyone and everything, including the camera, with a steady gaze of ownership.

For an invisible boy I formed quick friendships: with the *listiros*—the shoe shine boys who worked the bars. With the maids, both ours and those of our neighbors. With the coolies who ported goods on their heads, who spent whatever they made to get drunk on *tej* and *tela*. With the Arab shopkeepers who lived in the closet-size souks that sold everything from cigarettes to my little notebooks, and who spent all day sitting and chewing leaves of *khat*, planeloads of which were flown in—legally—from Yemen and Djibouti. The Koran did not forbid *khat,* and so every waking minute they plucked a few leaves and stalks from the pile next to them, and replenished the bulges in their cheeks. Sometimes they gave me a few leaves to chew. It produced a mild, speedlike high, explaining their ability to spend a life behind a tiny shop counter with such equanimity.

○

Twice a week, in the evenings, Mr. Swaminathan gave me and three other children a group lesson, one hour on the courts of my school, the English school, courts that had been installed for the British teachers and their friends. First we stood in a line like marionettes, Mr. Swaminathan in front and slightly to one side of us. He had us follow his movements, a dry run in slow motion *without* the ball: the candy cane, looped backswing, then the knee bend and pivot as we transferred weight into the stroke, front foot stepping into the ball, and then a full follow-through that brought the wrist up to face level and the racket above the head. He peered over his shoulder to inspect our poses. Once he was satisfied, he would cross to the other side of the net.

He used no ball buckets or ball hoppers or hampers, but instead used his pockets and his left hand, which could hold five balls in a pyramid. He was restocked periodically by the two Ethiopian ball boys. The balls, like most products in Africa, were imported and therefore quite expensive. The nap on them was worn to a mud brown, the original white color just a memory. They came off the racket with a flat, squishy sound quite unlike the *thock* of today's high-pressure balls.

Mr. Swaminathan's Dunlop Maxply racket had a face that would seem microscopic by today's standards. The secret was timing. The long, supple strokes began in the feet and were fed by knee, hip, and shoulder turns, and culminated in the racket face meeting the ball at just the right moment in time and at the geometric center of the racket head to send it off precisely on its path. It was a minimalist style, beautiful to watch, a contrast to the grunting, hopping-in-place, windmill hyperactivity of a Monica Seles.

He would drill us with forehands, then backhands, then line us up at the net for volleys, then it was time to point our left hands to the sky to track down overheads, and after that to serve. Then he paired us up for a quick doubles game, each person serving just once, and with that the lesson was over.

How I relived those lessons in the dark, within the confines of my mosquito net: a ball coming at me from another racket and not from a wall, my backswing, the shuffle of my feet, then contact and follow-through, the ball sailing away and kicking up clay at the baseline. My notebooks now had equal parts spy material and tennis. Mr. Swaminathan's casual asides were weighty aphorisms to me, recorded with more diligence than any schoolwork. *Racket back as soon as the ball leaves your opponent's racket. Meet the ball in front of you. Hit through the ball.*

Soon, on weekends, a scrawny, brown-skinned boy carrying a tan Slazenger racket rested his blue Hercules against a fence and watched the white folks play, fantasizing that a fourth would be needed and he would be the only person available. I even ball-boyed alongside the Ethiopian ball boys in the hope of being invited to play. I was better than a good number of the players there, tactically smarter. Hit short, bring the opponent in, lob over them. If they got it back, simply do it again. But the invitation never came.

Instead, I discovered that the father of one of the girls in my class was having an affair with one of our teachers. Her husband was an athletic, handsome man, a favorite of all the children, particularly the Indians, because he staunchly supported our cricket club. So it pained me to describe in my notebook the intimate glances, the stolen asides between the two lovers. One day after tennis I saw them leave in his car. He had not opened the door for her. When he was behind the wheel, he kissed her hungrily and quickly, like a man trying to eat a meal in one swallow. Months later, when the couple ran off together, abandoning their spouses, she pregnant with his child, the news rattled the expat society. I wasn't surprised. Tennis was so much more than a game. What you saw—four people, a ball, and lines that determined whether a ball was in or out—was but an illusion.

I showed promise with my lessons and picked up the game quickly. My parents were not particularly athletic, and had no reason to nurture a tennis dream. No, for people like us, tennis was a social asset akin to contract bridge or playing the piano. And even that was debatable; look what tennis had led to: an affair, divorce, the breakup of two families.

○

Years later, during my internship in America, where courts and partners were abundant, I rediscovered tennis, took it up again with a vengeance that I was too ashamed to explain. I played for hours on end, setting up matches back to back. And in that frenzy, something else happened: The restless and secretive boy who shunned interiors, who loved the outside, who worried that he was an alien, reappeared. My wife, Rajani, enjoyed tennis and we sometimes played together, but the time I was spending on the courts was excessive. Other men, she pointed out quite correctly, weren't out there anywhere near as much.

That comparison brought back the whirring sound of my bicycle wheels, made me retreat further into secretiveness, made me aware again of a surface, of the contrast between the appearance of things and what lay underneath, how I was once again trying to stay afloat, to appear to be swimming with everyone else, when all the while, the murky depths beckoned me.

4

Just a few weeks after Rajani and our two children, Steven and Jacob, moved to El Paso, an Indian restaurant opened in town. It was located on Airway, a well-traveled strip that led from the airport to I-10, a visitor's first glimpse of El Paso. To the mix of car dealerships, hotels, and strip malls now came the Delhi Palace.

Its front door opened to a reception area and bar. An elderly Sikh, distinguished-looking in his turban and gray beard, presided behind the cash register. His son, the maître d', also turbaned, led us through an arched doorway into the dining room. The four waiters wore black pants and rumpled white shirts with narrow black ties. But despite the uniform, I thought their faces had the insouciance and complacency of servers in a Bombay durbar. None of the bubbly "How're-you-all-doing-today?" of an Applebee's or a TGI Friday's.

Painted directly on the pink walls of the dining room were three scenes: a Taj Mahal, an elephant, and, finally, a woman with a tiger. I wondered if there was an enterprising Indian muralist who made a living reproducing these scenes on the walls of Indian restaurants from Toronto to El Paso. Instant India, but really not India at all. The music playing in the background was Kishore Kumar oldies from Hindi movies of the seventies. The menu announced that there were Delhi Palaces in Phoenix, Tucson, and a few other Southwest cities, all presumably owned by one extended family.

It was a formula that worked well: a location in a strip mall on a busy road. A clay tandoori oven from India. An owner who with his family as his employees, all living together in one or two apartments, no days off, no hassles with benefits, overtime, or that sort of thing, could make a notoriously difficult business into a sure thing. They came in at ten and fixed the lunch buffet, went home at three, returned at six, and closed whenever the last customer left. The lunch buffet didn't vary from day to day—rice, *mutter panneer, dal,* chicken curry, vegetable *kofta,* cucumber *raitha,* and *gulab jamun* for dessert. When you had served yourself and sat down, two pieces of tandoori chicken per person and *naan* were brought to your table. The tandoori was delicious but the other dishes suffered from the spice. The same stock *masala* went into every dish, whether meat, fowl, fish, or vegetable.

As we sat there, soldiers in camouflage gear descended noisily on the place, in two groups of ten. They were coarse, conversed with each other in Arabic, were short with the waiters. The idea of a buffet line was anathema to them, and they happily muscled in to get at the particular dish they were after.

Steven, who was seven, and Jacob, who was five, were not particularly enthusiastic about the food, their tastes for hamburgers and fries too well ingrained. But they were effusive, tripping over each other's words in their rush to tell me the plot of the "If You're So Smart, Why Aren't You Rich?" *Batman and Robin* episode they had watched after school: "And then . . . and then . . ." Jacob said whenever Steven paused for breath.

The waiter and I struck up a conversation. Rajani raised her eyebrows as I slipped into an easy familiarity with this cocky Goan.

"And who are they?" I said, nodding toward the raucous military crowd.

"Buggers from the Gulf," he said contemptuously. Steven and Jacob sniggered at this word, one that their daddy sometimes used and that their mother disapproved of. "Now that America kicked Saddam's ass, these guys are our new allies, you know? Free F-16s, free tanks, bring them to El Paso to teach them to shoot Patriot missiles, send them home with suitcases filled with rockets. Same bloody stuff America gave Saddam ten years ago. Ten years from now it will be pointed back at America, you watch," he said, wagging his head.

From their table a man yelled, "Hey, boy!" at our waiter.

"You see? They think they're talking to their *deshi* houseboys." Thousands of Indians, Bangladeshis, Pakistanis, and Filipinos worked in the Gulf in menial occupations and were looked down on by the locals. "Can't say anything. Bad for business."

The soldiers ate with urgency, heaping prodigious amounts of food on their plates and going back for seconds of equal proportion. Before they left they hit the buffet once more, cramming the Styrofoam takeout containers to overflowing. Fort Bliss could give them weapons and training but, clearly, not food that was to their taste.

○

One evening, no more than a few weeks after the place had been in existence, two black males came into the vestibule, brandished a gun, and stuck it in the face of the elderly Sikh cashier. The patrons eating in the dining room next door were unaware of what was happening. The manager put up no resistance. The robbers took the cash register and prepared to leave. Then, for no obvious reason, they shot the old man in the chest and made their escape in a Camaro.

I happened to be in the hospital that night, finishing up a late consult. One of our Pakistani interns was speaking to a distraught Punjabi lady in Urdu, trying to console her. Also milling around the corridors were other Indian faces that I recognized from the restaurant. The trauma team worked on the old man for a time, but his wound was fatal.

The dead man's son and his family left El Paso. A new contingent, perhaps from one of the Delhi Palace branches in another city, took over. The murder was never solved.

5

Clubs in the backseat of a hatchback in the doctors' parking lot. A putter resting in the corner of one office and FootJoy shoes hidden behind the door of another. A photograph of the good doctor and pals in duffers' caps at St. Andrews, at Pebble Beach, at Palmetto Dunes. The pharmaceutical salesman talked wedges, woodies, long par fours with doglegs in them. Nowhere did I see evidence of the callus over the inner aspect of the thumb that bespoke a serious tennis habit. I had always resisted golf, secretly sensing I would love it and become addicted. As years passed, and as golf became almost an icon for medicine, my resentment of golf culture only grew.

One of my colleagues in internal medicine, Hoi Ho, stuck his head into my office.

"What, Hoi? No costume?"

He laughed. It was Halloween, and many employees wore costumes to work for a contest to be judged at noon in the cafeteria. Hoi, who was originally from Vietnam, was Texas Tech's most avid Dallas Cowboys fan, his office filled with Cowboys paraphernalia. Hoi spotted the Arthur Ashe photograph in my office, a photograph displayed discreetly, so that casual visitors rarely saw it.

"You're a tennis player, huh? One of our students plays," he said. "Let me think . . . where is David Smith from? Let me see . . . Australia, I think."

An Aussie! I recognized the name: David Smith was an "extern" assigned to my ward team the next month. Externs were fourth-year medical students given almost as much responsibility as interns.

"David came to Texas on a tennis scholarship. Then he played on the pro tour. After that, he came to medical school," Hoi said.

This Aussie was clearly out of my league. Still, I was curious to meet him.

That evening, I joined the exodus to the parking lot from Texas Tech, just as the light was fading. Tech and Thomason employees were heading home, their witches' caps and fairy wands drooping, their makeup fading, but their mood still festive. A young man fell into stride with me, slouching slightly, a backpack draped over his shoulder, He had blond hair, thinning on top and worn long at the back. He grinned as he took in the Hershey's Kiss walking in front of us, a woman who was trying to look graceful when her already generous behind, now swathed in aluminum foil, had been tripled in size. He was shorter than I, about five feet nine, with the narrow hips and light tread of a dancer. And yet he walked with a side-to-side sway, as if he were walking on the outer edges of his soles. His backpack was the co-op model that the medical students carried, but he seemed older than the average medical student. Perhaps almost my age—late thirties. There was no watch on his wrist, nor a pale shadow there to suggest he had forgotten to wear it.

I had come to think that medical-school society in America was divided into people who made eye contact and those who didn't. There were stars in their own orbits who saw you when they wanted something from you, but otherwise never so much as glanced at you. I used to be envious of this trait, misinterpreting it as a kind of confidence that I seemed to lack.

And then there were people like me who walked around with largely unjustified and well-concealed paranoia, who saw everything but went unnoticed, hoping not to be discovered, as though any minute *they*—the powers that be—would jump out and say, "Aha! We're on to you; you thought you had us fooled!" When they came to get me, I thought I would not protest. I'd go quietly. I'd wonder what had taken them so long. Clearly, this sentiment had its roots in my being a foreign medical graduate in a two-tiered system where foreign graduates were treated as second-rate.

Now that I was a full professor at the age of thirty-seven, as high up in the academic ranks of a lesser medical school as I had ambition to reach, my perception had changed little, if at all. It had come out of the subconscious and become a habit. If you subscribed to this classification, it came with an ability to recognize those who were like you. You surreptitiously scrutinized each face for the secret signs. You looked for reassurance, hoping to form an alliance, to find strength in numbers in anticipation of that moment when "they" jumped you. It was those kinship signals that I picked up in the man who walked alongside me, almost as if he were a foreign graduate. We nodded at each other. Before I opened my mouth and introduced myself, I was certain this was David Smith.

He pronounced his name "Daay-vid." He too was aware that we would be working together because he said, "I'm on the green team with you in December."

"Heard you played tennis on the pro tour."

He laughed, a nervous titter—a sign of the fear of discovery. He had clear blue eyes and they showed alarm. You don't want to believe people are actually talking about you or, worse, that they know too much about you.

"How did you hear?"

"Word gets around."

"All misleading, I'm sure. I mean . . . well, I was on the tour. Only lasted a few months. On the satellite circuit in Europe, really . . ." He was retreating from even my attention.

"Still," I said, persisting, "I doubt there are too many doctors who have that on their CVs."

"I'd be more inclined to put it on my CV if I'd won a match! I never got past the first round."

Fine wrinkles around his eyes became exaggerated as he laughed. He produced a self-deprecating, muffled, half-swallowed guffaw. I think he hoped this would close the door I had opened. I waited and continued to look him in the eye.

"It was a totally different level of competition," he explained. "Fun. But so expensive. If I could've afforded it, I would have continued for a little longer. But you have to win to have a career as a pro. I'd ha' starved . . ." After a moment, a sturdier punctuation. "Ah, well . . . Do you play, then, Dr. Verghese?"

His Aussie lilt was fetching, deeply ingrained and unblemished by his time in America.

"Since I was a boy," I said, "but I'm definitely not at your level— I'm more of a club player."

We walked on in silence. I already wanted to tell him about the wall, Mr. Swaminathan, my compulsive TV–tennis viewing, my tireless reading about theories and strategies . . . But it was not the sort of thing you confessed at a first meeting to a former professional tennis player—or to your medical student.

We had come to where my car was parked. Perhaps the subconscious mind, sensing that the gatekeepers in the brain would not let certain thoughts pass uncensored, created a short circuit to my tongue: "If you'd like to go out and play sometime . . ."

As soon as the words were out of my mouth, I regretted them. "Never ask a better player to hit with you," Pancho Segura says in his instruction book, in the chapter on court etiquette. "You will either be turned down or the better player will sulk while he ungraciously hits with you." My mind flew right past the fact that I would be overseeing David's clinical performance the next month and that it would be difficult for him to say no gracefully. It could be an exercise in frustration for a top-flight player to hear "sorry" with every other shot as the balls skyed out of the court or hit the bottom of the net. Suddenly I worried that I had overstated my tennis skills, implied a semblance of parity or at least a bridgeable gap that I knew wasn't there. I'd be able to keep the ball in play with David, but *he* would have no way of knowing that till we got on the court. And it was too late to take that statement back, or to qualify it, because, after only a beat, David said, "Certainly."

I was drawn to him then. He was, I felt, nothing if not a gentleman, too polite to refuse.

And I was proud of myself, as if, finding myself in a new schoolyard, I had approached another boy and found commonality, brought about a connection, found that he too hoarded marbles, had been looking for someone to share this passion with.

David was bashful now, surprising me by saying, "You wouldn't have an extra racket I could borrow, would you?"

○

At home, Jacob and Steven were in their Batman and Robin costumes, bursting with excitement, hopping in the driveway, waiting for me to take them trick-or-treating. We made the rounds of the houses on our street. I was proud of the way they said, "Thank you," and, as if they had rehearsed this, "Have a happy Halloween."

Steven, garrulous at seven, said to a few householders, "We're your new neighbors from down the street," which made the reception considerably warmer.

There were all manner of goblins, witches, grim reapers, skeletons, and Scissorhands on the sidewalk. But as we crisscrossed the street, me racing to keep up with the boys, I became concerned by the number of cars that had suddenly appeared on this otherwise quiet street. A convoy of pickup trucks, station wagons, sedans of ancient vintage, all with Chihuahua state plates, was inching up the road. I watched as eight children and a few adults descended from a pickup truck, joined by an equal contingent from another car, and started to go door-to-door. The drivers of the cars kept abreast of their parties.

No sooner had we returned to our house than we were assailed by a steady stream of these trick-or-treaters. There were cute, polite children, many in vampire costumes, but behind them were adults who looked too old for this, thrusting their treat bags forward.

Steven and Jacob were doling out the candy, admiring costumes and asking questions like "Who are you supposed to be?" or "Can you tell who I am?" but not getting much of a response. I closed the door when there was a lull in the action. But then the bell rang again and Steven opened the door to two heavyset Hispanic women in their forties, in no costume of any sort, standing there looking sheepish. Steven waited, unsure. Finally, one of them nudged the other, who reluctantly said, "Thricoh-threeth," and with that, Steven, hearing the magic word, dispensed the last of our candy, thinking nothing of this strange encounter.

We turned off the porch and front lights and peered through the curtain. Fresh caravans of cars were arriving from Juárez, and clusters of figures went from door-to-door. More and more of our neighbors had turned off their porch lights and the lights in the front rooms of their houses. I imagined that they were, like us, peeking out from behind drawn curtains. It was nearly midnight when this traffic from across the bridge finally eased.

6

At Wimbledon, they used white balls for the longest time.

The white ball was difficult to see on television. At times, during a point, your eyes lost it completely. Still, when that happened, your mind projected ahead, gave the ball a position in space based on the location of the player, the speed of the swing, the tilt of the racket face at contact, the sound of the ball coming off the strings, and the shape of the follow-through. But you could never define exactly where it was. If you said it was there, you were wrong as soon as you said it. It was always in flight; like Zeno's arrow, it was never there. As you thought, There, it was gone.

What relief then when the ball, after this disappearance of a few milliseconds, appeared again. And if you knew anything about the game, if you understood its vagaries, the ball materialized in the exact spot that your mind and eyeballs had assigned it. It was as if seeing and sensing had taken leave of each other, executed a loop the loop, and then come together seamlessly to resume controlled flight. I loved this separation-and-reunion feeling. It reminded me of what I loved about medicine: how a patient's words and the clues the body gave you were coordinates for a disease lurking below. The art of diagnosis was to plot the trajectory of the invisible disease and then, like a mongoose, feint, coax the serpent into striking, sidestep the fangs, and seize it behind the head, where it could do no more damage.

What magic in this representation of a two-and-a-half-inch, two-ounce ball on a screen, this trick with pixels that created another trick on the rods and cones of your retinae which, in turn, created a trick in your brain—the idea that you were seeing the ball.

    And meanwhile, the actual ball was across the ocean, thousands of miles away in the town of Wimbledon.

    And even there, when the ball was in flight, it wasn't there.

○

In 1986, The All-England Lawn Tennis and Croquet Club, Wimbledon, finally changed to a yellow ball.

7

The night before I was to meet David for tennis, I tossed and turned rest-lessly on my futon. Kernels of memory ballooned to form tubercles that germinated, offshoots and fronds leading me everywhere but in the direction of sleep. The wind howled outside. When I heard a cracking sound from the back porch, as if from a revolver, I got up with more relief than trepidation to investigate. A flowerpot had been bowled over and its contents littered the porch.

Our new house on Stonebluff Drive sat on a slope of the Franklin Mountains, one of a row of houses whose backyards overlooked a deep arroyo, a steep-walled, water-carved gully. Not water, but wind now came whipping down through the arroyo.

In the boys' room, Jacob was burrowed under the covers, fast asleep, only his mop of hair peeking out. His older brother had thrown all his sheets off, his limbs akimbo, snoring softly. Their physical attitude in sleep matched their personalities: Jacob, thoughtful and careful with his pocket money, full of a million questions for which he wanted tidy answers ("Where does the pic-ture go when you turn off the television?"); Steven, impulsive, expansive. On Steven's bed was the Calvin and Hobbes comic strip anthology called *Something Under the Bed Is Drooling* that we read before they went to sleep. The three of us identified totally with Calvin and his life with Hobbes the tiger. Typical of the narrow, con-stricted, and literal world of adults, Calvin's parents saw Hobbes as a stuffed, inanimate tiger, and thought Calvin suffered from too vivid an imagination.

I bent over Steven's bed to restore his limbs, remove toys, straighten the sheets. With a shudder I remembered the woman I had seen kneeling over her child's grave in the Evergreen Cemetery adjacent to Thomason. It was the weekend after Halloween, which in El Paso was *Los Dias de los Muertos*. There had been vendors in pickup trucks lined up at the entrance selling plastic flowers, floral crosses, and diaphanous images of Jesus or Mary. Families were streaming in to tend the graves of children—*los angelitos*—on the Saturday; the graves of adults would be tended to on the Sunday. I had been looking down from the sixth floor of the hospital. One woman had come with a blanket and seemed to be in long conversation with her dead child, her hands gesticulating, as if she were telling a long "and then . . . and then" story in the manner of Steven and Jacob. I imagined she was explaining something to her dead child, perhaps using adult words, not talking down, not holding back. It had frightened me to see her. And now, in my sons' room, it frightened me to think of her. Would that I had the chance in my sons' lifetime and my own to one day explain to them all the forces that moved me.

No light showed from under the door of the master bedroom where Rajani slept. I retreated back to the spare bedroom. The futon had been my bed since the time of our arrival from Iowa, and for a year and a half prior to that in Iowa. The wind's wail seemed accusatory, as if to ask, *Why has it come to this?* Like a dog worrying a bone, my mind went back once again to examine the marriage, looking back for clues to its dissolution, for a unifying explanation.

The first image to come to mind was the old colonial house with the white siding and wood floors set on the grounds of the VA hospital in Johnson City, Tennessee. That was the town where we had lived the longest as a married couple—first during my internship and residency, and then for a second stint in 1985, after we'd returned from Boston, where I had specialized in infectious diseases. Unexpectedly, on my return, I had quickly accrued a sizable AIDS practice, mostly hometown boys who had left the town years before for the big cities, and were then coming back to their rural homes, to their families who were discovering for the first time that their sons were gay. And had AIDS. This was before the era of Ryan White funding, before the solid emergence of activists, of consortias—at least in small towns—that could have eased the burden. To be "the AIDS doctor" in the rural South was not a popular position. I had felt alienated from the rest of the medical community. Lacking any meaningful therapy for HIV in that era, I engaged with my patients in their houses, got to know their families. I crossed the traditional boundaries of clinic and hospital. I was caught up in the incredible life stories of my patients and thought it ironic that these men whom many dismissed as sissies were, in fact, the most courageous souls I had ever met. We were, I recognized, aliens traveling in opposite directions: I, the foreigner, looking to blend in, to provide for my children a geography more permanent than mine had ever been. My patients, despite looking the part of hometown boys, despite knowing all its little rituals, were hiding the secret of their sexuality, a secret that would always leave them feeling more alien there than I ever did.

The large numbers of patients, the long hours, the unrelenting deaths, each of which seemed to cost me personally, made me feel as if I had crossed into another world, where everything was relative, no rules held. It was a world that Rajani couldn't easily enter. The minor differences in our two personalities—me willing to smoke the occasional joint, to try moonshine, to be fascinated equally by the genius, the fool, and the misanthrope, to be inclined, as one of our friends put it, to "find strangers on the street and say 'Come in, let's talk,'" she, more careful, cautious, level headed—became more exaggerated every year, as if we were driving each other to the polar extremes. At dinners and get-togethers we presented a united front that belied the discord and unhappiness when we were alone. The gloom of that Abyssinian church had reentered my life.

I decided, as an act of self-preservation, to leave for a sabbatical at the University of Iowa in Iowa City. The only way to do this was to cash in my retirement to fund the time away. Rajani didn't disagree with my leaving, but she had debated to the last minute whether to come with me. After all, *she* was not the one who felt the need to escape from Tennessee. But finally, at the urging of her parents, she did. We had arrived in Iowa City on New Year's Day. And there, in that new landscape, surrounded by strangers, there was no need to put on an act for anyone. And when the pretense was gone, there was nothing left.

In no time at all, though, Rajani took the boys to stay with her parents in the hill station of Coonoor in the south of India. It was a town of quaint bungalows and tea estates and a vigorous social life revolving around the country club. Her father was a tea broker. Our wedding, ten years before, had been in the same town, with all the tea planters and estate owners and even a few straggling Brits in attendance.

○

Alone in Iowa, I had longed for the boys' voices, for the rumbling thunder of their footsteps overhead as I worked in the study below, for the feel of their breath on my face, their fingers on my ear as they wrestled with me. But the only sounds were the echoes of my own movements around the house, the clink of the kettle and its familiar whistle as I made cup after cup of tea, the shriek of the wind that rattled my solitude and seemed intent on prying off the roof of the house.

Rajani and the kids returned from India after a while. I drove down to Chicago, to O'Hare, to pick them up. The boys were tanned and exhausted from the long journey. For one second, as they emerged from customs, they looked at me without recognition. Then they came to me, reached for me, held me, and made me feel whole again. They frolicked in the cargo space of the station wagon as we drove back to Iowa City, delighted to be back in a predictable world of McDonald's and Blockbuster videos. Rajani was cool. Much later, when we talked, she said she wanted a divorce. The magic was gone. We were too different.

And since it didn't seem to matter anymore, since we were talking so pragmatically in the past tense about our marriage, when she asked me, I told her that when she had been away, I had had an affair. Such pain for her to hear that, for me to admit it. More than anything else, it felt as if those words were what had sealed the ending.

We made one last joint decision to move to the same city when the sabbatical was over, so that we could raise the kids together. As much as we loved Tennessee, neither of us wanted to play out the endgame of the marriage in the fishbowl of Johnson City.

○

For the remainder of our stay in Iowa, I was firmly entrenched in the downstairs study. She kept her counsel behind the closed bedroom door upstairs, had separate phone lines installed. Tennessee friends stacked up on both sides, hers ready to tell me how fortunate I was to have someone as beautiful, steadfast, stoic, and grounded, and to count my blessings. And mine to tell her how my eagerness, my boyish interest in everything around me, my passion for different causes (they wanted to say lost causes) were not a liability. Only the boys brought our trajectories together at mealtimes and for outings to the park.

At the end of the sabbatical, I found my new teaching position, at Texas Tech in El Paso. Our plan was to buy a house for her and the kids in El Paso, settle them in, and then, in a few months, I would move out.

We began again in Iowa the ritual of packing, cataloguing our belongings—the fifth move of our married life. We stepped outside together and looked critically at the old Ford LTD station wagon. Its odometer had stopped registering the miles after the first hundred thousand. The car had been loyal, faithful—the fifth member of our family. Should we risk loading it once again to its gills and crossing the country? Despite its size, Rajani had taken to it when I'd first brought it home, a car that another family had discarded. When Jacob was born two years after Steven's arrival, it was tough to imagine any other car accommodating the four of us and the strollers and paraphernalia that went with us. Now, it sat parked in the Iowa driveway, staring back at us, a talisman from better times, a motorized scrapbook of family memories. We could not part with it, and it had, as if recognizing this, carried us faithfully past the El Paso county line before dying.

In this new El Paso house—her house—there was one more chance to spread out the belongings of eleven years. I skinned my knuckles assembling the giant platform bed, a crude and inexpensive structure that she had disliked but that we had bought together in Boston. I carried in the expensive tile-and-wood dining table she had ordered during the more stable married-with-one-child stage of the young academic in Tennessee, a table I had never cared for. Its chairs had become rattly and loose after the move. I couldn't resist a comment that brought a sharp rebuttal from Rajani and then a listing of all my many follies.

○

The shock of arrival in El Paso, the newness of the land, new folk-lore to digest ("a Mexican elder tree outside the bedroom window of your daughter means she will not marry"—we had three Mexican elders but no daughters) allowed us briefly to defer what was coming. Our conversations revolved around the boys' schools and their adjustment.

Steven and Jacob knew we were having problems, but they didn't show it. I was envious of the boys, wishing I could feel their simple pleasure in Arctic Batman or Deep-Sea Batman, wishing I could lose myself in *Winnie the Pooh* and watch the video again and again, the way they did, without any diminution in their pleasure. I remembered how my bicycle and my tennis racket had done the same for me.

Steven came home from school with his first project, a papier-mâché pencil holder. He summoned us, made us sit down, and said, "This is for *both* of you. You have to share." Each night in El Paso they took turns camping on my bed and then hers before they were carried to their own.

Sitting at the backyard picnic table, shortly after moving into the new house, we had finally told the boys.

She began: "Daddy and Mommy are not getting along—"

Steven's face froze, as if he knew where this might lead.

"You haff to get along," he said.

She looked at me, for me to continue.

"Daddy and Mommy are not going to live together anymore. In a few weeks, Daddy will find an apartment close by—"

"But you boys will still see both of us all the time, we'll still do things together—"

The words sounded idiotic even as they came off our tongues, a pathetic explanation to an intelligent child. But it was too late: Steven had tears well out from his eyes, trickle down his neck, silently pleading with us not to let this happen, reducing us to tears. I thought then that children of his age understood and perceived everything. What they lacked were the words to describe what they felt.

Jacob had looked on, his face blank. His was an orderly, cloistered world, and even when he was in a silver station wagon driving into a landscape such as he had never seen, he had felt no concern, he had trusted us to be there. He was young enough to believe that we would continue to be there. Whatever it was we were talking about, he couldn't envision it. We had hugged the boys, a collective, tearful hug, a hug that seemed to promise that we would hold together even as we were coming apart.

Such pain that night in my chest, pain that I wished would have been physical, amenable to aspirin or ice packs or nitroglycerin.

After that conversation, with every moment that we continued under the same roof, it was possible for us all to believe that the choice had *not* been made and that there was still a chance to fix it. "When can we go to Disneyland?" Steven had asked.

○

It was after midnight now and I was still awake. I turned on the light and started to plow through the still unpacked cartons in my room. What I found first was a tiny scorpion, which I dispatched with the nearest thing handy, a dictionary. The corpse looked like a miniature lobster. Our neighbor had said that when you killed a scorpion, you could expect to see its mate within twenty-four hours. I was watchful.

Finally I found what I was after: a carton full of spiral notebooks. What fell out of the top one was a photograph I had as a child razored out of a library book and taped over my bed. In the picture, a young Pancho Segura, in long pants, was in full flight, his racket outstretched, his forearm muscles like cables under the skin, the flesh under his eyes taut, his hawk's gaze locked on the prey, a tennis ball that was out of the photograph but whose location on my wall I knew.

The little notebooks of my spying days had given way to these large spiral ones of which there were now several volumes. Their covers, once shiny and glowing, now had a mosaic of cracks over them. Ostensibly, they were my tennis journals, but they were clearly also diaries, tennis and everything else intertwined on the pages the way they seemed to be in my life. If Rajani was aware of them, she had never shown much curiosity about their contents. Flipping through them I could see how my handwriting had taken on different shapes over the years. The basic elements—the lack of a loop on the *y*s or *l*s—remained the same, but one year the words were giant and slanted left, and another year they were smaller and tilted to the right, as if reflecting the different skins I was trying on and rejecting. In the latest volume, the writing was upright, neutral, medium-size script, as if I had tired of pretense?

Bill Tilden, arguably the greatest player ever, did more than keep a notebook. He wrote a thick, squat textbook that I owned: *Match Play and the Spin of the Ball*. Its ancient bindings were coming loose, but its advice was timeless, covering every possible exigency, such as how to play Pete Swattem or Joe Form or the "goat-getter par excellence, the Pat-Ball artist, in other words, Old Joe Gettem, who never misses anything . . . a particularly deadly enemy to young players who have more strokes than brains . . ." After winning Wimbledon in 1920 at the late age of twenty-seven, Tilden did not lose a match in the next six years—a feat of domination that is inconceivable in modern tennis. Like a slugger batting a thousand for six seasons.

René Lacoste, the "Crocodile," perhaps the man most frustrated by Tilden, filled a notebook with lessons from those losses. He spied on Tilden as Big Bill took on other challengers. He diagrammed strategies in his notebook in the manner of a chess master penciling out new gambits. In defeat, he went back to the paper, amended his observations, reevaluated his written strategy, tweaked it in a different direction. In 1927, after innumerable attempts, he finally beat Tilden three different times. He did it by using a strategy of impeccable defense, a defense so complete that it was, in effect, offense. "A mathematical science," one observer called it. Lacoste took the ball early and on the rise, thereby rushing Tilden. He kept great depth on his ground strokes, came in to the net on approaches down the center, recognizing that Tilden loved to hit passing shots when stretched on the flanks. I loved this story. That words from a page should translate to a physical act on court was an affirmation of my years of keeping journals.

My notebooks were, without intending to be, a record of the changing philosophy of tennis as viewed and practiced not by a hacker but by someone who fantasized about being one of the greats. Bill Tilden's philosophy, with its emphasis on spin and placement, had given way to Jack Kramer's percentage tennis—"the big game"—where the odds were with the person who got to the net first. When the more powerful graphite rackets arrived, the percentages at the net didn't work that well—Lendl almost dared people to come to the net so he could blast the ball past them. And then followed the Nick Bollettieri philosophy of tennis: a power forehand that you run around and hit inside out to your opponent's backhand, a guileless strategy that had nevertheless propelled Arias, Krickstein, and Courier to the top, but which in its lack of variety may also have contributed to their downfalls.

Early heroes and the newspaper clippings of their triumphs in my notebook gave way to new heroes. Lendl was a constant, though, plenty of clippings of him in his argyle-patterned T-shirts, a reflection of the geometric precision in his game. Lendl was to me the Ted Williams of tennis, the way he used a brand-new frame and new shoes with every ball change during a match, the way each racket was strung with genuine gut at exactly seventy-two and a half pounds, the way he would toss a ball to the umpire when his fingers detected a drop in pressure that no one else had noticed. David Halberstam in *Summer of '49* describes how once when Ted Williams struck out at Fenway, he came to the dugout raving that the home plate was out of line. The next day, to humor him, they measured the plate. It *was* out of line. Lendl gave just the kind of attention to detail that would have made him a great clinician, and yet, like Williams, he didn't suffer fools well and was not a popular champion.

I had entries recorded while viewing Grand Slam matches on TV, or in person, transcribing the brilliant and insightful comments of a Mary Carillo or a John McEnroe. Once, out of frustration with Cliff Drysdale, who I felt talked too much, I copied down one of his impossible, loopy, chasing-its-own-tail sentences: "You cannot, Fred, on any given day, count this man out, regardless of his past performances this summer and I refer of course to losses to players ranked well below him, which all said and done, in this day and age, the caliber of players being what it is, count for very little when it's break point in the ad court, and when, no matter what you say, experience, particularly in Grand Slam situations, will always triumph over . . . yadda, yadda, yadda." I meant to send it to ESPN along with a letter of complaint, but I never did.

The shots my regular opponents most disliked were carefully recorded. It was my belief that one had to personally validate the tips that worked for you, snatch them out from the great universe that swarmed with maxims and rules, a new one appearing as a special feature in each issue of *Tennis* magazine, a million others offered in the how-to books of which I had every single one published in the English language. Vic Braden said to swing up at the overhead, Ashe said to simply smash it like a serve; Trabert recommended a closed stance when hitting the forehand and yet Agassi and Courier all hit from an open stance; Stan Smith said never to drop the racket head when volleying and yet McEnroe broke this rule with every volley . . .

At the annual infectious diseases meetings, the pharmaceutical companies organized a tennis camp, flying in pros like Ilie Nastase, Tracy Austin, Tony Trabert, Virginia Wade, Stan Smith, Vijay Armritraj, Marty Riessen, and others. I had faithful logs of these lessons and had pasted in the notebook a photograph of myself, sweaty and exhausted, standing with Tracy Austin and my friend Stuart Levitz.

o

I turned now to a page titled "Forehand"—the first stroke we all learn. When the forehand goes awry, it is cause for despair. Once, after a month-long spell of hitting errant forehands, I had mysteriously come out of the slump, found the stroke, felt its pieces come together and flow as automatically as the motion of lifting a glass to the lips, or opening a door. I could hardly wait to record the insight I had gained—or regained:

> *Abe, when your forehand vanishes it's because you aren't laying the wrist back, not keeping it laid back throughout the stroke. Look at any slo-mo of a pro hitting a forehand: The racket head t-r-a-i-l-s the handle. At the moment when the ball contacts the strings, the wrist is AHEAD of the ball. Abe, for God's sake remember to LEAD WITH THE BUTT OF THE RACKET when you swing at the ball! Swing through the ball completely! Don't poke at it! Don't push at it! Choke up on the handle if you have to. By picturing the butt of the handle beginning the stroke, you ensure that the racket head trails your wrist. Remember how when you were hitting against the wall as a kid, you discovered*

the laid-back wrist, almost accidentally, by necessity, as the only way to be consistent? Remember? Huh?

And some months later another entry about the forehand:

But don't get too close to the ball. And be sure to let the racket hit through the ball and finish in front of you and around, all the way to your left shoulder. FOLLOW-THROUGH!

Beneath this entry I had pasted a picture from a tennis magazine of Lendl's follow-through after a forehand, his right wrist almost at his left shoulder, the racket head pointing at the sky even as his legs danced to get into position for the next shot.

Many more entries on the forehand. Some with blank pages after them, anticipating that in a lifetime of playing, there would be inserts, more occasions when the shot would disappear and have to be reconstructed. I turned to an entry on the serve:

Before you serve, Abe, lean forward from your waist, your weight on the front foot, your hands in front of you and held together, so that the ball rests lightly against the throat of the racket, your wrist so loose that the racket head points at the ground—like Johnny Mac. At this point, pick the spot where your ball will land. Now, rock first, forward slowly. Then rock back. If you do this, then the other elements all work well: the ball toss, the knee bend, the shoulder turn, and so on. But it all depends on that first movement! Rock forward. DON'T FORGET TO DO THIS, ABE, EVERY TIME YOU SERVE!

This physical mantra for some reason ensured that all the mechanical elements of a serve—the toss well in front of me, eyes on the ball, not dropping my left shoulder, not dropping my head—came into play. It was revealed to me on a stifling summer day in Tennessee when I never lost my serve in two sets and served brilliantly. I had scribbled down the little insight in the car, while still parked at the courts, fearful that if I waited, it would, like a dream fragment, vaporize, and be lost. Later I transcribed the entry into my notebook.

The cryptic entries in my book would make little sense to anyone else, probably wouldn't work for them. Look at the way Pete Sampras begins his serve, his weight on the back foot, then mysteriously lifting up the toe of his lead foot. That toe raise serves no purpose, and yet it's everything.

Nail Pete's toe down and his serve wouldn't be the same.

○

I heard footsteps in the hallway, but had seen no light. Rajani, on her way to the kitchen, or perhaps to investigate the noise, looked in. She saw me with my notebook, recognizing it for what it was.

Perhaps the same thought occurred to both of us: If I had paid as much attention to the marriage, if I had kept notes on love, if I had tuned my act each time there was a discordant note, a flubbed move, if I had recorded the things that worked, perhaps we could have saved the relationship, moved to a higher level, made it as effortless and automatic as lifting a glass to one's lips . . .

I put my notebooks away carefully. I didn't want her to see them in my hand when she walked past the doorway again.

8

The Franklin Mountains were solid and immovable, startling in the way they suddenly rose from the flat desert basin. In the mornings, the ledges, spines, saddle backs, and deep gorges were ocher, turning brown-green at midday and burnt orange in the evening. When a cloud bank came spilling over the top of the long ridge, roiling and cascading like surf, the mountain turned gray. The Franklins irrefutably divided El Paso into west and east sides, the town wrapping around the mountain like a V, with downtown at the junction of the two limbs.

The El Paso Tennis Club sat in the shadow of the Franklin Mountains, closer to downtown and to Texas Tech than to the house. It was a workmanlike club, built in an arroyo so wide that its upper reaches were an almost impenetrable wilderness park. The tennis courts were spread out behind a simple clubhouse, newer courts tagged on as membership swelled, so that the property, surprised by its own success, had wound up with a jagged perimeter. It had no golf course. There were no flower beds or lawns between courts, just concrete walkways. To one side of the clubhouse was a large swimming pool.

The locker room was just off the lobby. I peeked in, but no sign of David. I had come directly from the hospital and I carried my Prince tennis bag with me. I walked past the pro shop, trying not to be noticed by a short, stocky man stringing a racket. I wasn't a member, but David had assured me that it would be fine. I walked through the lounge, past the juniors sprawled on sofas and watching TV, past the plaques on the wall with the names of club presidents and tournament winners—Men's A Singles, Men's Doubles, Mixed B Doubles—past faded black-and-white photographs of kids clutching trophies, the dates on the legends indicating a club history that went back to the 1940s.

David was outside the clubhouse, on a patio, looking over a teaching court, still in his work clothes. He was talking to a taller man wearing a broad-brimmed hat and wraparound shades. David waved me over and began to introduce me to Ross Walker, the head pro at the tennis club, but just then Ross was called away. He shook my hand and jogged off in one single motion.

On the way back to the locker room, David told me that Ross was from England, and had, like David, come to America on a college tennis scholarship. He had played on the pro tour—for longer than David—before turning to teaching. A few years before, Ross had won a national thirty-five-and-over tennis title, and now, David told me, he was setting his sights on the forty-five and over.

The locker room was small: one wooden bench surrounded by three walls of lockers, with a shower area beyond. A few men were in various states of undress and, till I caught myself, the naked flesh tugged at my eyes to inspect for signs of disease. On one man I saw a profusion of seborrheic keratosis. My mind leapt to form the words "Leser-Trelat sign"—a rare condition in which a sudden increase in the usual seborrheic keratoses is a marker for an underlying malignancy. It didn't matter that I had never seen a case, or that only twenty-seven cases had ever been described, the pathway to the words "Leser-Trelat" was grooved in my brain from repeating it to students whenever I saw flesh studded with keratosis. Only by hoarding such minutiae might I one day diagnose the twenty-eighth case.

And what, I wondered, as I peeled off my hospital clothes, if one of these naked men were also an internist and subjecting me to the same scrutiny? Love handles, scars of bilateral hernia operations, high-arched feet, three scattered moles that I had watched closely for years, hair that started at the neck and only spared the soles of my feet, but was increasingly abandoning the top of my head . . .

I stuffed my clothes into my racket bag while David, who had stripped to his underwear and had simply carried his sneakers, shorts, and T-shirt in a plastic grocery bag, hung his clothes on the one free hook. The carpet felt soggy. I did my best to avoid letting my bare feet touch it.

I was embarrassed by my new green-and-black Puma warm-up suit. But having pulled it out of the bag to get at my shoes, I felt obliged to put it on. It had struck me over the years that one's tennis game, at least at the club level, was inversely proportional to the elegance of one's tennis attire. And here I was, as David led the way out of the locker room, a perfect example of my own adage.

David had only half-pulled on his T-shirt before heading out. He had the classic tennis player's physique, a slim but not wiry build with shoulders that were unexpectedly broad given his narrow, boyish hips. Unexpectedly for being so thin, he had a little belly, a gentle protrusion below his navel that I suspected would disappear if he didn't slouch so. His head was thrust ahead of his torso as he walked, his body playing catch-up, giving the impression of constant forward motion. I scurried to keep up.

Court one was a doubles challenge court where you hung your racket on the fence and waited to play the winners. The courts next to the clubhouse were used for Ross's private lessons. We walked past these and down a narrow alley between backstops to a court on the edge of the property. Each court was fenced off from the next, except near the net post where a shaded bench and a water fountain were shared.

There were two junior girls playing next to us, pounding the ball, their strokes loose and fluid, keeping the ball deep. Their two-handed backhands and their wristy, Western forehands made them appear, but for the difference in their costumes, like clones of each other.

A low hum filled the air as the court lights, set to a central timer, came on. The sky turned red, then purple. But it was still pleasant, a far cry from November in Iowa.

I handed David my spare racket, a Prince Graphite. He fingered the grip and held the racket out, weighing it in his hands, checking its balance.

"Is it okay for you?"

He gave a short, sharp laugh. "Oh, I could play with any racket around," he said. "It was never really a big deal—" In midsentence, David spat on the palm of his right hand, then gripped the racket handle and twisted it, as though he were trying to unscrew a jar. I'm not sure that spit ever actually landed on his palm or on the racket.

It wasn't the deliberate expectoration of an Olympic gymnast getting on the parallel bars, more like a pantomime of spitting, a subconscious gesture. "—*getting* to the ball and selecting the right shot was more critical to my game . . . though with these new wide-body rackets . . ." I nodded, half-listening to him, the mantras from my notebook rattling around in my head. *Please, God, don't let my game fall apart today, let me get my racket on the ball consistently.* He was making me as tongue-tied as a schoolboy at his first dance. He didn't mean to sound arrogant, but he had a confidence here that I lacked completely.

The court was an older one and its surface was gritty, painted green inside the lines and tan around the perimeter.

David moved onto the court and I followed until we faced each other at the center strap. He looked up as if to see where the sun was, repeated his spit-and-handle routine, examined the center strap, looked to the net post as if debating whether to adjust the height. Then he startled me by smacking the top of the net with the edge of his racket. For a moment I wondered if he was upset. No, he was checking the net tension.

He put a hand on his head and pulled his head toward his right shoulder. He repeated this with his other hand, stretching his neck the other way. Now he worked on his shoulder. His ritual seemed automatic and instantly right and I tried to mimic it without being too obvious. I could have had my pregame warm-up done in a few minutes but David showed no haste in actually hitting the ball; he had just begun on his lower back.

Finally David looked at me as if he suddenly remembered that we were here to play, not to stretch. "Start with a little dink'em?"

I nodded, as if I understood. Dinkum? Wasn't that an Aussie expression for "the real thing"?

He took a position at midcourt, on the T between the service boxes. My confidence, already very thin, now vanished. Did he think I was *that* bad a player, that he wanted to find out if there was any point to our hitting from the baseline?

"Great way to warm up," David said, feeding the first ball to me, a gentle push—a dink—that landed on my side, well in front of me.

I hit it back too hard.

It flew straight at his chest. He was forced to volley. He softened his wrist just as the ball met his strings, cupping the ball and taking the pace off it. The ball floated back in a delicate arc, landing comfortably in front of me at about the same spot he had put the first ball.

"Gently," he said, which only flustered me further and made me rush the next shot. This time my ball did bounce, but almost on his shoelaces. He had to half-volley, his racket sweeping the ball up just after it met the ground. Again the ball bounced comfortably in front of me.

My third shot was much better.

"Dink'em helps you find the center of your racket," David said. He let out a soft grunt each time the ball hit his strings. He was dancing lightly on his feet. "It gets you used to meeting the ball in the center of your strings . . . helps you practice *seeing* the ball right onto your racket . . . warms up your 'feel' for the ball, your feel for your racket face. . . . It's also a good way of practicing your drop shots, your touch shots."

If this seemed a bit silly to me at first, the grace and control he showed didn't make *him* look silly at all. I had worried that the girls hitting next to us might laugh at two grown men playing ping-pong tennis. But now I was into it. It took a certain skill, a feather touch, to be able to play mini-tennis, like riding a bicycle very slowly.

"Back a bit, now," David said. We retreated, making our shots longer, until after a few minutes we were eventually behind our baselines, driving the ball. The dinks had become full-blooded strokes. I wasn't just warmed up, I was in a groove. My shots felt smooth, effortless.

I put more pace on the ball, exploring a few angles, not hitting *at* him so much. David had a quick first step and great anticipation. Shots that would make most opponents scramble, he returned effortlessly. If my ball misfired in depth or direction and if it sometimes wobbled off my racket, David's stroke applied the necessary correction and the ball came back restored, landing in my court with reliable depth.

I was focused on my own performance, keeping the ball in play, and yet I was drawn to watching David's game. It was a pretty game, smooth and flowing, his racket preparation early, his body always positioned sideways to the ball at the moment of impact, his balance perfect. He stepped into his shots, the way one was supposed to do. Compared to the windmill strokes of the juniors beside us, his strokes were compact and efficient. It was an old-style game, the kind Mr. Swaminathan taught in Ethiopia: the forehand hit almost flat, with very little topspin, a slice backhand, and not much grip change between the two shots. He hit well out in front of him, never getting caught on his back foot.

My strokes, by contrast, were much less orthodox. I hit the forehand with a Western grip, my palm almost under the racket, a shot that would have made Mr. Swaminathan wince. He had taught us straight out of Tilden's book: A traditional "shake hands" grip for the Eastern forehand; a slight rotation of the grip counterclockwise for the backhand. Although his admonition had been to "hit through" the ball, it often felt as if you were pushing the ball, guiding it. When I came to America, that style of play, David's game, was starting to wane. Only a genius like John McEnroe could still pull it off. In its place was a new baseline game made fashionable by Bjorn Borg, a game of extreme topspin. You pounded the ball, not just pushed at it.

Standing in front of our television in the living room in Tennessee, I had shadowed the new forehand, just as I had shadowed Mr. Swaminathan's strokes. Rajani had worried that I would break the lamps. I had seen how the high school kids with their odd-looking grips, the palm almost under the handle, smacked the ball full face, clearing the net by several feet. When the topspin kicked in, it would grab the ball and drop it just inside the baseline. I had practiced the shot again and again on a backboard, inspired by the story of how Bill Tilden had spent a whole winter reworking his backhand, developing a new grip, a new swing, losing to much lesser players until he finally got it right.

Surprisingly, the Western forehand came easily to me. My conversion was so complete I could hardly recall, much less reproduce, my old forehand. But I was no Borg, and if my timing was a shade off, the ball went too high over the net and landed long, or else it was all topspin with no pace and it landed short, or else I framed it and the ball looked like a sacrifice fly to center field. Still, when it worked, the big topspin caused the ball to rear at my opponent after it bounced.

When I shanked yet another forehand, I looked at David and held my hands up in surrender.

"Try hitting your forehand a little flatter," David called out. "With that grip of yours, it's more critical than ever to hit *through* the ball more. Your racket must finish way out in front of you before it comes across your body. And keep the wrist laid back."

The laid-back wrist! Of course.

He fed the next few balls to my forehand and I saw the problem correct itself. We took turns at the net and then practiced overheads and lobs, and finally came to the net to volley at close quarters, a quick-hands exercise that sharpened the reflexes.

After an hour of this, I felt I had been through the wringer. My breath was short and my thighs ached. David was sweating too, and I could tell he'd had a good workout, if only from chasing down my errant shots.

O

We sat high on the stone steps overlooking a show court, I in my warms-ups, David with a towel over his legs. Thirty-two-ounce sodas from the clubhouse sat at our feet. A doubles game went on below us, but it appeared that most everyone else had left. Some of the reserve we'd started with when we'd first met, and then in the locker room and on the way to the court, had slipped away. The tennis had seen to that. We didn't have to speak.

The men playing on the court below us were senior citizens, two of them wearing golfing hats. They seemed pleased to have an audience. They spoke in short bubbles: "Yes!" "Out!" "Lucky!" "Lucky, hell!" They all wielded the new oversized, wide-body rackets—caveman clubs. Their balls moved faster through the air than seemed possible, and though the players were as stiff and immobile as their age would suggest, their shots were unnaturally powerful. One long, entertaining point ended when one gent rifled a passing shot with no backswing, as though the racket had a trigger on its strings that shot the ball out.

"Nintendo tennis!" I said.

"Ping-Pong!"

"Wide-body rackets."

"Ban them, I say."

"Hear, hear."

We sighed.

"Well, I enjoyed that," David said. "It's been a year since I played. I must confess, when you asked me to play, I really wanted to say no—"

"I wouldn't have blamed you. You could have had a better match with someone at your level—"

"No, I didn't mean it that way," David said. He looked worried, as if he might have hurt my feelings. "I didn't *want* a match. College tennis, the brutal competition, took away my enjoyment . . . it was a relief to give it up. It's a pain in the ass to have people challenge me just to measure their game, you know?"

"God, I'd have loved to play college tennis," I blurted out. My childhood tennis fantasy had been about reaching the levels of the game David had already experienced. "I mean . . . I wish I'd had the chance to play more as a child and in high school." David was looking at me strangely. "I mean, there were so few courts when I was a kid . . . and then in college . . . I wonder if I would have been able to play at that level. But by then I was so single-minded about medicine that I missed out on a lot of stuff."

I surprised myself with this confession.

"Yeah, I was single-minded about tennis when I was younger," David said, shaking his head ruefully. "But in college it was . . . pressure. Win, win, win. Or lose your scholarship." His tone of voice changed at this memory, a somber note creeping in. "And matches were nasty—no line judges, a lot of cheating . . . Not like this at all."

○

In the parking lot, we exchanged phone numbers.

He told me his phone was in a hallway and I needed to ask for him as there was one other boarder. David rented a room on the northeast side of town, on the other side of the mountain, at the other end of Transmountain Road.

I noticed that his car, a beat-up black Isuzu, had cardboard in place of the glass in the passenger window.

"Where I live, the coyotes come down at night from the Franklins and look for fat little dogs." He pronounced it "kooyotee"—not kah-yoh-tee. "And then another species of coyote does that—" he said, pointing to the cavity where the cassette player once was, laughing at his own joke. "The larger ones eat tires. Every morning I hold my breath when I go out, wondering if the car will be sitting on its rims. Ah, well."

I started to ask why he didn't move, but then held my tongue. Most of the medical students lived in apartments on the west side of town.

We shook hands.

"Want to hang on to that racket?"

"Thanks! Yeah. And thanks for asking me to play ... Dr. Verghese."

"Please, call me Abraham. And thank *you*."

We drove off in opposite directions, different sides of the mountains. Perhaps it was because we were both from elsewhere, not natives of the land, more familiar with dingos and hyenas than we were with coyotes, that I had felt quite at ease with him. I liked his approach to tennis: plain old racket and ball, no head games, no gamesmanship, no artifice, no ego.

I was listing in my mind the many meanings of the word "coyote." In El Paso it was a person who carried people across the river. In an older usage it referred to a Spanish-Indian half-caste. And then David's usage of the word: On his tongue it was an urban larcenist who broke into cars and devoured them to their bones. To me, "coyote" also meant the most significant wild-animal reservoir of rabies in the Southwest.

As I drove home, up Thunderbird, I thought that it didn't really matter what side of the mountain you lived on, or why. You could hear the howl of coyotes from both sides.

○

The next day I saw David by the nurses' station on the seventh floor of Thomason, a floor shared by pediatrics and orthopedics. This was my first visit to the seventh floor. The orthopedists had consulted me about one of their patients, a colorful, tattooed ex-con whom I had just finished examining.

David smiled when he saw me, and came right over and shook hands. He leaned close and said softly, "Do your legs hurt, by any chance?"

"My calves are sore, my shoulder aches, my back is stiff, but otherwise I'm great. And you?"

He looked around, as if to make sure no one was in earshot. "My legs are killing me," he said, giggling even as he grimaced and rubbed his thighs. "I was so stiff this morning."

"Good! I thought it was just me."

"Didn't realize how out of shape I am. We've got to do it again. If we could do a workout like that, say, once or twice a week, it'd be great. That is," he said, his face becoming serious, "if you have the time."

I laughed. I had fantasized most of the previous evening that we might play regularly, since he was without question the perfect partner. But, like a boy eager to turn a first date into a romance, I was playing the game, not wanting to appear anxious, much less overanxious, and ask for another meeting too soon. I worried that I had already blurted out too much, exposed myself, and though he denied it, that he had agreed to play out of politeness. Still, when we parted at the tennis club, I felt we had found a sense of connection. Later, though, I conceded to myself that I might have been reading too much into it. This reassurance from him now flattered and excited me.

"Wednesdays and Sundays if you aren't on call?"

"I go to church Sundays," he said, "but if we're done by eleven . . ."

"It's a deal." He hadn't struck me as a churchgoer.

I showed him the chart of the patient I had just seen, a man with a week-old closed-fist injury. His opponent's incisor tooth had penetrated his knuckle joint. "Is this one of your patients, by any chance?" David leaned over and looked.

"Not mine, but someone's on our team. I've seen him on rounds," David said. "Apparently he felt his friend was making moves on his girl."

"Oh, I think it's more than that," I said, holding up the X ray for David to see. "He's got an old, healed, boxer's fracture on the fifth metacarpal of the same hand—see there? And he's got cauliflower ears, a flattened nose. And if he keeps it up, he'll get the slurred speech too. There's something he isn't telling us. Maybe he's a bouncer or a strong-arm man. I wasn't about to pry too deeply. He's got some interesting tattoos though. Tattoos usually come with stories, they tell a lot more than you think. *That* he's willing to talk about. He's game for me to photograph them, but I ran out of film."

The orthopedic team had been stumped by the growth of an uncommon bacterium in the knuckle joint. I pointed to the culture report that had just come back from the lab. "He's growing *Eiknella corrodens* in the joint fluid. What do you know about *Eiknella*?"

David's expression changed to a thoughtful one, his posture now that of the attentive student. I hadn't meant for us to switch roles so suddenly, or to *instruct* him, merely to point out something curious. I wondered now if I was showing off, asserting my role, my power here on this particular court.

His brain was searching its files for the relevant medical data. "It's . . ."—he hesitated, as if under normal circumstances he wouldn't hazard a guess, but he felt freer to do so with me—"part of the mouth flora?"

"Good! It is a mouth organism, but not the most common one. It must have come from his victim's mouth. The 'corrodens' part of the organism's name comes from the way it burrows into the agar on the culture plate in the lab. But if fits the clinical picture too, 'cause he'll need surgery to debride the knuckle joint. And two to four weeks of intravenous antibiotics after that. *Eiknella* can cause indolent infections. Lots of pus. Sometimes the need for repeated drainage of the wound." David nodded his head, impressed, I think. "The mouth is such a cesspool of bacteria, you know. From a microbiologic point of view, you could debate whether it's preferable to plant one's lips on the oral or the aboral end of the gastrointestinal tract."

David's explosive laugh attracted glances from people milling around the nurses' station.

"And do you know about *Eiknella*'s association with a certain behavior?"

David shook his head, perhaps not sure if I was about to deliver a lesson or a punch line.

"People who shoot up Ritalin* get infected with *Eiknella*. They 'skin pop' or else they miss the vein and the Ritalin extravasates into the surrounding tissue; it burns like hell. And then—"

---

*methylphenidate—a kind of speed

"They put their mouth to it?"

"Exactly. Something about Ritalin changes the redox potential in the wound. And that change favors *Eiknella* over all the hundreds of other species in the mouth. Bingo: *Eiknella* abscess of the forearm."

David looked at me strangely and shuffled his feet. As if he was bothered instead of intrigued by this bit of medical trivia.

○

Years ago, when I was moonlighting in emergency rooms around Boston, I tried unsuccessfully to resuscitate a young white ruffian who had been shot in the heart. Three of his former friends had chased him down an alley, up some stairs that led to a locked door. He was cornered and then shot. I say he was young, but he was my age then—late twenties.

On his right bicep he had "Born to Die" tattooed elegantly in an Old English font; the other arm had skulls and crossbones. In the emergency room we managed to intubate him, get a big-bore intravenous line going, but his blood pressure was unrecordable. A thoracic surgeon cracked open his chest on the stretcher and oversewed the hole in the heart—all this within twenty minutes of his arrival. I was assisting but I was distracted by that tattoo and the way it sat on his bicep. Even as my bloody gloves held lung aside, I was thinking about the old anatomy theaters where the words "Nascentes Morimur"—born to die—were inscribed on the walls, perhaps to justify the audacious act of dissecting a dead body. Now that same slogan, born to die, sat on the skin of this all but dead man, mocking our efforts to make him live.

When we finally pronounced him dead, I had to go out and break the news to his younger brother, who also had long, scraggly hair, a tank top, and tattoos. I was subpoenaed to testify in the trial of the men who did him in, but they pleaded guilty before I was called.

I think it was this incident that sealed my interest in tattoos, frequently made me pull out my camera and ask permission to photograph. The tattoos in El Paso were different from what I had seen in Iowa or Boston or Tennessee. They were of two types: store-bought from one of the tattoo shops on Dyer Street, or homemade. The former were fine lined, black and gray, often elaborate or brightly colored and chosen from one of the patented patterns ("mild to wild") in the catalog.

The second kind of tattoo was a cruder, blue tattoo that with time would fade to slate gray on brown skin. Its edges were splotchy and uneven, pointing to an instrument other than a professional tattoo gun. Some, like the four dots Enrique had on the web of his hand, were very likely made at home. Others were jailhouse tattoos. There, "ink" was produced by setting fire to a Styrofoam cup and then collecting the thick smoke by inverting a brown paper bag over the burning cup. The soot was then scraped off the paper bag and made into a paste. A sharpened paper clip taped to a pen delivered the ink into the skin. Religious figures abounded: the Virgin of Guadalupe above the buttocks, so that the sodomist's penis would shrivel at the sight of the mother of Jesus. One of my patients—a murderer, in handcuffs, being treated for heart-valve infection—had a giant Christ on a crucifix on his chest. Psychiatrists would call this "reaction formation": a deep, subconscious urge, in his case for murder and mayhem, countered with a conscious reaction in the opposite direction—the religious tattoo on the chest.

Other jailhouse tattoos were whimsical: a girlfriend's name, a picture of boxing gloves, or the words "El Paso" or its street version, "El Chuco" in place of the simple *pachuco* cross on the back of the hand. Or else they were deadly serious: a teardrop tattooed at the corner of the eye was said to signify a killing.

The pugilist with the closed-fist injury and the *Eiknella* infection had a striking jailhouse image that I had seen on several patients now. It was that of a woman, a *chicana*, who, like a Hindu goddess, had many forms. The original mold must be housed somewhere in the penal system of West Texas, passed on from one inmate generation to the next. In some versions she was clothed, but most of the time her chest was bare, and her nipples pointed upward in the gravity-defying manner of a young teen. Her deep-set eyes and high cheekbones reminded me of the painter Frida Kahlo. Her hair was worn long and flowing. At times she wore aviator glasses, sometimes a fedora or a sombrero.

On my patient's skin, I was seeing her full figure. Her pubic hair was a wild, dangerous tangle. She was a proclamation of his heterosexuality, his machismo. I thought of her as a mythical, idealized figure, re-created and restated on the skin of so many men.

And indeed, from time to time I had seen her in the mall in baggy pants, wearing black lipstick, hanging out with a disrespectful, giggling cluster of her teenage friends. I had seen an older, sophisticated version of her in a downtown restaurant, dressed to the nines, breathing in the admiring looks that came her way as if they were the oxygen without which she would wilt. Another time she had stared at me out of a low rider, a powerful but sneaky and surreptitious glance, because in that car she was a possession, a fixture valued as much as the velour interior and the thin chrome wheels. One could see shades of her in the works of El Paso's best-known painter, Luis Jimenez: part *puta*, voluptuous and unsettling, and part Virgin Mother. She seemed to have sprung to life from the deep subconscious of the *frontera* culture, an icon for the idealized, *pachuco* era of zoot suits and patent-leather shoes that originated in El Paso before blossoming fully in L.A.

The label *"cholita"* did her an injustice; she was not just a pretty *chicana*, she was WOMAN, *border* woman. Dangerous, deadly, irresistible, and omnipresent.

9

On the first of the month, newly assigned teams of interns and senior resi-
dents searched for their patients, while the doctors rotating off took
leave of theirs. At a cubicle behind the nurses' station, a bedraggled
intern furiously scribbled a "sign-off" note that should have been
completed the previous night. I looked over his shoulder: The handwriting, bad to begin with, had deteriorated to indecipherable at the
bottom of the page. Not the best day to be admitted to a teaching
hospital.

The nurses, in contrast to the doctors, were as steady as the tides,
their routine the same from month to month. The night-shift nurses
were leaving and the morning-shift nurses swept in, needing fresh
orders, wanting to alert the doctors to changes in their patients. I
watched them bounce from one white-coated figure to another, trying to determine to whom to report.

My fledglings, I found, were not on the sixth floor but on the second floor, assembled in a conference room off the intensive care unit.
With the exception of Sergio, my senior resident, and David, the
extern, they looked like condemned prisoners. "Good morning," I
offered, but though their lips moved, no sounds reached my ears.
Ward service was stressful—they would routinely put in seventy-plus
hours a week—and all the while I would be evaluating their performances. Still, I thought their apprehension was excessive.

David wore a white coat over a blue shirt and a mustard-colored
tie. One wing of his collar had lifted up. He was grasping his clipboard against his chest. On the tennis court, he had been relaxed, in
control, capable at any moment of overwhelming me, but here his
footing was less secure. When it had been just the two of us on the
seventh floor, discussing the man with the closed-fist injury, our con-

versation had bridged tennis and medicine, and had had a pleasant, collegial air. But the balance had now shifted noticeably. Unlike the two third-year medical students, David's role as a fourth-year medical student, or extern, would be to function as a mini-intern. For the first time in his short medical career, he would write orders (to be countersigned by me or one of the interns) and manage patients.

"Good morning," I said again, pointedly, trying to shake them out of their solemnity.

David chuckled.

"Good morning, Dr. Verghese," they murmured now with one diffident voice. Sergio leaned forward to hand me a pack of twelve index cards, each stamped with the name and medical record number of patients we had inherited from the last team. "And thirteen," he said, handing me one more card for our new admission, Angelina Cortez, who was still in the emergency room. New teams tended, if only subconsciously, to resent the "inherited" patients. So much easier to care for someone whom *you* had admitted from the emergency room, evaluated, and then followed through the various stages of the hospital stay.

Sergio settled back in his chair, giving me a conspiratorial wink as if to say, "Don't mind the fact that the young pups are peeing all over themselves. I've got everything under control." Sergio had a Buddha-like serenity and a figure to match. He looked dapper in his spit-shined shoes, dark trousers, beige shirt, and psychedelic tie, a deluxe Proctor Harvey–model stethoscope draped around his neck to top off the ensemble.

My two interns were from Palestine and India. This was their third month of internship. Their faces said more than they wanted to reveal.

The two third-year students had no particular reason to be tense, but they had picked up the mood of their seniors, as if this were the right posture to adopt. So far the students' only introduction to clinical medicine had been a physical diagnosis course in Lubbock; for practice they had, for the most part, examined one another. Lubbock was the Texas Tech mother ship where all the medical students did their first two years before a third of them came to El Paso, another third went to Amarillo, and the rest stayed in Lubbock for the last two years. Now here they were with brand-new coats, their pockets stuffed with flashlights, stethoscopes, reflex hammers, and little "peripheral brains"—condensed versions of the bigger tomes they were supposed to read at night. They looked much like first-time skiers who had managed to get onto the ski lift, but now, as the crest of the mountain appeared, still had to figure out how to get off and not fall flat on their asses.

I closed the door to the conference room. "Please turn your beepers off completely for a few minutes."

They reacted as if I were a sheriff asking them to part with their firearms. One by one they reached down and fidgeted with the instruments clipped to their belts.

I studied their faces. If I was an unknown commodity to them, they were equally unknown to me. Over the years I had encountered brilliant students, a few exceptional interns. I had also seen my share of those who had decompensated from the stress. One man had taken me aside and asked me to examine his finger. It looked perfectly healthy to me. "See how it is bleeding furiously?" he'd said, when not a drop of blood was in sight. Another had sunk into a life-threatening depression. And I had run into two true psychopaths who had made it through medical school only to have their traits fully revealed during their internships. Undoubtedly, there were others like them who had slipped through our hands, too smart for us, and now let loose on society. It was the oldest joke in medical school: What do you call the guy who graduates at the bottom of the class? *Doctor!*

"Osler," I began, wondering if my practiced spiel was a mistake with this group, "Osler said, 'to learn medicine without textbooks is like going to sea without charts. But to learn medicine without patients is like not going to sea at all.' Well, we *are* going to sea this month. My job is to be sure we are going to sea with good charts. You guys," I said, turning to the two third-year students, "as well as you, David, are, for me, the most important people here—after the patients. I want to make sure that you pick up good bedside habits. Good habits will last you for a lifetime. You can add the knowledge of disease later, but the technique of examining patients, of getting a good history, of milking the body for every clue it offers about the underlying disease is going to be my emphasis with you. Technique is everything." As I said this my mind was suddenly picturing my forehand, my wrist perfectly laid back as I met the ball.

"We're going to train your eyes to see, to notice everything. Let me ask you, what does it say on the outside of this door?"

Their eyes automatically went to the closed door, as if they might have suddenly developed X-ray vision.

"'ICU Conference Room'?" volunteered one of the third-year students.

"There is no sign there. I looked for one. Only reason I knew where to come was because the door was open and I saw all of you sitting here. From today on, I want you to observe everything. If you get on a hospital elevator, don't get off without making at least one diagnosis on your fellow travelers. The interns and Sergio already have their habits, good and bad. There's not much we can do for them. Oh, we'll polish them and maybe disabuse them of *some* bad habits, but for them the die is cast."

I smiled as I said this. Sergio smiled back, the smile of a poker player whose bet has been raised. The two interns became more apprehensive. This was not going the way they had hoped. I pressed on.

"As far as possible, we'll spend the least amount of time we can sitting in conference rooms like this. We'll spend most of our time at the bedsides, in the patients' rooms."

I pulled out my pocket-size six-ring folder from my coat. It had little tabs separating pages. It was well-worn and had the faint impression of my fingers on its blue vinyl cover.

"Every time we see a patient, something will come up that I realize I don't know much about or that I have forgotten or that I haven't read about in a while. I jot it down on the back page of this book, together with the patient's name. And so, by the end of the day, I have about ten things written down next to ten patients' names. And I never go to sleep at night without getting out my yellow highlighter and looking up those ten things in *Harrison's Principles of Internal Medicine.*"

The interns looked at me as if I were crazy. They were so busy with intern chores, the thought of reading at the end of the day was anathema to them. I wasn't being quite truthful: My *intention* most nights was to read the textbook before I went to bed.

"I'm suggesting you do this too. You'll be surprised by how, if you keep this up every day, you'll find your knowledge coalescing. There will be very few sections of your textbook that are not highlighted in yellow."

I was committed now to this sermon. "In addition, every day, I'll ask a couple of you to look up something that arises in the course of our rounds and make a mini-presentation back to the group. We'll start right now. David, I want you to look up coarctation of the aorta. For tomorrow. I'll explain why later."

David quickly wrote down his assignment on his clipboard. If he was curious as to why, he didn't make any sign.

"For your presentation to be digestible it must take no more than three minutes. We'll time you. It must fit on an index card, even if the material you looked up occupied thirty pages. And as you speak, the rest of us will take notes on our own index cards. You'll be amazed by how much we will all learn by the end of the month, not just by our own reading, but by the three or four mini-presentations we'll hear each day. That will be about twenty mini-presentations a week, close to one hundred for the whole month."

I saw one of the interns eyeing my blue book. "What I have in this blue book is the stuff that's useful for me. Things that I've looked up and had a hard time finding or that I know I want handy. The dose of epinephrine for anaphylactic shock, for example. It's my own personal manual. If you haven't got one going already, I suggest you start one. Its contents will change as you go through different stages of your training. But I'd be lost without it."

The female medical student, Sherry, was well-equipped. She brought out a stack of index cards from her pocket—I could tell she was going to start her little blue book that night. The two interns eyed her cards with fury.

As much as I wanted to impose my system on them, I didn't tell them that I had found that it was *patients* who lingered in my memory; the dry synopses of diseases on index cards never did. When I thought of a given disease, what first popped into my brain was the words and the tone of voice a patient had used to describe a symptom of that disease. Sometimes I recognized that same inflection in another patient's voice and it became a scent that led me down a diagnostic path—not necessarily the correct one. The index cards that I had accumulated, boxfuls now, worked like a database. I always knew I could find them in the filing cabinet, just as I knew what was in my tennis notebooks. Still, my instincts often ran ahead of my accumulated index cards, just as on the court one had to produce shots before there was time to deliberate about them. Perhaps that was why I often kept one hand in my pocket, on my blue book.

10

No sooner was Thanksgiving over than the houses in our neighborhood began to sport Christmas lights, strung on the edges of roof lines, more lights trailing through the pines and Mexican elder trees in front yards.

One evening, just before the light faded, I set out to look for an apartment. It was a depressing task. I felt I was too tired to start like this again, too old for apartment living. An El Paso housing guide in hand, I cruised from one complex to another. My only criterion was that it should be on the west side, close to the boys. I found only sadness in the banners and come-ons: POOL! FREE CABLE! LAUNDRY FACILITIES! CLUBHOUSE!

○

It was close to midnight when I returned home. The children were asleep, and their mother was watching television in the living room. Rajani must have seen in my face a reflection of my feelings after the apartment hunting.

"Nothing out there?"

"Oh, plenty out there."

"But . . . ?"

"What I realized tonight is that when I move, *I'm* the one the boys will think abandoned them."

She turned off the television.

"They'll never think that of *you*," I continued, "even though this is a mutual decision—"

"Did you want *me* to leave, then?"

"Picture the boys watching when the movers come and start taking things out."

I could see her visualizing this, putting herself in her sons' shoes. Her features, which had been set for a fight, softened, and she looked away, out of the window into the backyard. Pity is a poor reason to change one's plans. But, ever so softly, I heard her say—out of pity—"You don't have to move right away . . ."

Which would solve nothing, only postpone the inevitable.

"We could . . . ," she said, as if trying out the words, "resume counseling . . ."

"Is that what *you* want?"

"Only if *you* want to . . ."

After a silence, I said, "All right, then," hearing the skepticism in my own voice, but still saying the words and feeling some relief. Anything, it seemed, to avoid the pain of what we were planning. How much simpler it would be to live and be content with the mother of my children, the woman who jointly owned my every asset.

We sat around that night, drinking hot chocolate, giving wide berth to the momentous decision we had just made. We caught up on what had been happening with the other. "Who's this you're playing tennis with?" she asked, curious about the person who made me scribble entries in my journals late into the night. I was quick to tell her he was in the medical field, that we had some common ground. In the past, this had been a point of friction: that my tennis buddies had very little in common with me (or so she thought) other than the tennis.

I asked after her parents, her brother, since I knew she had been getting letters from India. A piece of news—gossip, really—made me burst out laughing, which made her laugh too. We hadn't laughed together for so long. That laugh, but nothing else, seemed to carry the promise that this might work after all.

I realized as I sat with her that I had been angry with her for a long time and that I had found it necessary to be angry because I knew I was at fault. It was so much easier to be angry with her than with myself. She had been the steady, consistent one in the marriage. It was my ambition, my profession, and my arrogance that kept me bouncing off walls, made me impossible to live with. "Why do our envelopes and bills lie around, between newspapers? Is it too much to have some order here?" when the order I wanted and needed was in my head, not in my house. And when, in the end, she had been faithful but I had not, that too had made me angry, resentful of her right to be righteous, whether she exercised that right or not. All these thoughts passed through my head, but now, despite this truce, I was unwilling to come clean.

When it was time for bed, I went to my futon and she to the platform bed. It was too soon, too sudden for us to conceive of taking this reconciliation—if that was what it was—much further.

And a good thing too.

By the cold light of morning, things deteriorated again: a small incident, so small that it defies memory, immediately found us retreating to our positions, to our familiar tones of voice. Out came the same old artillery, the same old barbs, her anger and mine now matching perfectly. The idea of counseling went out the window.

Back to square one.

o

On the tennis court the next day with David, I was tired, puzzled by the strange dance Rajani and I had done around each other, grateful that I had at least this tennis date to look forward to.

But I was perplexed as to exactly how to play with him. There I was, a flyweight, an amateur at that, going into the ring against a seasoned professional middleweight. This was only the second time we were meeting to play.

I strutted out of the locker room with him, proud to be his hitting companion, the fear and anxiety of our first tennis meeting a thing of the past. Once we started hitting ground strokes, adrenaline rose, and I pictured myself as Lendl incarnate, hitting the ball harder than ever. When David offered a rare short ball, I pounced on it and hit a screamer to one corner that pulled David off the court. He went off chasing it and I charged the net. He retrieved the ball but didn't try to pass me. Instead, he strummed under the ball with his beautiful slice backhand and lifted it to perfect volleying height, back to me. I angled the ball away sharply, giving him no chance.

"Good shot," he said, but I felt ashamed. Here I was hitting winners, while he was a ball machine, feeding the ball to me, feeding my ego, letting me vent my frustration. He had eliminated all competitiveness from his game, while my competitive instinct kept surfacing. In boxing terms, I was flailing at him, banging away, while he absorbed the blows, declining the counterpunch that could have set me flat on my ass.

Already I felt I had known this smiling young Aussie for a long time . . . from childhood. As if all childhood friendships between boys have common building blocks, the same in Africa as in Australia. I saw in him (perhaps he saw the same in me?) elements of my actual childhood friends. Maybe this was how adult friendships were formed, by recognizing and seeking out the archetypes of those we found comfort with in our youth.

Regardless of its origins, I wanted this nascent friendship to grow. David was easy to be around, and I sensed that he was very comfortable with me. If others who approached him to play tennis were intent on competition, or else were angling for a lesson, he had no such fears with me. In the hospital, he was proving to be an eager and able medical student, a sponge for whatever I had to offer. He had heard my introductory spiel on the wards, seen me in *my* pro mode, watched me in full flow at a bedside, engaged in my craft. I think he had a new respect for me, valued my company for that reason, just as I valued his for his skill on the courts. But the time had come to define the terms of how we played.

I was tempted to tell him about the events of last night and the morning, as explanation for the emergence of this killer instinct in me.

I stood at the net, my hands on my hips.

He walked over.

"Sorry," I said.

"For what?"

"I guess I should ask you what we're trying to do out here. Should I try to go for it? Hit winners?"

"I don't mind . . . that was a good rally there."

"But—"

He was amused, but he understood my dilemma.

"Why don't we just think of these sessions as extended practice, hitting as many balls as we can, keeping it in play. Consistency is what we're after. And fitness. That's my main goal, anyway. Besides," he said, gently mocking my earnestness, flipping a ball at my chest, "it's just great to be out here."

"Yes! Okay!"

I understood now.

O

We walked out of the club together and stood on the steps talking. A car pulled in, and only when it was right alongside us did I realize it was there for him.

"Gloria. My girlfriend. She's home from New Jersey," David said.

She rolled down her window and David introduced me, then walked around and sat in the passenger seat. Her sudden arrival left me speechless. Before I had even registered the wavy, thick black hair that reached past her shoulders, the disarming smile, the dusky eyes against fair skin, the soft hand that had touched my sweaty one, the image of the woman in the tattoo popped into my head. David's blond, light-skinned, sun-bleached appearance exaggerated her dark looks. She was without a doubt the embodiment, the quintessence, of the refined, elegant woman aspired to by the crude tattoo, the fantasy that, for most men who sported the tattoo, would never come true.

That was how I remained, mouth agape, rooted to the steps as they drove away, as if I had just seen an apparition.

11

Angelina Cortez had her bed propped up and the curtain pulled away from the window, allowing her a magnificent view of Juárez. Though her lips were still, a rapid dialogue in Spanish emanated from her, as if she were a ventriloquist. The audio from a soap opera playing on the wall-mounted television was coming out of the speaker clipped to her pillow. Flowers, probably from the room of a patient recently deceased or discharged, sat on her bedside table. A get well card taped to the wall had flopped open and it read, *"Para Papá*—We Miss You—*Que te sientas mejor."* She had transformed her half of the room into her salon. Her neighbor's half was, by comparison, dismal.

Angelina was thirty-nine, and all that was not hidden by the sheets was lovely. She bore no resemblance to the woman we had seen in the emergency room just a few days before on the first day of this rotation. The ER had been backed up, with gurneys spilling into the hallways and a drunk screaming and a child wailing. The trauma team was busy with a drive-by shooting. The air in the cubicle where Angelina lay had borne the mingled scents of an unwashed body and cheap perfume. She had been disheveled, with grimy nails and with sores festering on her legs. When I had tried to talk to her, she'd shaken the side of the stretcher in protest, whining and pleading for a shot of Demerol, even specifying the dose—150 milligrams—that she required for her fever, the pain in her chest, and the pain in her joints. She carried nothing with her except what she knew we needed: her name, social security number, and date of birth. Even if Angelina had no permanent address, no box of prized possessions, she was sure of one asset: a two-volume Thomason chart. It's orderliness, the tabs separating different admissions, the typed-up opinions of the various consultants who had seen her were in contrast to the disorder of her personal life.

The tranquil woman now holding court was a testament to modern medicine—and to methadone's ability to blunt the tremors, the runs, the pains, and the bitchiness of withdrawal. Angelina had reapplied a brilliant red nail polish ("FM" red she had told me on a previous visit, and when I'd looked puzzled, she had explained: "fuck me" red), matching lipstick, and theatrical face powder and mascara. Her bare arms were slender. A mother-of-pearl rosary, brought by the chaplain, was intertwined between her fingers. Her hair, blond at the tips and black at the roots, was parted in the middle, and arranged on the pillow on both sides of her. She had doubled up on the hospital gowns, tying one at the back in the prescribed fashion, and wearing the other one over it as a dressing gown, open at the front. Even with no flesh showing, her posture, the set of her arms, the curve of her cheeks, the arch of her penciled eyebrows, the way she had outlined her lips seemed to hint at a carnality, a *furor uterinus*, that didn't feel quite hers. Rather, it was a painted-on, generic, girlie-magazine sexiness. If Gloria was the epitome, the zenith of the idealized woman represented by the jailhouse tattoo, Angelina, despite all her efforts, could not transcend the image of the tattoo. She was rougher than the tattoo itself.

As we assembled around her bed, Angelina put on a practiced look of seduction and helplessness. "Good morning, Dr. Barrio, Dr. Smith," she said, her eyes touching each face and naming each person, even calling the medical students "doctor" before settling on me, the *jefe*, "and Dr. Verghese. How are you all this morning?"

Angelina's clinical illness was straightforward. She was an intravenous drug user. Pus had welled out from injection sites on her leg. She had a loud heart murmur, and the conjunctivae of both her eyes showed tiny red dots—emboli. A raised red lesion on the pulp of her middle finger—Osler's node—was evident, together with "splinter" hemorrhages in the nail beds. Her spleen was enlarged. There was blood in her urine. These disparate clues, if viewed as true and related, were relatively simple to put together. She had endocarditis, an infection of the heart valves.

A normal heart valve is a smooth, glistening, pliable surface that seals off and then opens to the chambers of the heart with every beat. Blood glides over the normal valve. Angelina's repeated injections of intravenous drugs with their particulate impurities had roughened her heart valves, rendered them sticky, causing platelets to adhere to them like flies to flypaper. From one of the boils on her legs, bacteria had swept into the bloodstream and lodged on the platelets stuck to the valve. The bacteria replicated there, made the surface even rougher, and more platelets arrived, forming a conglobate mass from whose crumbly surface little bits broke off and carried infective clots into the lungs, the kidneys, the joints, the conjunctivae, and the spleen.

After sending samples of her blood to the microbiology lab, we had begun Angelina on antibiotics. By the second day *Staphylococcus aureus* was growing in the blood cultures. Endocarditis used to be a fatal infection in the pre-antibiotic era, but with six weeks of intravenous therapy, Angelina would recover. It was possible that one of her heart valves would need to be replaced.

Angelina worked the room, charmed the medical students. This town was still fairly new to me, the hospital not totally familiar, but Angelina herself was timeless. I had seen her in other hospitals in other cities. At that moment, elsewhere in the building, a thirty-four-year-old man with a previous partial amputation of the right arm from gangrene developing at an injection site was in danger of losing his left arm for the same reason. And on two other medical ward teams there were patients like Angelina with heart-valve infections completing their course of antibiotic therapy. In the intensive care unit was a "mule"—a thirty-two-year-old carrier of heroin who had ingested tightly wrapped, drug-filled balloons and walked across the border, but who had had the misfortune of having his cargo rupture within his bowels and get absorbed into the bloodstream before he could take his priceless crap. And there were many others—patients with gunshot wounds, strokes, respiratory illness, AIDS, and survivors of motor vehicle accidents—whose problems were directly or indirectly related to drugs.

In infectious diseases folklore, Angelina had a special place, a fond place, even. The propensity of people to stick needles in themselves and inject drugs directly into the bloodstream had given birth to a colorful medical subspecialty. Countless scientific papers, including a few of my own, dealt with the problems of infections in intravenous drug abusers, or IVDAs. They had launched many an academic career. One of my publications as a fellow in Boston had come from studying infections of the major veins of the neck and thorax—the vena cava, the innominate, the subclavian. Pus within one of these veins—suppurative phlebitis as it was called—was fatal if untreated; the usual treatment called for was complete surgical excision of the vein. Easy enough in the forearm, but a brutal undertaking in central veins—veins that led from the neck into the chest. We had shown that in certain patients with infected central veins, prolonged treatment with heparin, a blood thinner, along with a lengthy course of antibiotics, could salvage some patients without the need for risky surgery.

What made Angelina and her fellow IVDAs fascinating was that they were as committed to their *method* of drug use as they were to the drug itself. Being willing to deliver a drug through a needle into a vein, have it shoot through the heart and hit the brain—the "rush"—put them in a fellowship different from those who sniffed, snorted, smoked, or swilled. The vein was central to their existence. Its penetration was mystical, magical, so much so that in the absence of drugs they would sometimes shoot water into the vein, as if they were tapping into a primitive ritual, much as the Kikuyu in Africa open a vein for their initiation ceremony. The advent of AIDS, the risks of hepatitis B and hepatitis C, malaria, tetanus, syphilis, abscesses, and heart-valve infection had done little to disrupt the habits of the committed user. The crack epidemic hadn't tempted hard-core IVDAs like Angelina away from the needle. Instead, crack had spawned a new subculture, with its own paraphernalia and terminology, and now its own repertoire of telltale symptoms and signature illnesses—"crack keratitis," "crack thumb," "crack hands," and a Parkinson's-like tremor and movement disorder whose name was coined on the street: "crack dance."

One of the two interns on our team reported on Angelina's progress. Angelina was a ready teacher, someone who had been in the system so many times that she had a proprietary interest in bedside rounds. And she was finally well enough to participate in this exercise.

"Angelina," I said, when the intern was done, "would you mind if I point out a few things to the students as I examine you? I'd—"

"Sure, Dr. Verghese. Any time."

"What's your drug of choice?"

"*¡Ay!*" she sighed. "Both. Heroin and coke. Started when I was eighteen. I stayed clean for many years. I had a family and two kids . . . *y luego* I moved to L.A. Then I had problems there and got back into it. So I came here to get away, but the man I met was into it. I was speedballing—mixing coke with heroin."

"Tell us, if you don't mind, how you get the heroin, how you inject, the steps . . ."

"Okay. First I buy it, then—"

"Where?"

"On Dyer. Or downtown if I want speedballs—so many places." Dyer Street paralleled Fort Bliss, on the northeast side of town, a street with an abundance of nightclubs, hookers, motels, and bars. The press often reported shootings and stabbings that had taken place on Dyer. I had driven down it in the daytime, to eat at a Korean restaurant. It had looked benign then, but its character changed at night.

"How is it packaged?"

"In little rubber *botas*. Different-colored balloons for different prices."

"And then?"

"Dissolve it in water."

"From where?"

"Evian. Tap, sometimes."

"A drug has to be dissolved before it's injected," I said to the students. "Any drug you can dissolve, you can shoot. Actually, that's not quite true—even gasoline can be injected. For years, IVDA meant heroin. But now it can be coke or speed and all the various combinations. The drugs you buy on the street are 'cut' or diluted by the supplier. The 'fillers' probably cause some of the chronic heart and lung problems we see.

"Cocaine dissolves at room temperature. In the movies, they often get this wrong—you see them heat the cocaine. Some shooting galleries may have sterile saline. Most have 'clean water' for injecting—and a jar of 'dirty water' for rinsing needles and syringes. If there's no running water, the user might carry a bottle. Or use saliva, or toilet-bowl water."

Sherry was looking puzzled. She had spent all her life in Lubbock, where the only shooting gallery was sponsored by the NRA.

"Shooting galleries," I explained, "are places where, for a cut of your drugs, a shooter will inject the heroin or coke for you. Often these 'block docs' have some medical training, maybe as an army medical corpsman or a nurses' aide—"

Angelina was nodding. "Or else they learn in the hospital, watching you guys put needles in," she added.

I tried to take the reins back. "They make the customer strain down as if working for a bowel movement—a Valsalva's maneuver, in other words—and then they shoot the neck veins."

"Shooting pockets!" Angelina said.

"I've seen infection in the conjunctival veins, sublingual veins, the dorsal vein of the penis, hemorrhoidal veins . . ."

Angelina wrinkled her nose. "*Nunca, nunca*," she said. Still, she was looking at me with new respect. She hadn't credited me with this much knowledge of her world.

"Some of the infections that are associated with certain cities," I continued, "may relate to unusual practices among the addicts there in the way they prepare their fixes. For example, *Pseudomonas* infection is common in Detroit, *Candida* in New York, *Serratia* in San Francisco—"

"Okay," Angelina said, jumping in to pick up the narrative and recapture her audience, "next you take a piece of cigarette filter—a tiny piece—and drop it into the spoon. Then you suck up the fluid into the syringe through the cigarette filter."

"Why?" Sherry asked.

"Keeps all the shit out! You have to keep the shit out." Angelina glanced at me, as if to ask where we got such a *pendeja*. "If you don't, you get real sick."

"It's a filtration step," I said. "Some people will deliberately *not* filter in order to experience a 'talc flash,' particularly with tablets that are not crushed properly."

Angelina gave me a look of annoyance. I resolved not to interrupt her. "Okay, then I use diabetic syringes. None of this eyedropper shit you see on TV. And then," she said, settling back on the pillow, "you find a vein and pop it in."

When I was sure she was done, I rolled back her sleeves.

"Venous access is the name of the game," I said. Angelina had no tracks on her right hand, but several track marks on the left. "Cocaine generally doesn't leave tracks, and if it does, it is a depressed track from the vasoconstriction cocaine produces. The nondominant hand is usually where you see it. This is a typical heroin track," I said, tracing with my finger a dark, linear line, the width of a pencil, extending down from the crease in her elbow. "The chronic inflammation in the vein causes the skin overlaying it to become hyperpigmented. And if they sterilize their needle with a flame, they inadvertently carry soot into the skin, making a tattoo. Once in the vein, then you 'boot.' Can you explain 'booting,' Angelina?"

"See," she said, turning to Sherry and demonstrating with an imaginary syringe in her hand, "you get into the vein and then you pull back some blood into the syringe; it mixes with your stuff and then you inject a little bit into the vein and then pull back some more blood, then you inject a bit more, and again and again . . ." Her body was gently undulating as she demonstrated.

"Why?" Sherry again. She seemed caught up by Angelina and her story.

"Because," and she paused here, realizing that in that question and in her answer lay the difference between her world and that of this young *güera*, "because it feels good, *mi'ja*." After a noticeable pause she spoke again, but this time as if from a distance. "The drug hits your brain and hits you again and again. That's why you boot. The rush. That's what it's all about. That's why my life went like this . . . always looking for the rush one more time."

She stopped as though she had caught herself. Talking about the rush had triggered the ritual in her brain that led her to get a fix. With cocaine, where there was not as much physical dependence as psychic dependence, environmental clues could suddenly trigger the urge to use. I had a patient who was driven to use every time he heard a pay phone ring. He associated the sound with his paging his dealer and the dealer calling back.

"But no more. This time it really scared me. I was so sick before I came to the hospital. I have to get clean. I almost died."

"How come you never used your arms much?" I asked.

"I didn't want my arms to look ugly. I'd seen the girls with the puffy hands, and scars . . ."

I gently drew back the sheets. This was a difficult moment for Angelina. As long as her legs were covered, she did not have to acknowledge them, she could play the vamp. But now Jezebel's spell was broken. For beneath the sheets, her legs looked like the swollen trunks of two Mexican elder trees, her skin having undergone a hide-like thickening. The exterior was dry and flaky. Scattered over the surface were sores the size of quarters. Some were scabbed over, others were recessed scars with concentric rings of peeling skin around them. All semblance of a pretty calf or a shapely ankle was obliterated by a jelly-roll swelling. Her tiny feet emerged from a puffy collar.

Angelina stared with shame at her lower limbs. If she could have, she would have traded them for the old woman's in the next bed.

"Skin popping," I explained softly to the students, "is often the method of choice for women. Especially if the superficial veins of the feet have clogged up."

I covered her legs back up. I examined her heart, looked into the fundi of her eyes, felt her spleen, and then stepped back.

It was then that I became conscious of David. He was at the foot of the bed, his hands folded over his chest, his face pale, his eyes opaque, and his expression one that I barely recognized, as if something painful had welled up within him. The story seemed to have affected him even more than it had Sherry. I had focused the session on Sherry and the other student because I knew that Sergio, the interns, and David had all seen patients like Angelina before, even if they didn't know all the details she and I had come up with. If there had been no one else in the room other than the two of us, I might have asked David what he was thinking.

He became aware of my gaze. One side of his face twitched and he uncrossed his arms as if to break the spell that had come over him. The expression I had seen flickered like a faulty fluorescent light, and slowly, the David I knew reappeared and he put on a contrite expression. As if I had caught him daydreaming.

"What about the result of my AIDS test?"

I pulled my eyes off David.

"We're waiting for it. Have you had a test before?"

"A year ago. It was negative. But I want another one."

"Have you shared needles?"

"No, only years ago with my first husband, who died. But you know . . ." She trailed off, embarrassed.

"Were you . . . ?"

She seemed relieved that I had guessed this rather than her volunteering it.

"Yes. But you know, all I did was blow jobs. Or hand jobs."

"Blow jobs with condoms?"

"All the time. I'm really scared of AIDS. Just a few times I didn't use condoms. They say you can't get it that way, right?"

"It's maybe less likely. I'm hopeful that your test will be negative. But you really have to get away from drugs. When we see you next, we'll talk about rehab, getting you to stay drug-free."

Angelina was content to let us go.

We left, all of us somewhat subdued. It was impossible to leave that room without being awed by the power of the needle, how it had taken a pretty young woman and made her life and her livelihood orbit entirely around it.

I looked at Sherry to see how she was doing. She was an empathetic student and Angelina was a first for her. She seemed on the verge of tears. I thought it better to talk to her separately, later.

David's face was inscrutable now, his clipboard at the ready, prepared to present the next patient to us, a man with pneumonia in the ICU.

12

We missed tennis on Sunday because David was on call, and by midweek
I was itching to play. The air outside was still and it was, incredibly,
in December, in the midsixties.

I picked up the phone and paged David. "Dr. Smith," I said when
he called back, "a matter of great importance has come up regarding
your patients." It was four in the afternoon.

"Yes?" I could hear the anxiety in his voice.

"It appears that you have discharged two of your patients, so by
my calculation you have no patients till we are on call next—"

"Sergio told me to—"

"—and therefore there should be no obstacle to your slipping
away for some cardiovascular endurance training with racket and
ball?"

I heard him breathe, and then begin to laugh softly. He might
have been tempted to call me a choice name, but instead he said, "I
just have a few loose ends to tie up."

"Page me when you're heading for the parking lot. Put in six-zero,
and I'll know you're leaving. If for some reason you can't make it,
put in zero-six."

"Got it." Since it was my idea to slip away, I imagined I had
absolved him of guilt.

When my pager displayed 6-0, I went to the parking lot. He was
behind me as we left Alameda, but once on the freeway, he sped
past me on the right side. I shifted into a lower gear and reeled him
in, winking at him as I sped by, but he surprised me by heading for a
downtown exit that surely was too far east of the club. I changed
lanes and followed him. The chase was on now; he wove through
back roads, climbing up toward Pill Hill, then left on Schuster

where antiabortionists, looking bored, held up signs outside a clinic. I lost him at a light but caught up again at Stanton, and then made a right turn on Robinson, which brought us directly to the tennis club. I resolved to look up this route on the map.

The previous evening I had come by the club and signed up as a member. I didn't think David was a member. He told me that he had participated in a couple of pro-am fund-raisers for the club. Perhaps he was welcome to play whenever he wanted to.

○

David had opened two cans of balls. "I was trying to remember some of the drills we used to do with John Newcombe," he said. "Classic Harry Hopman drills. I'll show you."

It started off simply: crosscourt forehands, crosscourt backhands, down-the-line shots, ten minutes or so of each. And then the killer drill: David hit crosscourt, swinging me from side to side while I returned down the line. It was only possible for me to keep this up for a few minutes before needing to catch my breath. Then it was my turn to swing him around. Other than the briefest instruction for each drill, we conversed little. I could see that David was working on a topspin backhand, and he could hit it well. But when rushed, he always fell back on his slice backhand, a much more reliable shot for him and so pretty to watch.

When I hung my head, gasped for air, David giggled and sent a ball right at me, before I could even straighten myself. I understood that this was punishment for scaring him when I'd first paged him at work.

"Harry Hopman? Didn't he have both his hips replaced?"

"C'mon, then," David said. "Show some life. Let's get on with it."

I was ready to quit after about forty minutes, but David, who looked equally tired, kept calling, "Last three balls!" It was only when we ceased that I became aware that some of the club players had stopped to watch us. And to realize that the sounds from our court had been like that of a metronome, a contrast to the chaotic sounds from adjacent courts.

"Bloody slave master!" I said.

"That is, in fact, what the green team has been saying about our fearless leader."

"They have not! . . . Have they?"

○

I slumped on the bench. David filled six of the small, disposable conical cups from the cooler with water, setting them one after the other between the strings of his racket, then swung the racket toward me like a tray.

"Inventive and elegant," I said.

"The small but important things one picks up on the pro tour."

○

The sky was clear, streaked only by jet trails from planes that had passed long before. With my head resting on the bench, my legs extended in front of me, I felt light, exhilarated. If hunting for apartments had made me feel old and weary, the kind of tennis we had played made me feel youthful and virile.

"Coffee? You been to Dolce Vita?" David asked.

I was in no particular hurry to get home that day. The kids were out Christmas shopping with Rajani.

In the locker room, David stripped off his clothes. I was reluctant to shower, never entirely comfortable with mass nakedness, or perhaps my own nakedness. So much better to scrub and sing in the privacy of my own home, my own shower. But since David was already naked, I undressed too.

Soggy carpet led to cold tile. There were other men in the communal shower, all of us pretending we were unaware of each other, lost in our soapy world. Momentary confusion once again: My eyes, so trained to look at flesh clinically, had to be held back.

When we were toweling off, I told David about this: the brief disorientation when I saw naked flesh in a nonclinical situation, and how my eyes, from habit, looked for disease.

"Are you serious?"

"Yes."

"As a matter of fact, I've been trying to practice," he said. "The other day I spotted a goiter in the hallway—"

"A *patient* with a goiter."

"A patient with a goiter. And I looked at the eyes to see if they were protruding, and they were. I was pretty proud of myself. In fact, I've made up a set of index cards for common skin conditions I might see."

"Tell me," I said, dropping my voice, "do you think male obstetricians get distracted when they make love? Do they have to push out the thought about the pelvis being too narrow for a baby's head? Do they register the position of the cervix? Do they try and decide if a uterus is retroflexed?" David was giggling and looking me as if I were weird. "I'm serious!"

"Yeah. As serious as a whore at a christening."

We dressed silently, putting on our work clothes again, save for the neckties.

○

Dolce Vita was an avant-garde coffee shop on the strip of Mesa Street that ran past the University of Texas at El Paso, UTEP. The double cappuccinos came in what looked like soup tureens. If El Paso was unlike any other city I had lived in, the crowd at Dolce Vita was not. They could have been transplanted from a coffee shop in Seattle or Iowa City. Almost everyone had papers in front of them— UTEP professors correcting essays, poets waiting for the muse, songwriters scribbling notes. No one ever seems out of place in a coffee shop.

We chose raised bar stools along the picture window, sitting shoulder to shoulder rather than face-to-face at the small tables. We were both observers, spies, if you will, with, but not a part of, the crowd, having drawn our own invisible circle.

"You know, when I was little—" David started but was distracted by a gorgeous brunette, tall and as beautifully awkward as a giraffe. He swiveled to follow her with his eyes as she went behind a curtain marked EO. The curtain stayed closed, the brunette hidden. In that instant, the one door that David had opened to his past closed as if blown shut by a breeze. When he picked up his place, I sensed he was taking me into another, safer room. "When I was little, I loved Laver. He was small, like me, you know. But he had the strokes, he was aggressive. As a professor of mine is fond of saying, 'It isn't the size of your instrument but how you use it that counts . . .'"

"Seriously? Laver?" I asked, ignoring his teasing.

"Styled my game completely on his. The grip I use, for example," he said, holding his hand straight in front of him, as if he were about to pick up a hammer, "and not changing grips for different strokes—that's Laver. But I never developed the topspin backhand he had. Serve and volley was my game. Groundies were merely a way to get to the net. Couldn't overpower anyone with my ground strokes.

"Did I tell you I worked as an assistant at John Newcombe's tennis ranch in New Braunfels? Yeah, for a couple of summers. At the end of the day, we'd play serious matches—just the coaches. Everyone would come watch. Once, when I went into the clubhouse after some match that I'd won, Newcombe was at the bar, and he turns to me and says, "'Ere comes the most aggressive *pusher* of the ball the game has seen! Give that man a beer.'" David laughed at this recollection. "He'd diagnosed me. That's really what I did—push the ball back and get to the net. Live or die by my net game."

"Hey, it worked well enough. Got you a scholarship. Got you on the pro tour."

He shook his head. "That was just a lark. Couldn't make a living like that. I knew it before I started."

Thank God for the study of medicine in my life. And his.

"But I can't blame my game alone," David said, catching himself. "If I'd'a had enough money to stay on the tour, to get the *experience*, I could have gone quite far even with a game like mine. I know that now. Not that it does me any bloody good. Brad Gilbert's a perfect example. He's a counterpuncher—no big shot and a serve that's a joke. But he's been out on the tour long enough to have figured out how to win. It's as simple as that—he's figured out how to win. He's the cleverest player on the tour. What he does is make the other bloke play badly. Look at some of his wins: He owned Becker. And he made McEnroe go into retirement. Didcha' see that match at the Master's?"

I nodded. "Where McEnroe told him, 'You don't deserve to be on the same court with me'?"

"Right. McEnroe wasn't playing his best. And Gilbert's game *looked* so pedestrian. Still, it's sometimes tough to beat a player you're *supposed* to beat. Right off the bat, it puts pressure on you. And when you see that you might lose, it puts even more pressure on you. What Gilbert did that day was to take away McEnroe's lefty serve in the ad court, the wide serve that swings out to the right-hander's backhand and pulls him into the stands."

People watching us must have wondered what we were talking about as David made chopping movements with his left hand and pointed in different directions.

"See, Gilbert camped in the doubles alley, waiting for that serve, tempting McEnroe to go down the middle. But Mac kept missing with the down-the-middle serve and so instead he'd take something off his second serve and it would come to Gilbert's forehand. At which point Gilbert was in charge of the point! It was an amazing match for me because I looked at Gilbert's game and *I* thought I could beat him. And yet, if I had Gilbert's game, I'd never have been able to imagine beating a McEnroe. I'd have lost the match in me head before I started."

The brunette, wearing an apron now, came out and asked us if we were ready for refills. I asked for water.

The direction our conversation had taken opened up old wounds for us both. From being animated as he described Brad Gilbert, David was subdued now, as if he felt he had offered too much. It was a sad thing to realize that your childhood dreams weren't going to come true. In my case, the tennis dream became a fantasy so early that it never cost me any time. David had come much closer.

If we had traded places in childhood, if I had been given as much opportunity to play and develop, would I have had the courage to pursue tennis as a career? Would I have found a way to make it on the pro tour?

I said, to pierce the silence, "When I came to America, when I was getting back into tennis, I was Lendl's number-one fan. No one else seemed to like him but me. When he first came up, he had a ferocious forehand but only a slice backhand. He learned a topspin backhand. Hell, he invented the idea of off-court training. And so finicky about his rackets weighing just so, being balanced just so, . . . it showed there was another way to get to the top: hard work. And the pivotal moment in his life,"—the waitress had come back with water, catching me with my finger in the air—"the pivotal moment, after he had been in so many Grand Slam finals without winning, always a bridesmaid, never a bride, was the French Open final against McEnroe. 1984. Did you see it?"

David shook his head no.

"Roland Garros packed, ready to see the first American since Tony

Trabert in 1955 win the French. McEnroe ahead, six-three, six-two. Completely in control. They were one-one in the third set. It looked like Lendl was going to lose again. I couldn't bear to watch. But McEnroe begins to gripe about a TV camera as Lendl starts to serve. Lendl is down, love-thirty, and now McEnroe is bitching about photographers. Lendl manages to hold serve, and by now the crowd is down on McEnroe, calling out stuff and booing. Lendl breaks McEnroe, serves out the third set. Lendl wins the fourth set seven-five.

"By this time, I'm a wreck. Fifth set in a Grand Slam is when Lendl chokes. And *my* whole life seemed to depend on his finally winning, you know what I mean? I had my lucky shirt on—same argyle pattern as his. I had my lucky tennis shoes on, my racket in my hand—that year I played with an Adidas, just like his. And I didn't let it touch the ground the whole match. I'd figured out that one corner of the living room was lucky, and I had to stand right at that spot or else he'd start making errors. I was standing whenever they were on the court, sitting only when he got to sit. But Lendl didn't choke. He went on to win seven-five in the fifth. Man, I was in tears, I was exhausted. I think I was happier than Lendl himself. And the rest is history. He went on to win eight Grand Slams! Two Australian Opens, three French Opens, three U.S. Opens!"

David was laughing his braying laugh. People were looking at us: a couple of oddballs, they figured. He shook his head, as if in amazement.

"There's something I don't understand . . . ," he said, trailing off. He leaned forward, his expression one of concentration as he formed the question, as if he were trying to frame it in a way that didn't give offense. We were sitting in neutral territory, neither at the hospital nor on the courts. He was entitled to ask me anything.

"It's like, this . . . you're as passionate about tennis as you are about medicine. It seems like . . . *one* of those would be enough." I must have looked blank, so he went on. "I mean, you know the students are in awe of you. When you go to the bedside and start demonstrating all these physical signs . . . it's as if you're pulling off blindfolds. Coming up with and connecting things to make a diagnosis. It's spectacular and . . . and you rattle off facts, but not just facts, you seem to thrill with those medical stories, the history behind it . . ."

He leaned back now. "And meanwhile, see, for me . . . all I could excel at was that one bloody thing, tennis. And even that . . . When it was over, I had to find a life, didn't I? Had to come back to the real world . . . I mean, you act as if tennis is just as consuming, as interesting, as medicine."

I was flattered by what he was saying.

"I wish you could have seen my first instructor, Mr. Swaminathan."

"Why? Was he an inspiring teacher?"

"You know, I'm not sure if he ever loved the game. He was . . . distracted by our lessons. As if the lessons required only a fraction of his intellect and physical skills, so he kept his mind and body in reserve. But even so, there was something about him, a wonderful grace to his tennis, a grace to the way he walked off with his rackets stacked on top of each other, the handles under his armpit, his hand under them like a waiter holding a tray. As though you couldn't play such elegant tennis without it affecting the rest of you—your carriage, your walk, your every movement. It was Mr. Swaminathan who first made me feel that tennis players were a . . . different breed."

I wanted to tell David that I saw some of that style in him. And very much so in Ross Walker at the club. It was there in the way they walked, the way just then that David had used his hands while talking about McEnroe. *Keep the ball in play. Keep your eye on the ball. Follow through.* These were admonitions for both tennis and life, and they spilled over from the one into the other.

But I didn't say this to David. Because what I did not see in him off the court was the confidence or the poise I had assumed came with a tennis life. Its absence was the most striking thing about David.

13

My senior resident, Sergio, had once been a used-car salesman. He had come to Texas after medical school in Guadalajara and a brief stint in Brazil. When he was studying to pass the requisite qualifying exams to pursue a residency here, he made money by buying late-model, big American cars and driving them down to South America where he sold them for a profit.

When he showed up in my office, twenty minutes before rounds were to begin, wearing an orange shirt, matching tie, and dark, crisply pressed trousers, there was nothing to suggest that he had been up all night and had admitted seven patients from the emergency room.

"Everything is under control," he said as he did every morning. He was still a good salesman. As we walked across to the hospital together, he told me that one of the admissions was in the ICU, assigned to David. "I don't think David even left his side to pee," Sergio said. "He went with me to admit him from the ER. He wheeled him to radiology and up to the ICU himself. He's been there all night."

I was proud to hear that David had so fully immersed himself in his patient's care.

We were stopped in the hallway by a laboratory worker. After a hurried conversation in Spanish, Sergio whipped out a pad from his back pocket and wrote an antibiotic prescription for the man's wife. "These are the people who really run the hospital," he said, not apologetically, but by way of explanation. Sergio was clearly *in* with all the hospital personnel. The measure of one's effectiveness as a resident lay in working the system, so you got the CAT scans and endoscopies you needed scheduled ASAP and your blood work run right away. Sergio had the machinery well-oiled. He greeted people in the hallways with the confidence of a labor boss. People who saw us walking together might have assumed I was his understudy.

○

The staff in the ICU was routinely cheery. I thought of them as fairies at work inside a womb. They handled impossibly complex machinery, kept untangled the umbilical cords that fed patients, patients who were largely unconscious or unaware of the perils they faced.

A pretty nurse who had taken wonderful care of one of my HIV-infected patients in the ICU pulled me aside. "Dr. Verghese, can I ask you something? You know your tennis buddy, Dr. Smith? Do you think he'd be interested in going to a rodeo?"

"Rodeo?" I said, surprised that our tennis link was so quickly common knowledge. "As a matter of fact, I know he's been dying to go to a rodeo."

She looked skeptical, unsure if I was putting her on.

"You sure?"

"Positive. Just the other day he said, 'I'd love to go to a rodeo.'"

"I wanted to ask him out for something different, you know? Not a UTEP basketball game, or dancing." The clinician in me told me that this was no playful banter; she was seriously smitten with my Aussie friend.

"But he's got a steady girlfriend," I said, and then regretted it.

"So?" she asked, her body stiffening, as if this was of no great consequence. But her eyes told me that this was news to her. "He told one of the other nurses that he'd come to the nurses' Christmas party."

"Maybe I got the girlfriend bit wrong."

"God, I hope so."

○

Mr. Rocha was one of the few ICU patients who was awake.

"Mr. Rocha is thirty-four years old and presents with a chief complaint of increasing shortness of breath and a fever of five days' duration," David began, speaking softly. The chief complaint was like the title of a short story, an indication to the audience of where to turn their minds' files as they heard this tale.

David looked fragile, anxious, as if he were all too aware of the responsibility Mr. Rocha's illness put on him. David's age showed about the eyes. He hadn't shaved, but it didn't matter, because it took four days for him to develop the kind of five-o'-clock shadow I developed by noon. The green-and-yellow freebie pharmaceutical company pen in his hand, the same one he had used since the beginning of the month, was beginning to look ragged at its end where he had chewed it. Given how these pens lie around like bait for mice, it was touching to see David hold on to this one pen as if it were a priceless Mont Blanc. And while the other students had spent a good bit of money on shiny manuals and handbooks and recipe books—pocket libraries that stuffed their pockets and made them waddle like penguins—David had only his stethoscope in one pocket, and a stack of index cards held together with rubber bands in the other.

"Mr. Rocha speaks no English," David paused to explain. "I obtained this history with Sergio . . ." He cleared his throat as he began the HPI: history of the present illness. His voice was hoarse. "Mr. Rocha was in his usual state of health until five days prior to admission when he noted the onset of shortness of breath and low-grade fever. He works as a stable hand for a horse farm just across the state line in New Mexico. He continued to work for one or two more days after the onset of the fever but the shortness of breath progressed . . ."

Medical students and interns often adopted a depersonalized jargon when working in ICUs. I was sure it was a macho affect to mask their fear, a form of self-protection. But David's voice trembled.

○

Mr. Rocha was a short man, portly, with hooded eyes, bald on top but with a profusion of Nerolike curls on both sides of his head. There was a coarse stubble confined to his chin. His cheeks and chest were hairless. He was sitting up, his arms propped behind him like rigid struts that supported his heaving chest. The musty scent in the room brought to mind the image of a frightened blood horse. He looked out fearfully over the green muzzle of the oxygen mask.

When David was done, he held up Mr. Rocha's chest X ray, the ticket that earned him direct admission to the ICU from the ER. It showed a diffuse, opaque, ground-glass pattern over what should have been the blackness of his lungs. Since the mideighties, this was a pattern, when seen in a young male, that was *Pneumocystis carinii*, ergo, AIDS until proven otherwise. But David had established from his history that Mr. Rocha had no obvious risk factors for HIV infection. Blood had been drawn in the emergency room for a rapid HIV test. It was negative. This was not AIDS, and yet it was no ordinary pneumonia.

When David and I were alone, without an audience, we usually stood close to each other, and spoke sotto voce, coconspirators. But now, facing each other across Mr. Rocha's bed, our roles were more formal. I nodded twice at David, and from the smile that flickered on his face he knew I was proud of his presentation.

"When a patient comes in with pneumonia, it's the history—the epidemiology in particular—that leads you to suspect an unusual cause of pneumonia and begin treatment. That's critical because it may take the lab several days to isolate the pathogen responsible—if it manages to isolate it at all."

The students had their pens and index cards out.

"If Mr. Rocha had been hunting or skinning rabbits, what would you think of?"

"Tularemia," Sergio said when no one else volunteered an answer. "I asked, and he denies that."

"Did you ask him if he cleaned out a chicken coop or chopped down an old rotted tree trunk? Or has he been digging or excavating? Exploring caves?"

David shook his head.

"If he had, you'd think of histoplasmosis or coccidioidomycosis. Did you ask him about tick bites? And has he traveled outside the area lately?"

"No travel outside the area. Denies tick bites."

"Has he noticed dead rats around? 'Rat fall' is an antecedent to plague in humans. There are scattered cases of plague reported every year in New Mexico. And has he eaten *queso de cabra*, unpasteurized goat cheese, from Juárez?—the usual mode of acquiring brucellosis. It's a disease that I have never seen and yet I know it is endemic to the area. Does he own a pet bird? A risk factor for psittacosis pneumonia."

As Sergio quizzed the patient, David looked sheepish. He leaned close to me and murmured, "Sorry, I should have asked about that stuff."

"That's precisely why I'm here."

Mr. Rocha answered all Sergio's questions by shaking his head.

I examined Mr. Rocha from head to foot, telling the students what I was looking for and why, pointing out things that I noted on the way. Mr. Rocha had parotid gland enlargement, gynecomastia, diminished axillary hair, and a pubic hair distribution (the escutcheon) that looked female: a triangle with the apex pointing down. I said to David, "I think he is underreporting his alcohol consumption." Chronic alcohol ingestion and the resultant liver damage made the liver less efficient at metabolizing the estrogens that males normally produced.

David now read off the values for the various laboratory tests he had ordered. None of them was particularly helpful. Influenza season was upon us, but a rapid DNA probe test for influenza was negative. "The most significant laboratory abnormality is a low-oxygen tension in the blood, and this morning's blood gas is even worse, even though he's on a hundred-percent non-rebreather mask," David said.

"All right, then. You've worked him up. We've formulated a differential. Now, Dr. Smith," I said, "what do you think we should do?"

"Well . . ." David looked to Sergio for reassurance, color rising in his cheeks. Sergio nodded encouragement, the senior salesman prodding the novice to deliver his pitch. "We've begun treating him empirically for community-acquired pneumonia. We are covering Legionnaire's disease and the pneumococcus with erythromycin and ceftriaxone. We didn't think about some of the things you mentioned . . . but he doesn't really have risk factors for them. But meanwhile, he's on the verge of respiratory failure, so when his carbon dioxide level goes over fifty, we'll have to breathe for him."

I looked at how hard Mr. Rocha was struggling to breathe. "I wouldn't wait that long. He's tiring out already. The moment to breathe for him is now, before he crashes."

I asked Sergio to explain this to Mr. Rocha. I could follow most of what Sergio was saying: He told him about the ventilator, said we knew it was frightening, and that he would not be able to talk with the tube in his trachea, but that we would sedate him throughout to minimize his discomfort. He told him not to give up, to be strong willed. We would do everything in our power for him.

Mr. Rocha, as scared as he was, said, *"Esta bien."* He let his gaze linger on David. There was fear and urgency and pleading in that glance, as if to say he was putting all his faith in him. David put his hand on Mr. Rocha's shoulder and nodded, as if to say he'd be there with him. This seemed to reassure Mr. Rocha, who then put his own hand over David's.

We had many other patients to see, but this could not wait. Mr. Rocha glanced briefly at the ventilator the nurse was wheeling into the room and then looked away. It resembled a fancy, top-loading, digital display washing machine.

We paged the anesthetist and stepped out to free up space.

○

"Did you see how Mr. Rocha looked at David? Did you see how his touch reassured him?" I asked the group. "Picture yourself lying on that bed. Go on . . . picture it." They shuffled their feet. "It's a terrifying experience. It's important that you realize that every illness, whether it's a broken bone, or a bad pneumonia, comes with a spiritual violation that parallels the physical ailment. A doctor has to be more than just a dispenser of cures, but also, to use an old term, a minister of healing. That's what that touch is about. Recognize this ability in yourselves, think of it as a potent instrument. Sharpen it and learn to use it."

They had the uh-oh look, the concern that we were straying into touchy-feely territory, an area of medicine that was not fashionable, particularly in an ICU where it was as if the high-tech gadgetry stood in for the spiritual, the emotional. What they wanted to hear were aphorisms like the rule of five tubes: A patient in the ICU with more than five tubes in him will die.

○

Now David and Sergio reentered the room, removed the headboard from Mr. Rocha's bed, and persuaded him to lie flat, a difficult thing for him to do. The anesthetist arrived, and he and David put on gloves and positioned themselves behind Mr. Rocha's head, checking their intubation tray to see that everything was in order. David now pushed the needle of a Valium-loaded syringe into the intravenous tubing and slowly injected the drug. Mr. Rocha's eyelids fluttered closed, his whole body relaxed visibly, and his breathing became shallow.

Using both hands under the jaw, David tilted Mr. Rocha's head back, taking the curve out of the airway. With his left hand, he lifted the tongue up with the blade of the laryngoscope until he could see the epiglottis and the vocal cords below it. Then, with his other hand, David slid the endotracheal tube past the tip of the laryngoscope and on into Mr. Rocha's trachea. His hands, I had noticed on the tennis court, were not coarse, but expressive and delicate. Gloved, the fingers looked even longer, and his touch was sure.

"Perfect!" the anesthetist pronounced after listening with his stethoscope to make sure the breath sounds were equal on both sides of the chest. The nurse stepped in and taped the tube and connected Mr. Rocha to the ventilator.

David was more skilled with his hands than the average senior student.

14

"Bend your knees, not your back!"

We had started off taking turns serving, playing out a few points. David consistently returned my serve low, at my shoelaces as I rushed in to volley, taking away my offense, my very purpose in being at the net, forcing me to let the ball bounce and hit a half volley.

I served once more, came in, hit the half volley, but it was short and sat up. David stepped in and passed me easily. He ambled over to the net, trying to look stern. At what point had this become a lesson?

"Abraham, the secret to the half volley is never to have to hit it!"

"You're no help. You keep chipping it back so low!"

"Move your serve around, then. Change the pace. Keep me off-kilter. If my returns land at your feet each time, then you just have to get to the net sooner, get the ball in the air. But if you have to hit a half volley," he said, demonstrating, "then lower your butt to the ground by bending your knees, keeping your body as upright as you can." I watched with a thrill as he ran up and executed a mock half volley, showing the grace of a ballet dancer and perfect balance. "Don't just bend over at the waist," he said, imitating me in what I thought was an exaggerated fashion.

"My knees complain; that's why I use my back."

"And just block the ball on the half volley. No swing, just a straight follow-through. A scoop, is what it is. The ball hits the ground, then racket in one motion—it should sound like this: *rat-tat*."

"Is that one of your Aussie reptiles? A coolibah creature?"

He shook his head as if I were a hopeless case. He went back to the baseline. "Some more serves, please."

My half volleys were deeper, more penetrating, forcing David to work a little harder to pass me. I mistimed the last half volley and it sat up for him. I faked hard to one side and moved to the other. But David didn't buy it, waiting —"holding the ball on the racket" as they would say on TV—and passed me cleanly on the other side. Players like David managed to expand and magnify the moment of contact, as if time had a different frame of reference at that level of the game. It reminded me of boxing, the slow-motion replay of the knockout blow, the brilliant counterpunch. Simple enough in slo-mo, but always leaving me in awe that a boxer could wait for a punch to be thrown and time his counterpunch to the opening so perfectly.

"You did the right thing," he called out as he walked forward. "If you're a sitting duck at the net, you might as well guess and go to one side. But don't move so early. Wait at least until the ball bounces on my side." He sniggered at his own joke.

On my next serve, I had faked as if I were coming to net. But this time, I stayed back. His return would have given me a difficult half volley but instead now it was a short ball. I ran around my backhand and pounded the ball deep to David's backhand corner. It reared up, forcing him to hit an awkward slice backhand, at shoulder height. I had the momentum now and I hit one more forehand to the same spot. I was pushing the pusher back. I was teeing off. I hit my third shot for all it was worth, back to the same spot. This time, it sailed long.

"Remember," he said, grinning, "the one with the fewest errors wins. You overhit."

Oh yes, I did overhit. But for a while there I had him looking awkward. I had seen the chink in his armor. I knew the entry in my notebook that night would record his pearls about the half volley, the *rat-tat*, the need to use my knees to lower my body, keeping my trunk erect. But I would also record how by attacking his beautiful slice backhand with my heavy and deep topspin, I had reduced it to a defensive shot, one that he had to cut so fine each time. It was important to stand way over to the left, to try to keep his return to my forehand, keep him pinned down in the backhand corner. The one word I knew I would put in the center of the page and underline would be "patience."

○

In the parking lot, I told David I had something for him. "I brought you a review article on Adult Respiratory Distress syndrome. Might be relevant to Mr. Rocha. Make copies of it for Sergio and the others if you don't mind. Perhaps you can make a brief presentation on ARDS to the group, tomorrow, or the day after."

David nodded his thanks for the article.

"And . . . ," I said, pulling from the trunk of the car a copy of *Harrison's Principles of Internal Medicine*, the latest edition, which a pharmaceutical company had given me, "an early Christmas present." Other students often ported their big textbooks around in their backpacks, but David never did. I'd seen him use the reference books in the library. I suspected he did not own his own textbooks.

His eyes grew huge, as if he had been shown the crown jewels. His lips curved up.

"And . . . ," I said, "knowing you're such a sucker for drug company goodies, I dug up this knee hammer. You won't mind the logo on it, will you?" I had put a Christmas ribbon on it.

He was grinning like the Cheshire cat, sputtering his thanks. It made me wish I had gift-wrapped the book.

"Say . . . if you're not doing anything tonight, you want to come home and meet the boys?"

It was a simple invitation, like asking David to play tennis. He had no idea what he was getting into. I hadn't mentioned the marriage meltdown, but perhaps I was tempting him to discover it. I was like the patient who would rather the doctor deduce what ailed him than come out and confess the extramarital quickie that had left sores on his pecker, or the swallowing of condoms filled with cocaine that could explain the belly pain, the raised heart rate, the dilated pupils.

"I'd love that, actually," he said.

If he was surprised by this invitation, he didn't show it.

○

David was the first person in this new town that I had asked to visit the house. There were Christmas lights haphazardly strung in a bush—Steven's idea. When they heard the cars, Steven and Jacob came running out, hesitating when they saw the stranger with me. "Dad, there's a Charlie Brown Christmas special tonight!" Steven said. I introduced them, and they shook hands with David. As we neared the front door, the boys, despite our visitor, jumped on my back. I struggled into the house, explaining to David that this was the way Hobbes (Calvin's imaginary tiger) pounced on Calvin whenever he came back from school.

The Christmas tree was lit in the den, and Santa's mechanical band chimed and clanged below it. We went first to admire that, and for Steven to point out those wrapped presents that were his, and what he thought they were.

Once we were seated, Steven brought his Batman figures from his toy chest and, hesitantly at first, stood near David, waiting until David asked, "What's that?"

"Deep-Sea Batman . . . and that's Arctic Batman," he explained. Jacob followed Steven's cue, dragged in the Joker and Parachute Batman, plopping them silently on David's lap.

"And these?" David asked. Jacob offered no explanation, merely looking at the carpet, until Steven spoke for him.

○

Rajani must have heard us, realized there was company. She emerged after a while, regal and striking though dressed simply in jeans and a sweater. David stood up, stammered a formal, "How do you do," and they shook hands.

"Please sit," she said. I could see he was taken aback by her. "Did Abraham offer you something to drink?" I was drinking a beer, but David had wanted nothing.

Steven was telling David about Parachute Batman, Jacob whispering further details into Steven's ear to be conveyed to David.

Rajani must have wondered what David knew about our marital state. She sat, slightly wary but full of pride in her sons. We were both seeing them through the eyes of our visitor: handsome fellows with matching Beatles' mops, round, expressive eyes, and long eyelashes. They were so much more reserved, I thought—at least when there was company—than other children their age. But they had taken to David. Steven said to David, "I just can't wait for Christmas."

Jacob's first words to David came bursting out, because he couldn't help himself: "Me either!" and then his face lit up in a glorious smile.

We laughed and Jacob got shy again.

"David?" Rajani said, glancing at me first, "I was about to serve dinner. Would you care to stay? There's plenty of food. Really. I don't know if you like Indian food?"

"If you're sure it's not too much trouble . . ."

"Oh, it's no trouble at all," Steven said.

I could see David taking it all in, filling in the blanks. He liked the boys—it was difficult not to. I remained in the background, watching. If my perception was that Americans were quickly comfortable in most social situations, David had more of the colonial reserve. He reminded me of my own behavior when one of my professors in Boston had invited us to a swim party years before. I had been anxious about it, and I remember being envious of my fellow trainees who seemed so quickly at ease in his pool and around the barbecue. They had held forth on politics, on movies, as if this ritual of dining with staff was exceedingly familiar—almost expected.

The boys, who had already eaten, settled down to watch their TV special.

The three of us moved to the dining room. David ran his fingers over the tiled surface of the dining table, expressing admiration for it.

"Thank you!" she said. "Abraham doesn't care for it much." It was a special order from Hickory, North Carolina, she explained, bought when we were living in Tennessee.

She brought out the food, South Indian fare: rice and *sambaar*, *papad*s and yogurt and pickle. Not the sort of thing that one usually tried out on Westerners, but David ate with relish. Rajani stood up periodically to serve him more.

It was a cozy and comfortable scene: the guest at the family table. David addressed us as a couple, and it forced us to reply with the voice of the marital collective, a voice that was raspy from disuse. And yet, as things stood, it was a false scene, since I was back to looking for an apartment, the reconciliation of one night just a mirage.

"How did you two meet?" Rajani asked, and I let David stumble through our encounter in the parking lot.

"I heard you played in the pros? What are you doing playing with Abraham?"

David stammered through his explanation, how it was just the satellite tour, how it hadn't lasted very long. "Abraham's not half bad—" he added.

"Gee, thanks!"

"—and I'm rediscovering the pleasure of just going out and hitting the ball. No pressure."

He looked to me, and I knew he genuinely meant this and it made me proud.

"How did *you* two meet?" David said now, a mischievous smile on his face as he deflected the attention from himself.

We looked at each other. Which one of us would tell this story? And would our versions be similar?

"At a wedding," Rajani said. "That was some years before he began to pursue me. He was busy chasing other women in the intervening years." David thought this was hilarious.

"Not true—" I said.

"Then we ran into each other again, and he came after *me*," she said, warming up to this tale.

"And you dated for how long?"

"Dated? The kind of dating Americans take for granted is frowned on. We met, I think, three or four times"—she looked at me for confirmation—"and the marriage took place a month after that—"

She stopped suddenly, as if the tape had been cut off. It had begun with the portent of a charming story, and when it reached the point where we should have been looking lovingly into each other's eyes, reality burst the bubble.

"So it was an arranged marriage, then?" David said.

"Nooo . . . ," she said, but I could see her decide to come to a defense of the arranged marriage system. "Nothing *wrong* with arranged marriages, though. People here think it's primitive. But it's really an elaborate version of the dating system, not particularly different from a blind date, and better than hoping to find a life partner at ladies' night or happy hour—"

I jumped in to explain: "In India, 'good' girls you don't meet, because, by definition, parents don't let 'good' girls out of the house. When the girl reaches a marriageable age, they arrange for her to meet a suitor, go out to a movie, maybe a couple of movies, and then you have to say yes or no. And if it's no, then you start again . . . "

"Was that how you two did it?" David asked.

"No. When we went out, her parents didn't know. She was very eligible. Her parents were trying to match her up with a bunch of different guys—"

"Not true. I saw two guys."

"Three guys."

"Did you like any of them?" David asked her.

"No—"

"She was tempted by one of them, a big-time cardiologist in Florida—"

"I was not."

"—who makes more in a day than I make in a month—"

"He was a bore."

"—and so I had to move fast—"

"Ultimately," Rajani said, giving me a glance that shut me up, "there is a belief in India that it's your family, your upbringing, and your education that determine who you are, and parents try to match those qualities for their son or daughter. That's what you bring to the marriage. After that, it's your *commitment* that counts, not some magic chemistry that guarantees it will work forever." That was the point at which she and I did exchange meaningful looks. "Love marriages are no guarantee of success. Maybe they are even a predictor of failure."

This I took to be her admission that at one time she had been in love with me. I had been a lowly intern, but she'd seen more promise in me than the fuddy-duddy cardiologist.

"Yeah, I think that's true," David said. "As a society, we put too much stock in the chemistry."

"So, do you have a girlfriend?" Rajani asked.

"He does," I said. "I saw her briefly in the parking lot of the tennis club. She's beautiful."

David blushed.

"Gloria and I met here. We've dated for almost two years now. She's finishing up her pharmacy degree in New Jersey. We've"—his voice squeaked and cracked like a little boy's—"*talked* about marriage. But it's scary, you know? We've had our ups and downs . . ." He let out a little sigh, and hearing himself, he blushed some more and laughed. I could see a new set of neuroendocrine messengers come pouring out, altering blood pressure, muscle tone, heart rate, a first-rate chemical display, completely beyond his cognitive control. It was as if there were women, and then there was Gloria. She was a cosmic body separate from other mortal women.

Rajani and I were silent, in awe, envious perhaps, but not wanting to add to his obvious embarrassment. Besides, neither of us felt expert enough to offer advice.

I was tempted to tell them both about the tattoo and how Gloria seemed the embodiment of that dream, but I thought it might be in bad taste to link his girlfriend with a penal-system tattoo.

O

"He's nice. A gentleman," Rajani said when I asked her what she thought of David after we saw him off. Of course, I took that to mean that the problem in the past had been that my friends were not always gentlemen. Should I take the bait and fight?

"Do you know if he has somewhere to go for Christmas?" she asked. "He looks half starved."

15

David spent almost all his time with Mr. Rocha. We had a tennis date on a Sunday morning, and I had shown up on the court only to have my beeper flash 0-6, telling me that he couldn't make it. I had gone home disappointed.

Mr. Rocha's lungs had become boggy and stiff. Whatever the inciting infectious agent that had caused Mr. Rocha's pneumonia, it had gone on long enough to trigger ARDS—the Adult Respiratory Distress syndrome—a condition in which the fine capillary network that carried blood through the air sacs became leaky. We had to juggle the ventilator setting to provide enough oxygen and to remove carbon dioxide that built up. But if the pressure driving air in got too high, the lungs would pop like balloons. Fluid and caloric requirements had to be calculated and provided in the form of intravenous dextrose and through a gastric feeding tube. Sergio and David had floated a Swan-Ganz catheter into Mr. Rocha's heart where it sat measuring filling pressures so that we could straddle the fine line between pouring in enough fluid into the vascular system to maintain blood pressure, but not so much that the lungs would get boggier.

David made careful entries in Mr. Rocha's chart, morning and evening. He had subheadings—cardiovascular, respiratory, renal, hematopoietic—under which in clear, almost childlike cursive script he documented how he was supporting each failed organ system. David had become possessive about Mr. Rocha, unwilling to delegate his care to anyone else, staying in the hospital on his nights off, or, as he did when he canceled tennis, staying after weekend rounds. This, I thought, was good for both patient and doctor, and for a week I didn't broach the idea of tennis again.

O

Ten days after Mr. Rocha had been admitted, I went by the ICU in the late afternoon to check on the two of them. David was standing outside the room, shoulder to shoulder with Jack Peacock. Jack was in scrubs, a mask dangling from his neck. Gray hair peeked out from under his surgical cap. Jack had served as a combat surgeon in Vietnam, and was enormously experienced. He had a quirky sense of humor, loved to teach, and was adored by the students. I had seen Jack talking with David several times before. I knew them to be close. Now, as I saw Jack laugh and elicit a wry smile from David, I felt startling jealousy.

"Here's the man with all the real answers," Jack said when he spotted me.

I stepped up just behind them and we all stared at Mr. Rocha's latest X ray. The opacities in the lungs had become less coarse and more diffuse.

"I've got no answers, Jack."

A shrill beep went off from a ventilator alarm and David moved into the room to check on it. David had a cold and was wearing a mask when he was around Mr. Rocha. Jack and I stood, watching.

We could see David's stethoscope move back and forth from right lung to left lung, trying to decide if the endotracheal tube had slipped down past the point where the trachea divides into two, and if it was lodged in the right bronchus, if that was what had triggered the alarm. As a reflex, Jack held up the X ray one more time and we both looked again. The tube seemed to be sitting well above the bifurcation on the X ray.

"How's that young man doing?" Jack asked, using the film as a screen.

"Magnificently. He's got great hands and a sharp mind—all the ingredients to make a good internist. The other kind we encourage to go into surgery." Jack laughed as he walked away, saving his rebuttal for another time.

O

David and I waited, listening to see if the ventilator alarm would go off again. It didn't. Whatever was wrong, David had fixed it. The wrinkles around David's eyes seem more pronounced. He seemed

lower in spirits than I remembered ever seeing him. He was func-
tioning as Mr. Rocha's support system. It was as if Mr. Rocha were
his creation, a bionic man he kept alive. Not surprisingly, David's
mood had now become tied to Mr. Rocha's progress. I had seen this
phenomenon before.

"You're doing everything you can. Now you just have to keep the
ball in play." He smiled wanly at this metaphor.

"I'm serious, David. That's the essence of his care now. There may
be no magic bullet. But if we just keep him going, the body will
eventually heal, the ARDS resolve. His youth is a big advantage.
Nothing like good underlying protoplasm. The game might be over
if he were a seventy-year-old with concomitant heart disease and
diabetes."

David coughed and held his chest.

"Are you all right?"

He shook his head no, and grimaced.

"Go home and rest. And if you aren't feeling well in the morning,
let me know. I'll tell Sergio. Don't worry, we'll take good care of Mr.
Rocha."

"Don't think Sergio will like it very much if I don't come in."

"I'll talk to him."

○

I called David early the next morning. The phone rang for a long
time and finally a rude male voice answered. "David! Phone!" I
heard the man yell, and then there was the sound of a fist banging
on a door. When David came on the line, he sounded hoarse and
nasal. He said he felt weak and dizzy, but he was dressing to come to
work. I told him not to think of coming in, and to let me know if he
needed anything. Again he said he didn't think Sergio would like it.
I was getting vaguely irritated with this. I told him I would take care
of it.

When I met Sergio later on rounds, he appeared a bit miffed by
the news that David would not be there.

"Are you sure he's sick?"

"He sounded ill, Sergio," I said, snapping a bit. "You saw him
dragging around yesterday, didn't you?"

Sergio shrugged. He was unimpressed.

16

With a map and a guidebook by our side, the boys and I explored the town. Twice we shot over the bridge into Juárez, encountering a scene on the other side at once familiar to me: vintage taxis held together by chicken wire, roadside vendors hawking their wares, aggressive shopkeepers, bustling crowds, a robust *mercado*, an even more robust red-light district, dodge-and-weave traffic—this could have been the Addis Ababa of my childhood, or the Madras of my medical-school years. Both times it took over half an hour to return. The boys were entertained by the narco dogs that sniffed our tires and wagged their tails at them as we inched our way to the customs booth. Once the barrier went up, we were back to the orderly streets of El Paso.

Though I didn't tell my sons this, I was scouting out apartments, getting a feel for their distance from the house. We used Mesa Street as our hub; Mesa ran east-west, parallel to I-10, parallel to the river, parallel to the border. From Mesa we knew how to find our way back to Thunderbird Drive, which led home.

Thunderbird Drive was named for a rust-colored rock formation, halfway up the mountain, shaped just like the mythical bird with its wings outstretched. To see that thunderbird against the limestone gray of the rest of the mountain was to be reminded of the volcanic eruption on the ocean floor that had given birth to the Franklins, pushing up seabed and lava to create this striated formation. The thunderbird rock formation itself was red, glassy rhyolite—lava rock—sandwiched between layers of ocean-bed limestone.

I described this underwater volcanic explosion to the boys. I think they found it deliciously eerie to look around at a landscape that begged for water and picture how water had once been everywhere, that the buttes and arroyos had once been canyons and gorges, that the cacti and creosote bushes stood in for coral and sea urchins, and the rattlesnakes lurking in the dry sand stood in for sightless deep-sea creatures.

"Oh," Jacob asked, tilting his head to me, "could it happen tomorrow?"

"No, it'll never happen again," I said with the utter confidence and unshakable authority of a parent who wills nature to spare his children.

In our ramblings in the car, the window down, I imagined that the whir of my tires sounded different in El Paso than elsewhere. As if the seabed still echoed beneath the desert skin.

Impulsively, I took the boys to the end of our subdivision. We parked near some luxury cookie-cutter zero-lot-line condos, and after just a few steps we were on the mountain face, staring up. Our eyes automatically traced a path to the top. It was not an impossible climb, and gravity would keep you applied to the rock face if you tried to ascend. But coming down, particularly if you had not chosen your route well, was dangerous, gravity now working to pluck you off. Better to go up the well-marked trails that led off Trans-mountain Road.

Still, we walked up about fifty yards. I paused to show them a creosote bush, pluck its waxy leaf and have them smell it. They were unimpressed by the fact that it might be one of the oldest plants on the planet, and so I didn't bother to tell them about its link to the common and potentially deadly disease—coccidioidomycosis—that their daddy was bound to see in the hospital.

"Look!" I said, bending down to point to a bare rock face that had cracked open or else been weathered down to reveal pearly, glistening, oval shapes the size of a baby's fingernails. "Fossils, boys." I pronounced this with the gravity of Batman finding the scent of the Joker, or a riddle left by the Riddler ("By the numbers on my face you won't find thirteen anyplace!"). "These are skeletons of shellfish from millions of years ago. From the ocean."

"Millions? Is that like zillions?"

"Even more!" When I told them it was possible to find sharks' teeth in these rocks, their eyes became huge with the magic of this new West Texas landscape that was now home.

We carried pieces of volcanic rock back to the car. The mountains had quieted the boys. They had no words for the immediacy of it, for the feeling it created in them, for the way the world of Kay Bee toys, cereal box freebies, Calvin and Hobbes receded, replaced by the touch of red rock that was linked to molten lava and to sharks. In the house, they were, like me, at times restless, irritable, glued to the television, with any interruption by us sounding like a nagging commercial. But at the mountain I sensed them retreat within themselves. I wondered now in the silence if they thought about their future, the rockiness of their parents' marriage. Did it loom over them as it did me, enormous and unspeakable?

17

The team and I went to see Mr. Rocha on the last day of the rotation. He had mastered his bed and TV controls. He had propped up both the head and the foot of the bed, as if he were on a recliner. Save for the fact that he was still chained to the ventilator by the tube in his throat, he looked not just comfortable, but firmly established. As we assembled around his bed, Mr. Rocha did not take his eyes from *Morelia*, the Spanish soap opera beamed from Mexico City.

His lungs were slowly improving, exchanging oxygen for carbon dioxide more efficiently. He no longer bucked the ventilator. In fact, the machine had the reins and Mr. Rocha followed, rather like a docile mule.

But this confinement to the windowless, unnatural ICU world, and his inability to speak because of the endotracheal tube, had brought about a distinct personality change. We were simply part of the scenery to him, as opaque as the machines with their digital displays and graphs that hovered over his head. He was as indifferent to our voices as he was to the beeps and alarms that punctuated his waking and sleeping. His only sense of time passing was the nurses' shift changes and the few hours when the television channels displayed test patterns. He stared at the TV, as if its prattle stood in for the activity of his mind, for his locomotion, for his life. David became the medium who spoke for Mr. Rocha, who imagined his discomforts, and who also kept the machinery of his body ticking.

"Mr. Rocha," David called, touching his shoulder. Mr. Rocha turned his head slightly in the direction of the sound, but kept his eyes on the screen. "Mr. Rocha?" Now a hint of exasperation in David's voice. Nothing. David sighed and lifted up, peeved. "I think he's depressed," he said.

David sounded depressed.

"He has no interest in anything," the nurse chimed in. "He doesn't ask for sedation. He just stares at the TV."

"I've asked for a psych consult," David said. "Though they won't be able to talk to him. They'll have to take my word for it."

"Is there any past psychiatric history? Schizophrenia? Bipolar disorder?"

"None at all."

"Don't call psychiatry, then," I said. "Give him a clinical trial of an antidepressant. It might help get him off the respirator sooner. Let the new team know what we're doing, because it will be a week or more before the antidepressant starts to work. If it works."

I picked up the clipboard on which the respiratory therapist recorded "weaning parameters" every morning. David momentarily kinked off the tubing leading to Mr. Rocha's mouth and we looked at the pressure gauge to see how much inspiratory force Mr. Rocha's diaphragm was generating. The needle made a good excursion.

"It won't be long now," I said to David.

David's head shake suggested he didn't really believe that. So soon the triumph of his patient's survival had slipped away from him. All he could focus on was Mr. Rocha's indifference.

○

We had one new admission to see. Raju, my intern, presented her to us: a sixty-six-year-old woman with sudden onset of weakness of the left side of her body of two hours' duration. When I examined her, she seemed to have all the findings of a stroke, and in addition, had bruits in her neck from narrowed carotid vessels. The wall of her radial artery felt as if it were made of concrete. Then Raju showed us her chest X ray. She had a small mass in the right lung. Nothing in the history or physical had pointed to it.

"I'm thinking cancer of the lung with a metastasis to the head," Raju said.

I found this hard to accept. She was a nonsmoker. And, as I now pointed out to the group, the mass in her chest appeared to have calcium in it—a sign that it was probably benign. And meanwhile, the CT scan of her head showed nothing, a common finding in the first days of a stroke. If she indeed had a metastasis to the brain from lung cancer, I would have expected to see the metastasis that was causing her left-sided weakness on the CT scan, and to see several other metastases in the brain.

"I suspect," I said, much to Raju's chagrin, "that this is a stroke in a lady with an asymptomatic and benign chest mass. It's an example of true, true but *unrelated*. As opposed to true, true and *related*." Raju looked puzzled, as did the rest of them. "You were right to try to link all the abnormalities she has, to try to tie them together with one hypothesis. What is the name for this principle?"

"Occam's razor," Sergio said.

"Good. Named after Sir William of Occam, a philosopher, not a physician. It's the principle of being parsimonious with our explanations, to tie things together with the simplest explanation. For example, if an elderly person presents with pain over the temporal areas as well as proximal muscle weakness, you shouldn't diagnose tension headache and bilateral rotator cuff syndromes. Instead, the one disease that would explain all these would be . . . ?"

"Polymyalgia rheumatica," David said.

"Good. By the way, Sergio, do you know what Sir William of Occam died of?" He shook his head. "*Multiple* causes," I said.

Only David and Sergio got the joke.

"Occam's razor is a great principle," I said to Raju, "but you have to be careful not to overdo it. You must make sure that the truths you are trying to tie together are, in fact, true, true and *related*."

Raju sulked. He thought he had made a brilliant diagnosis, which I had now shot down.

○

After rounds I took the team to lunch at the Delhi Palace, an economical and efficient way to feed a group this size. As soon as we walked in, I noticed that the wall between dining room and vestibule had been taken down, so that you walked into one big, open room. The faces of the waiters and maître d' were new. But the lunch buffet fare hadn't changed. There were, however, two laminated signs posted near the buffet: TAKEOUT BUFFET WILL BE PACKED BY OUR OWN STAFF and TO OUR BUFFET CUSTOMERS: PLEASE DO NOT WASTE FOOD. THERE WILL BE ADDITIONAL CHARGES FOR UNREASONABLE AMOUNTS OF LEFTOVERS.

The end of our stint on the ward made everyone, even Raju, our Indian intern who had spoken only when he had to, talkative. He was shy, reticent with women, but Sherry, by being his shadow all month, had managed to crack his reserve. It had been amusing to see her, tall and confident, towering over him as they walked down the corridors.

"First came ECFMG. Then they changed it to Visa Qualifying Exam—VQE, a two-day exam. Then it became a two-part USMLE: United States Medical Licensing Exam. But each part had to be taken at a different time of year. And not in India."

Raju was describing the hurdles he had to clear to come to America. The exam was moved from India to Sri Lanka, and, when that proved too accessible, to Thailand, the Philippines, and Singapore. Undaunted, medicos packed the twice-a-year charters that took off from Madras or Bombay, their heads buried in study guides.

"As I understand it, only a small percentage pass the exam," I said. "A larger percentage lose their virginity in Bangkok or Manila. Right, Raju?" He was mortified, shrinking into his chair, burying his smile in his napkin as Sherry stared at him with renewed interest.

Massoud, the Palestinian, said, "Hey, but even if you pass the exam, you have to get a visa. It's not automatic. For us, the visa was the most difficult part."

"Terrible!" Raju exclaimed. "The queue was a mile long outside the U.S. consulate. You had to pay a 'queue stander' for a spot. They stand in line overnight and sell their position in the morning to the highest bidder. Then, when you got inside, you had to prove you would not remain in the United States when the residency was over. I carried surety bonds, land certificates, bank statements to show I was doing fine in India, and that I would come back. Some people get relatives to transfer all their assets to them for twenty-four hours, so they can be rich for the day. Or else, there are "instant-wealth" agencies who give you papers, good for only the one day you are in the consulate."

"And so you are planning to go back?" Sherry said.

Sergio and Massoud laughed. "Nobody goes back," Massoud said. Sherry looked confused.

"The visa officer in my days in Madras was a black gentleman," I said. "Rumor had it that he hated his posting. I had a green card. But my classmates who were applying for study visas had to go through an interview with this man, to prove that they planned to return to India. One morning, he turned down six consecutive doctors and told the seventh, who happened to be my friend Vadivel, 'Spare me the crap about coming back with specialized knowledge to serve your country. Why do you really want to go?'" Sergio, Raju, and Massoud were howling at my imitation of an American accent. Sherry looked discomfited, either because she didn't know I was capable of such mimicry, or else because she felt the sovereignty of her country being threatened. "Vadivel was the meekest of the meek, but he had held on to his American dream for so long that he could speak with the passion of a visionary. 'Sir, craving your indulgence, I want to train in a decent, ten-story hospital where the lifts are actually working. I want to pass board certification exams by my own merit and not through pull or bribes. I want to become a wonderful doctor, practice real medicine, pay taxes, make a good living, drive a big car on decent roads, and eventually live in the Ansel Adams section of New Mexico and never come back to this wretched town where doctors are as numerous as fleas and practice is cutthroat and where the air outside is not even fit to breathe.' The consul gave him a visa. The eighth applicant, forewarned, tried the same tactic but was turned down."

○

David ate slowly and remained subdued. I wondered if this was because of Mr. Rocha or because, as I'd noticed after he was out sick for a day with his cold, he didn't say much when Sergio was around.

David had performed magnificently that month. His mini-presentation on coarctation of the aorta was outstanding, as were all the subsequent assignments I gave him. His care of Mr. Rocha had been superb. My bias toward him notwithstanding, I was giving him an honors grade. When we walked to the buffet line together to get dessert—*goolab jamun*—I let him know this.

"Great! I'm not sure I deserve it, Abraham, but . . ."

"Of course you do. Even Sergio told me he thought you had done extremely well."

"Really?" For the first time that day he smiled.

○

I met David on the tennis court that Sunday at three in the afternoon. The sun was shining, but when the wind blew it felt chilly.

We walked out to a far court, pausing to watch two of the club's best juniors in a heated baseline exchange. One of them finally approached on a short ball, and the other, trying to do too much with the passing shot, framed it. The ball sailed out into the arroyo behind the court. I waited for David to make some comment, but he merely shook his head, as if the ball sailing out was symptomatic of what was going on with him.

The stretch, the dink'em warm-up, and still silence. I wondered suddenly if the limits of the friendship had been reached. Had my wanting to play tennis with him become an imposition?

"Something bothering you?"

He smiled wryly, but said nothing, which only galled me further.

"Mr. Rocha?" I asked.

"I suppose, partly. And Gloria . . ."—the sigh now—"she and I . . . it just isn't working. Mr. Rocha is representative of the whole thing—" Here he gave a hollow laugh. "I'm pleased he's better. But I have no idea what was the matter with him in the first place. Makes me feel as if I didn't do my job. All the serum we sent out came back negative."

David's habit of opening doors to his personal life and then shutting them was already familiar. I was tempted to tell him that he was projecting his disquiet onto Mr. Rocha. It really didn't matter now—certainly not to Mr. Rocha—what had triggered his ARDS. What mattered was that we nurse him back to good health.

He surprised me by saying, "I guess it's more *my* problem than it is Mr. Rocha's."

David's forehand was lethargic, a hitch coming into the stroke so that it either sailed or found the net. It irritated him, and the more he focused on it, the worse it became.

Perhaps he found it difficult to withdraw from our twice-a-week arrangement. Perhaps he wanted more competition. Since I would no longer be his attending physician, he had no need to keep up the charade.

I too began missing simple forehands, catching the top of the net, throwing off our rhythm. My strokes were fragile constructions, and even as I tried to engineer the corrections, my mind wasn't there.

If David wanted out, why didn't he just say so?

"Let's really play. A set." I had used my hospital tone.

"Okay," he said, and I saw surprise on his face, as if he couldn't believe that I would challenge him.

He spun his racket. I called "up" and won. I warmed up with a few easy serves.

"These are good," I said.

I thought hard about where to serve. I tried to study David's position as I bounced the ball. He seemed doleful and needy, but I was angry. And it was that flash of anger and hurt—more so than any strategic planning—that guided my serve. David wasn't even close. I had aced him.

It was the only point I won in that service game. I hit good, deep serves and came in on them, but David's returns were either at my feet or went right past me. I hit one nice volley but David anticipated it and lofted a beautiful topspin lob that arced over my head and landed a foot inside the baseline.

At break point, I made the mistake of coming in on a second serve. David stepped in and teed off. I ducked as it swished past my left ear. There was an edge to that shot, an extra oomph to underline something—my hubris, his frustration. He raised his racket and took a step forward, penitent. I waved him off.

We changed ends. David won his serve easily and broke me again. I took a moment as we crossed the net to realign the strings in my racket and tried to concentrate on strategy and forget about who was on the other side of the net. Think Brad Gilbert, Abe. What I should do was step in and take his serve early.

It worked for one point. David raised his racket and brought it to the palm of his other hand to applaud a return that went whistling down the line as he charged the net. But he understood what I had done and made the adjustment. On the next point he served into my body, handcuffing me.

I was seeing him in full flow now and it was an impressive sight. Even as I was being defeated, losing track of my strategies and reminders, I was glad that I'd wakened him from his stupor, brought him out of his passivity, and could now see him do what he did best, do what he had spent the better part of his life perfecting.

His agility and speed of foot reduced his court to the size of a postage stamp while my side of the court felt like a football field. At one point, as he lunged for a volley, he displayed the extension that was captured in the photo of Pancho Segura that I had taped to my wall as a child. I had always associated that image with passion and joy. At that moment, though, David, for all the beauty of his game, showed no passion, no joy.

We were in uncharted territory. Our previous meetings had been an extended warm-up, an aesthetically pleasing practice session or a lesson that had no connection with the kind of tennis we were now playing. And yet the *mano a mano* metaphor was only marginally applicable, because, in a strange fashion, we were somehow still on the same side. I had unleashed my game, going at him, doing my best to win points; he had stopped being considerate. Still, in my mind at least, there was something cooperative about this competition. After all, he couldn't play alone.

Our handshake over the net felt different from those in the past. The air had been cleared. The month on the wards was behind us. I had never taken more pleasure in a loss. If we never played again, this was the way to end it.

"You played great," he said.

"You caught me on a bad day," I said. He laughed, for the first time that day.

"Sorry about my pissy mood, Abraham," he said. We sat on the bench, our silence no longer the strained silence in the locker room preceding the match. Then he uttered one word, "Women!"

I didn't reply.

"Coffee?" David said after a while. "Or do you need to get home?"

"Home? . . . Home . . ."

What followed wasn't planned. But the words came out.

"I'm moving out of the house in a month or so, David. I'm going to find an apartment."

He looked at me as if I had slapped him.

He made as if to say something, then stopped. His expression was pained. Perhaps he felt, as a friend, that he should have had warning, should have been allowed to know what was going on. Perhaps, in light of my trials, he felt shame for his own peevishness that day.

"When the time comes, perhaps you can give me a hand with the move?" I didn't really need the physical help as much as I needed not to be so alone as I did it. "I've decided not to take much. Just clothes and a few cartons of books, that's all."

"Sure. I'll help." He was still shell-shocked. We all form fictive pictures of one another, stories that we project onto one another. I insisted on seeing him as having had an adventurous, romantic tennis career, even though he had told me more than once that it hadn't been that way. And if the story he had projected onto me was one of stability and happiness, it was disappointing for him to find it not to be so. "I guess . . . I had some sense—don't know how—that all was not well."

I was tempted to try to explain, to give him the chief complaint, the history of the present illness, to line up the symptoms and signs and let him put them together and see if he came to the conclusion I wanted him to come to, that this was an irreversible condition.

"And the kids?"

"The kids . . ." To think of the boys, to think of their faces looking up at me as I had read them a scary story the previous night, to remember how their eyes had gotten wider, how their bodies had pressed against me, how their hands had gripped my shoulders as the tale went on . . . my voice briefly left me.

David looked away. When I could speak again, I told him how we had gone to a therapist in El Paso to get advice on how best to bring about the separation. The therapist had suggested we refer to the apartment I was to rent as a "time-out" place. I told David how this subterfuge had helped me more than it had helped the kids. A time-out place sounded better than saying a father was moving out, leaving two little boys behind. It eased my sense of abandoning them.

"God!" he said, shaking his head, scolding me, "I wish you had said something." I should have known that he would be nonjudgmental and supportive. I had told very few people because I hadn't wanted to hear advice or criticism. My parents, for example, wanted me to hang in there at all costs. That wasn't what I wanted to hear. I was doing a good job of beating up on myself without hearing the disappointment in their voices. My brothers were unconditionally supportive, but far away.

"And you and Rajani . . . can you still talk to each other?" he asked. "I mean, this didn't blow up last night or something?" I shook my head. "And the boys . . . you'll still get to see the boys all the time, right?"

The therapist had encouraged us to continue to do things together, all four of us, so that the boys would not feel they had lost a parent. She was agreeable to my going back every day at dinnertime, or at the kids' bedtime. And the boys would come camp out with me on Fridays and Saturdays—and as often as they wanted to and their schoolwork permitted. I wondered if he thought Rajani and I were screaming at each other, throwing things.

"The truth is, we don't really have harsh words anymore," I said. "Irreconcilable differences, as they say. After eleven years of marriage."

"Well, that's good about the kids . . . I guess," he said. He seemed to be at a loss for what to say or do. I could almost see him rehearsing several options in his mind.

Finally he said, "How about Dolce Vita?"

"I'd rather go grab a beer somewhere, if you don't mind."

"That's fine," David said, standing up. He reached over with his racket and tapped my shoulder.

○

The bar on Mesa Street was cavernous. The clicking of billiard balls and the clinking of glass against ice provided a soothing background. It was early and the UTEP crowd had yet to fill the place. We found a table in a corner under a neon Budweiser sign.

With each swallow of beer, a knot melted deep in my chest. Without David's asking, the tale of my marriage and its unraveling came spilling out.

"You look back at yourself, at something you did years ago, even one year ago, and you think, 'God, how stupid I was.' But by then it's too late . . . Marrying her was an affirmation for me. Acceptance from my parents, staying within the community, that sort of thing. And of course, I thought I was in love. Trouble is, when you marry with that kind of an objective—affirmation, acceptance, whatever— you lose steam when the circumstances change, when you find affirmation somewhere else, like at work.

"The first year was great. We knew very few people when we got to my internship. It was just the two of us. That isolation brought us together. But three years of residency changes you . . . you become a different person."

David was nodding his head, as if in recognition of events in his own life. The beer was making me garrulous.

"When I first met her, she was wary of me. I was a good student, a very serious student, but still a bit wild. I rode a motorbike, I hung out with a crowd that she was never a part of. And perhaps she found this marginally exciting. And I must say in my defense that the wildness, which I still feel, is not all bad. If people think that I'm a good physician, a decent teacher, then that wildness is at the heart of that. It's what makes me interested—no, fascinated—by people like Angelina Cortez . . . the side of me that might have seemed romantic when we first met became objectionable to Rajani."

I was conscious that the act of *describing* a marriage made everything that had happened seem deliberate and logical. As if this were a proof in geometry at the end of which I could write QED. In telling this story, I was very aware of what it did to David, how it seemed to open him up, and seeing that, changed or encouraged what I said next. To tell a life story was to engage in a form of seduction.

"There was a time—after the kids came—when she wanted us to go into therapy, to talk about the fact that the marriage wasn't working. But I was in denial. And by the time I woke up and looked around, we had two beautiful kids, but nothing else. I'd never take it all back, because it would mean not having my boys. But as a marriage it was or had become a sham. And too many harsh words have been said to retrieve it, to fix it . . ."

And then I was drained, out of words. "Didn't mean to unload on you," I said pretty much under my breath.

"No, it's fine. I'm . . . I don't have much insight into these things. I . . . should have insight." He looked up playfully, smiling as he said, "I've been married twice, you know."

He was enjoying my shock, hoping it would make me laugh. I felt as if I had pulled out a splinter when he was harboring a grapefruit-sized abscess.

"Kids?"

He shook his head. Gradually the smile faded and then he dropped his eyes. He took a swig of his iced tea and then hung his head, studying the water marks on the Formica tabletop.

"You don't really know anything about my past, do you?" he said, looking up.

He took a deep breath. From time to time, an involuntary twitch would affect David's face, wiping away his usual smile and pleasant expression, fleetingly bringing to the surface something darker, something wrenching and painful. I had seen this at Angelina's bedside. It was a surprisingly transparent expression, springing out as if the forces that restrained it had failed. I was seeing it again.

"The business with Sergio . . . he's suspicious of me because I was a big fuckup the last time I did medicine." He paused now, and then said in a flat monotone, "I'm a recovering cocaine addict."

He was studying my expression, watching how I would react to this news. I didn't move a muscle.

He took another sip of his tea. "This rotation in medicine was my *second* go-round . . . I had to repeat the fourth year. Worked with Sergio the last time. And he hasn't forgotten what I did . . . the stupidity of it. If you thought I did well this rotation . . . I should have. I had done it once before." His tone was harsh now, as if he were reciting a story about someone he detested.

What to say to this? I wanted to raise my glass to my lips, to take a huge gulp. But I was frozen.

"You didn't know?" he asked softly.

"I had no idea."

He shook his head as if he was amazed that I hadn't heard.

"I walk around with the feeling that everyone in the hospital knows."

He read my mind, because he said, "I wasn't just snorting it either. I was injecting it. As much as I could, as many times a day as I could. Buggering up my veins. It was bad. Filthy. When we were talking to Angelina Cortez?—her story is my story."

All traces of his normal affable manner disappeared, and the red neon glow in our corner made him look like a specter of the man I had just played tennis with. He loathed his past. To call up the memory transformed him. I understood now why he slunk around the hospital expecting nothing from anyone.

"But shooting up, David? How did you get into *shooting* up?" The words were out of my mouth before I could consider the propriety of asking such a question. He shrugged, as if the reasons still escaped him.

"The details you came up with when you were examining Angelina just blew my mind. It seemed like *you* must have tried . . ."

"I've tried just about everything else at one time or another," I said. "But not that. Not injecting."

The bar was filling up. The faces of the people walking in seemed relaxed, their lives uncomplicated by the sorts of things we had just traded across the table.

"When I came back from Europe, after my stint on the pro tour, I lived in Dallas. I met a woman at the tennis club where I worked as an assistant pro. She got me started. I was in the process of applying for medical school."

A hint of a smile flickered on his face at this memory.

"She was outrageous. I found it appealing, to be around people who had *energy*. She and her pals were so sure of themselves. I lacked confidence and she had it. Her secret was amphetamines intravenously."

He looked at his arm as if trying to remember what that first shot, the first rush had been like, as if the clue might be there in his ante-cubital vein.

"See, for me, tennis was like a drug too, for a while. Even if I didn't always enjoy it, exactly. It had its own excitement. Parties, women who liked the idea of a tennis pro—all that came with the territory. It filled a void. Let's just say that my childhood . . . I had a tremendous feeling of inadequacy. A deep pit that tennis filled, or at least covered up."

I understood that David was drawing a line as to how much he could or would tell. This childhood void of his would remain unexplored.

"And when the tennis was over, I was empty. I had no crutch, nothing to make me feel special. The world was gray and dull. When she offered me the needle, from the very first shot, I was hooked, it just seemed to fill the hole," he said, putting his fist over his chest. "Right here."

His story was spilling out with more urgency than the tale I had told him. There was a compulsion to his speech, as if it were causing him physical pain to talk about it, and he wanted to get it over with quickly. He had, he said, prided himself on his facility with the needle, his ability to use veins on the dorsum of the foot. When he was doing his master's in biochemistry, waiting for admission to medical school, he had learned to synthesize amphetamines. ("All you need to do is use red phosphorus to dehalogenate pseudoephedrine, and there you have it.") All that time he was considered a reliable, responsible grad student who worked incredible hours. There had been some unpleasantness when his little amphetamine factory was discovered. He had been lucky not to get arrested for a felony. After a while he tried cocaine—again intravenously. He had never snorted. He became addicted to that. The dose escalated. What it took to get him high also caused him to have seizures. He'd wake up with his tongue bitten in half, having soiled himself, and promptly head out the door to get more.

○

David straightened up in his chair now.

"I stopped when I entered medical school. Relapsed in my second year in Lubbock and had to repeat the year. Came to El Paso, in eighty-eight. Finished my third year without a problem. But then I relapsed in my fourth year here in El Paso. It happened after my parents visited me. No sooner had I dropped them at the airport than I went and got some and shot up."

I was curious to know what his parents had to do with it.

"I had been going out with Gloria. I was in love with her. My parents hadn't particularly approved of my wives. Here at last was someone decent, beautiful. I thought they would fall in love with her. But they were, like, 'Ho-hum, that's nice.' I had hoped Gloria would wipe the slate clean. I don't know. In any case, it didn't happen.

"And that relapse was a terrible one ..." He paused, as if it amazed him to remember it. "I wrote bad checks. I stole from my roommate. I did despicable things, was in and out of detox and rehab, but it never stuck. I hurt Gloria. I'm still making amends to all those people. Gloria finally shipped me off to Australia, literally marched me onto a plane. And once I was home, back in Armidale, away from it, I came back to earth. I practically begged her to fly out to Australia. She stayed a few weeks and then we came back together, for me to face the music at Texas Tech. I thought Dr. Binder would kick me out. But he didn't. He said if I went into a long rehab at Timberlawn in Dallas, and then if I stayed clean for a year, demonstrated my sobriety, they would take me back."

By this time Gloria had been accepted in pharmacy school in New Jersey. She had deliberately picked a place away from El Paso, so that she and David could be in a new environment. David did a three-month rehabilitation at Timberlawn and then followed Gloria to New Jersey.

"The rehab at Timberlawn was a waste of time. In the sense that I was already sober, committed to it once I got to Australia. Couldn't really relate to the others there. But I went through it. Then, in New Jersey, I worked as a phlebotomist, and meanwhile attended meetings and had urine checks."

At the end of a year, he returned to Texas Tech, presented the evidence of his reformation, his sobriety, and was allowed to reenter the fourth-year class in July of '91, just a few months before I'd arrived in town.

"I've got about a year and a half of sobriety now. Usually, I don't hesitate to tell anyone who asks that I'm a recovering addict. The twelve steps and AA and NA made all the difference for me. A day at a time. That's all I can do. Because if I think too much about the past or worry too much about the future . . . well, that doesn't get me anywhere.

"I go to NA and AA meetings twice a week. I have a sponsor who works with me. I have to submit to random urine tests at work. I pray a lot and keep busy. When I look at my refrigerator and I see it actually has *food* in it, I'm amazed. When I was using, it was completely empty."

O

I paid, and we went outside to our cars. It was dark and cold now and we were both shivering. I was still at a loss for words.

He turned to me. "I spent all the time I was drugging living hour to hour. I'm finding rituals to live by now. Gloria is central to my life, my well-being. So when we fight it's like the whole world ends. But I want to tell you, the tennis with you has the quality of a ritual, a good one. It's more than tennis. I see you as . . . stable. Someone with long-term goals . . . I see you as someone who's accomplished what I'm seeking to do. The fact that you are having problems . . . I'm so sorry."

I thought what he meant to say was that he didn't think someone like me *should* have problems. And how what I had confessed to him must have deeply disappointed him, unsettled him.

When he held out his hand, I reached for it with both of mine, as if this were the beginning of an examination.

Part II

The marrow of the tragedy is concentrated in the hospitals . . .

—*Walt Whitman*

18

The examination, for me, begins with the pulse. I reach for the hand in a manner more cautious than when I shake someone's hand.

My right hand supports the fingers, the fingers of my left hand slide down the ball of the thumb, down that familiar incline, into the groove between the flexor tendons, to the radial artery. If I were a cellist, this would be my fret board.

When I find the pulse, I look into my patient's eyes. Sometimes the pupils dilate, and the pulse itself quickens, as if recognizing that I have discovered its hiding place.

I need no watch to tell me the rate; this is my equivalent of perfect pitch. If the pulse is fast and the palm sweaty, I look to the eyelids to see if they are retracted, and to the neck to see if the outline of the thyroid is visible.

Now to the rhythm of the pulse. Is it regular, or irregular? And if irregular, is it *regularly* irregular, or *irregularly* irregular, as in atrial fibrillation where the atria do not contract but quiver like a bag of worms.

In my mind's eye now, I draw the contour of the pulse, the shape of its rise and fall, the little notch halfway down the descent. There are so very many abnormalities described: the *pulsus parvus et tardus* of aortic stenosis where a narrowed valve opening chokes off the blood as it tries to get into the aorta, delaying and prolonging the pulse contour. Also *pulsus alternans, pulsus bisferiens, pulsus paradoxus,* and my favorite, the Corrigan's water-hammer pulse. Here, a leaky aortic valve allows the column of blood ejected into the aorta in systole to plunge back into the heart in diastole. Corrigan, who was an Irish physician, named this sign after a toy called a water hammer, an evacuated tube of glass with a bead of water in it. A child's entertainment came from inverting the tube, the water falling through the vacuum to the bottom with a sharp snap, the exact feel of the pulse of aortic incompetence.

Now I occlude the vessel with one finger, milk it free of blood with another finger, and palpate. The empty vessel should be impalpable. If it feels hard, like a pipe cleaner, then the patient has arteriosclerosis and I picture the vessels in his brain, his kidneys, his heart, also like this, stiff and narrowed, harbingers of stroke, or heart attack, or kidney failure.

I know I linger too long on the pulse, as if wanting my hands to remain submerged in this subterranean river, feel it wash over me.

There is one last thing. I reach with my right hand under the elastic of the underwear or under the paper gown, to feel the femoral pulse in the crease of the thigh. It is, if done gently, not necessary to explain, for the patient realizes that I am now feeling *two* pulses—the radial with the left hand and the femoral with the right, stepping into the same river twice. Normally the pulse should register at the fingertips of both hands as synchronous, without a delay.

This last maneuver, checking for a delay between radial and femoral pulses, fascinates and haunts me, as if it were a song whose notes sound in my head though its origins escape me. It is a step in the examination often skipped or forgotten. The only reason to check for radio-femoral delay is to pick up coarctation of the aorta, a rare congenital condition where the aorta narrows acutely after it gives off branches to the head and upper limbs but before it feeds the lower limbs. Typically, coarctation is silent, goes undetected until the patient presents with high blood pressure. And even then, if the physician doesn't check for a radio-femoral delay, it is missed. Or, years later, the patient may present with a cerebral hemorrhage, the pipe bursting upstream from the narrowing. Or else they develop heart failure, the pump tiring of forcing blood through the constriction.

It is likely that in a lifetime of practicing medicine, a doctor will be visited by one or more persons with coarctation, lurking there among the coughs, the fevers, the podagras and sciaticas. They will be in the office for something else altogether. They will not know they have coarctation; it will sit there, part of the secret of the body, what the body does not tell.

This is my nightmare: that someone will pass through my office with coarctation, a diagnosable and treatable condition. That I will miss it because I skipped part of my ritual. And so I teach this, perhaps teach it excessively.

And when I forget to check for radio-femoral delay, I am tormented until I see the patient again. Once I called a patient back on a pretext because I thought if I didn't, he would turn out to have coarctation. And if I did check for it, then he would be spared.

There are so many other silent killers hiding in my patient's body, so many thousands—no, millions—of other bedside maneuvers that I could home in on. Why do I worry so about coarctation? It is an obsession as silly as not stepping on the lines between points during a tennis match. But it is out of such rituals that we carve lives for ourselves.

19

The day before the move, I took the boys to see the time-out place. It was, I told them, theirs as much as mine, a hideaway from the main house.

Jacob tilted his head to one side, looking up at me. I knew a question was coming. "You mean, like a tree house?"

I took off my watch and had Steven time the drive for us. Mountain Village apartments was just two miles down the road, due west of his mother's residence. It sat under the wings of the same familiar thunderbird that the boys could see from their bedrooms. There was, I pointed out as we drove, no highway to be negotiated, no thoroughfares, not even traffic lights. Just this curving, uphill, sleepy road at the edge of human habitation, a road that began a few yards from the spot where we'd found our first fossil. From there it ran along the side of the mountain, past stately homes, past the Coronado Country Club and its golf course, then a sharp turn down onto Los Cerritos and three stop signs before coming to Bandolero and the gate into the apartment complex.

"See, it's only five minutes away," I said, disliking this false cheeriness in my voice.

"Yeah, Jacob," Steven said, leaning forward from the backseat to speak into his ear, "it's just five minutes and twenty seconds away." Steven had slipped into the role of reassurer and translator for his younger brother. He deferred to Jacob in most matters—who was to occupy the front seat, who got to choose the video to be rented. He was determined to avoid conflict of any sort.

"Anytime you want to see me, or come over," I said, "just pick up the phone and—*vroom*—I'll be there."

○

Mountain Village apartments consisted of a series of free-standing brick buildings, each three stories high, spread out over a large land-scaped property. Giant oleanders with red and white flowers alter-nated with fir trees. The fir trees were as tall as the buildings. Brick-edged manicured lawns and carefully tended flower beds lined the circuitous walkways that led to the clubhouse and laundry room. Hundreds of gallons of water a day kept this appearance up, this Connecticut in West Texas. The backdrop of the brown mountain, however, close enough to touch, never let you forget you were in the desert.

I parked in a free slot in front of my unit. Metal stairs wound up the outside.

The boys first wanted to see the swimming pools. There were two of them, one on each end of the property. We went to the closer one.

"Are we allowed to swim here?" Steven asked.

"Of course."

"Now?"

"It's too cold now. In a few weeks."

"See, Jacob, our own pool!"

"Look, soda machines! Daddy, can we have soda?"

I could already see the ritual evolving, soda as coda to a swim. I fished for change and popped in fifty cents. Jacob went first, his fin-gers hovering first over one button, then another, second-guessing himself.

After they examined the pool, peeked into the pump room, explored the party room, tested the deck chairs, we walked back. The half-finished sodas were freezing in their little hands, so mine were pressed into service. My apartment was on the third floor. The boys clambered up ahead of me, their flip-flops chattering on the metal stairs. "Careful!" I said. "Careful" seemed to be the word most often on my tongue when I was with the boys. The more agile and mobile they became, the more my fear mounted.

I opened the door and the boys stormed in. "Look," Jacob said to Steven, "a balcony!" A sliding glass door off the living-cum-dining room led to a tiny sit-out, and this was what they wanted to see first. "It's like the cockpit of an Imperial Cruiser," Jacob said, his hands on the rails, peeking nervously over. Indeed, through the trees whose leaves had thinned out this time of year, there was an excellent view to the west. Back inside, they explored the small kitch-enette, which was separated from the living/dining room by a counter. They stood behind the counter, put their hands on it, tried to pull themselves up. "Excuse me, sir," Steven said, "can I take your order?"

The bedroom was tiny but offered a clear view of the thunderbird. The walls throughout were off white and the gray shag carpeting was brand new. Jacob discovered the walk-in closet. A naked bulb hanging from the ceiling had a pull switch whose chain he could reach by standing on his tiptoes. In its emptiness, the closet made a perfect hiding place. He summoned Steven and they had me wait outside while they shut the door. I heard them turn the light off and sit in the darkness till they lost their nerve and screamed and reached for the chain. It was a while before they tired of this game. When they came out, their faces were flushed.

The bathroom was between living room and bedroom. Jacob promptly inaugurated it, pulling his shorts to his knees, leaning forward to counterbalance his bottom, which threatened to fall in. "Stay with me?" he said.

Then it was time for them to peer up the fireplace, hear the echoes of their voices in the chimney as they called up. On to the pantry now, to shut the door and turn off the light, but the floor was linoleum and not carpet and a crack under the door let light in. Back to the Imperial Cruiser.

I stood watching them jabber excitedly on the balcony. Steven pulled Jacob's head close with both hands and whispered into his ear. Now Jacob whispered something back, again putting both hands on Steven's face and pulling him close, as if simply leaning over and whispering wasn't enough. There was something so intimate about this gesture.

They were firing on the enemy: passing cars. Despite the two years' difference in their ages, they were like twins, close to each other, leaning on each other, more so now that the world of their parents was so unstable. Their fantasy games had their origins in *Star Wars*, but they were secretive as to the specifics, conscious that adults had little capacity for suspending reality and playing along.

Their visit gave me a different view of the apartment, showed me possibilities in a place that before had held nothing but dread for me.

"So, do you boys like it?" I asked when they came back in.

"It's great, Dad," Steven said. "Don't worry, everything will be all right."

I reached for him.

"Yeah, look at all the place we have to wrestle," Jacob said, pointing to the sweep of the carpet in the main room, free of any furniture. He looked at me as I hugged Steven, then he let out a banshee wail, and charged me. I pretended to topple over and then curl into a ball while they sat on me and pounded me with their little fists.

○

That night, after the kids were in bed, I began to pack. I had not found the courage to tell them exactly when I would be physically out of their home. But they had seen the apartment, they had seen U-Haul boxes being repacked, they had seen the open suitcase that spoke of flight. I wanted to present the actual move as a fait accompli, not something they had to witness. I thought of Jacob and how his mind worked with metaphors: I didn't want him to witness the hauling out of furniture and books, didn't want him to say, "Like a captain abandoning his ship."

I told Rajani that I would move in midmorning, after the boys had gone to school. After eleven years, two children, five different homes that we had lived in, what was mine, what was hers? Or rather, what did I want? The suitcase was for the contents of my study desk. I spread out a bedsheet in the center of the room and cleaned out my closet, laying the clothes, still on their hangers, one on top of another into a pile and then tying the corners of the bedsheet to make a *dhoby* bundle. I made three such bundles. My books were still in their cartons, an amazing number of cartons. The wooden frame of the futon, which could be folded so as to be a sofa, had been taken apart. The mattress I would roll into a bundle in the morning.

Rajani appeared and stood with me, looking at the pile. She had stayed out of my way during most of the packing. "I'll set aside some cutlery, dishes, cooking vessels, stuff like that for you to take—"

"I don't need a thing," I said. "If I'm starting again, I'll take just the bare essentials."

And that was what now sat piled in the center of the guest bedroom waiting for morning.

"You'll need a chest of drawers," she said, which was true, because the apartment had closet space but no drawers. The chest of drawers belonged to my mother and it seemed fitting for me to take it.

"The table and chair?" she asked.

"Let Steven use it. I'll get another one." This room would soon be Steven's bedroom. Eventually I would buy a table and a chair and perhaps a bookshelf or two.

"What will you sit on?" she asked.

I looked at the futon. It would be cumbersome to wrestle it into the sofa position every day, and then back into a bed at night.

"I'll take my recliner." Mine, because I had been the one to pick it out and because she never used it.

"Take some of the living room stuff if you want to."

I shook my head.

We stood looking at that forlorn pile. Rajani went off to her room.

○

Later that night, the phone rang, David calling to say he was ready to help.

I explained that I wanted to move while the boys were at school, but I didn't want to pull him away from the hospital, from his new rotation.

"How will you manage your boxes and stuff? I can break away."

"I don't think either of our cars will do the job anyway."

He didn't argue. "The boys . . . ?"

"They're something else. I took them over . . ."

"Yeah?"

"So far they're doing better than I am."

○

Manuel, the mover, was in his early forties. Even with a bulky jacket on, he looked puny. His movements, like his speech, were brisk and efficient.

He quickly surveyed what items were going and then, with barely a pause, addressed himself to the chest of drawers, tilting it and turning it and bringing it to his body and then onto the dolly with the ease of an orthopedist reducing a dislocated shoulder.

His assistant was twice his size, and I heard Manuel call him El

Chino, and later just Chino. Nicknames were the rule in El Paso; the police most-wanted sheets listed them alongside the real names. Sometimes the origins were clear (*El Loco*, *El Chiquilin*) but others were more obscure. Mexicans think of Chinese as having curly hair—*pelo chino*—and so if you had curly hair, as Manuel's assistant did, you became *El Chino*. *Super Ratón* (Mighty Mouse) could in time be shorted to *Ratón* (mouse) and then, later, affectionately became *Rata* (the mouse becoming a rat), and his progeny could become *Ratoncito* or *Ratitas*. One of my residents, whose real name was Meza, was called *Tablito* since "Meza" sounded much like "Mesa," which means table in English.

El Chino was slow. There was more muscle in his boss's lean, wiry biceps than in Chino's big, flabby arms. We were loaded in no time. The van was small but it dwarfed my meager belongings. I took one last look around. Rajani remained in her bedroom and I called out to her that I would be back in the evening. "Good-bye, house," I said, under my breath, as I closed the door behind me and hurried out, feeling a sob rise in my throat, wanting this leaving to be over.

Manuel followed me in the van to the apartments. Unloading was more difficult because everything had to be hauled up the three flights of stairs. El Chino stacked cartons on the dolly, three at a time, then slowly wrestled the dolly up the stairs, while his boss worked without the dolly, carrying two cartons at a time and lapping El Chino.

○

"Divorcing, huh," Manuel said softly as he wrote out the invoice.

"Separating . . . You can tell?"

"You learn so much about people by moving their things."

"Like?"

"Like you, maybe you should have taken more stuff."

"Didn't want anything. Just the essentials."

He seemed to understand that sentiment, though his expression suggested that in time I would regret that. "You're a doctor, no? Well, don't worry. One day I'll move you to a bigger place and you'll be happy again. Or maybe I'll move you back there?"

"I doubt it."

"Where were the kids?"

"At school."

"Two boys?"

"Two boys."

"They'll be fine. You'll always take care of them, no?"

"You bet."

"You betcha. Mind if I use your bathroom?" I waved him toward it, admiring his clinical acumen. He paused as he was about to enter the bathroom. "You'd be surprised how many people don't want you to use their bathrooms. Can you believe it?"

○

The cartons were unpacked, the clothes put away. For the most part, I liked the apartment the way I'd found it, the previous occupant's traces painted over but visible in the liner in the kitchen drawers, a candle forgotten in the closet, plastic chairs left behind on the patio. There was something elemental about this, bending my head over the sink to drink water. Still, I would have to get things like a shower curtain, a kitchen trash can.

In the evening, I went back to visit the boys, played with them in their backyard. I sat with them while they had dinner. And then I put them to bed.

"Will you sleep over in the apartment?" Steven asked.

"Yes . . . but I'll see you guys when you get back from school tomorrow." My mouth was dry, my heart racing. Nothing seemed more important now than sounding confident for them.

Jacob sat up. "Are grown-ups scared to sleep alone?"

"No. You say your prayers and then you are not scared. And when I sleep, I'll know you guys are close by—just five minutes away. It's almost as if I'm sleeping in the room next to you."

"Steven is going to have his own room," Jacob said.

His thought process was like the knight's move in chess. You had to look carefully for the connection between sentences. I thought I could see where this was leading.

"Are you scared to sleep alone?" I asked.

His head righted itself. He looked forthrightly back at me and said, "A little. But if I get scared, I'll go into Mommy's bed."

"Me too," Steven said.

○

I tiptoed out of their room after a while, and then out of the house. Before Rajani locked the door after me, we wished each other good night. That was it, the only acknowledgment.

I drove back on the loopy mountain road, deserted and dark at this hour, picking up speed. I was too fast when I entered the sharp curve at Los Cerritos, a curve made more treacherous by the steep descent at its end. The tires squealed, then broke free. I was sliding. To touch the brakes would have sent me over the edge. I hit the accelerator, felt the wheels spin, the skid get worse, and then the tires held and grabbed asphalt. Now I was coming down the hill much too fast, fish-tailing. I flew through one stop sign, praying, gearing down, braking, the brakes and tires shrieking. The car stalled to a stop five yards past the last stop sign. I was pouring sweat, and aware that I must have roused the neighborhood.

I pulled into the apartment, still shaking. I sat there, my hands glued to the wheel, not yet ready to step onto the ground.

A few minutes later, I saw David pulling in to the complex in his strange, angular Isuzu. Its rakish front end didn't seem to go with its chopped-off butt. "It's a turbo, you know," David had told me once, since nothing about its sound or performance would have made me suspect that, "the same model that Jackie Chan drove in *It's a Mad Mad Mad Mad World.*" It listed slightly to starboard, creating the illusion that it was moving diagonally, crab fashion. He pulled into the space next to me, revved the engine a few times, popped the hood, and left the motor running, and we both stepped out.

"Hi," he said, smiling apologetically as he propped the hood up. "The accelerator was sticking. Scared the bejesus out of me coming down the hill."

"You too?"

"What?" He studied me. I still felt tremulous.

"Nothing."

"That's one steep hill."

"Tell me about it."

"I popped the clutch in and it stopped."

I peered under the hood with him to be sociable. David had bought the car for a few hundred dollars on the recommendation of a mechanic who had assured him that even though it had been wrecked and didn't run, the engine was a jewel. With a few hundred dollars of repairs, he would be getting more car per buck than if he bought one in running condition. This jewel-in-the-rust philosophy was widely subscribed to in El Paso, particularly in the two-mile stretch east of the hospital on Alameda where *carrocerias* and used-car lots ran one into another. In the late afternoon, when I headed home from work, men congregated on Alameda, next to the cemetery, under the freeway overpass, swigging discreetly from bottles hidden in brown bags. They leaned against their parked cars, hoods propped open, moving from one to the next, as if on rounds. I imagined each man a specialist in his own field—carburation, circuitry, suspension—offering expert consultations.

"It's a good car, you know," David said, looking at me across the engine. "It's just a step away from greatness."

When I made no reply, he shrugged, shut the hood, and turned the motor off.

Upstairs, I gave him the grand tour. The pantry was bare but the refrigerator held a six-pack of beer and a six-pack of Coke.

"It isn't half bad, mate," he pronounced. "It beats where I'm staying, that's for sure."

I had the recliner in the center of the room, a reading lamp next to it. A running border of books followed the wall and continued over the mantelpiece above the fireplace. The bedroom had the futon in the center, the chest of drawers against a wall, and more books propped against the wainscoting. It was the kind of decor only another male would approve of.

"How's it feel?" David said as we moved out to the porch and sat down.

I was sucking the beer down as if it were medicine. It was difficult to believe that this was where I would spend the night. "It was worse imagining this day than actually living through it." I thought about the hill and how I had almost lost it.

"I should have been there to help you move. I was worried about you—"

Suddenly, with a gurgle that made me jump, the sprinkler system came on below us, filling the air with what sounded like tropical rainfall.

"Relax, Abraham."

"I want to relax all over this floor," I said, reaching for a second beer.

"Thinking too far ahead," he said hesitantly, "or looking back, won't get you anywhere."

He had found my pulse and I listened.

"'One day at a time!' That's not just for AA folks," he said.

I took a deep breath, and we sat in silence.

"I feel relieved," I said, after a long while. "This weight I've been carrying is . . . it's less . . . I feel like I did when I went off to college, left my parents. Nobody to answer to. Come and go as I please. Smoke a cigar out here if it pleases me. Finish this six-pack . . ."

David was quiet, slumped back in the chair, his eyes squinting, studying me, as though he was suspicious of this simple epiphany. He had one hand on his face, the finger extended along his brow.

"Take your time," he said. "You have to experience the pain that you have to experience. You march through it and come out on the other side. When I came back to restart the fourth year, it was agony to walk into the hospital again. Everyone knew what had happened. It went on for weeks. It still goes on. But then I tell myself, 'It's painful because of what you did, it's not painful because they are doing anything to you.' But I hung in there. A day at a time. Now it's the source of my strength. The fact that I lived through the pain and discomfort."

His words didn't affect me as much as his simply being there. I wanted to tell him how precious his company was this night. I knew why I had wanted him to come: I didn't need help in moving or unpacking. But it would have been difficult to walk into the apartment alone after putting the boys to sleep. I had lied to Jacob—I *was* scared to be here alone. It was lucky for me that David had driven in just when I'd returned. And just like the kids, his take on the apartment as "not half bad" had saved me from seeing it as "not good." He was right: For all my bluster, deep down I felt forsaken, ashamed. Only his presence had saved me from feeling overwhelmed. But I didn't say any of this to him.

○

On Friday evening, the kids came over. I heard their voices, excited and high-pitched, and I heard their shoes slapping on the metal stairs, making the staircase vibrate and ring as they charged up. They burst in, both wearing backpacks, my two little campers ready for this adventure of sleeping at the time-out place. Behind them came their mother, carrying two rolled-up Mickey Mouse sleeping bags. I took them from her. She also carried a plastic grocery bag, which had two cereal bowls and small boxes of cereal, two spoons, and milk.

"Didn't need all this," I said to her.

"Where were they going to sleep otherwise?"

"On sheets, on the floor with me."

"Well, this is better. You might as well keep the bowls and spoons here. And the sleeping bags. For them."

She looked around at the flat. Her expression suggested that she thought this minimalist approach to living was unnecessary, as if I was posturing. And perhaps she was right. Nothing stopped me from getting a sofa and a dinette set.

I had no television, but the boys didn't seem to care, the apartment was excitement enough. We ordered pizza, and while we waited, we taped up and inverted one of my packing cartons as a dining table.

Afterward, we spread out the sleeping bags in the living room, said our prayers, and lay down, one boy on each side of me, their arms and legs thrown over me, immobilizing me. Their twitches, tics, and sniffles slowly gave way to sleep. I gently extricated myself and moved about the apartment, silently picking up.

I sat down with my notebook. The last entry in it had to do with coming to the net against David:

> *If David hits short, and you want to rush the net, don't. Your top-spin forehand, even when you hit it with good pace and depth, isn't an ideal approach shot. It bounces high and he can tee off, particularly if you hit it to his forehand. If you hit it to his backhand, he takes the ball so early, blocks it down the line more often than not, and it's past you before you're near the net. Even if you do anticipate down the line and cover it, it stays very low, and because of the underspin on it, even if you get your racket on the ball, the tendency is to dump it in the net. So if you want to rush the net on him, do it with a backhand slice. Better still, don't.*

Now, pen in hand, I made my first entry from Mountain Village apartments. Half an hour later I stopped, with the words "Not half bad."

O

I came awake to the thought that my existence now resembled David's. The apartment was my boardinghouse equivalent: a bare refrigerator, minimal furnishings. As for a circle of friends—he was it. He went to an NA meeting on Tuesdays, and to an AA meeting at the Arid Club on Fridays; those were the two evenings I spent with my sons. We met for tennis on Sundays and Wednesdays. It pleased me to think of his life and mine being parallel, overlapping, as if the sum of our two lives created a safer shelter than what we could construct alone.

20

Chemotherapy had helped Enrique, the young man with the pulmonary Kaposi's sarcoma. He had felt well enough to visit friends in Monterrey, Mexico, over Christmas, and had wound up staying there till mid-February, even missing some of his clinic appointments. Now he was back in El Paso and back in the hospital. He had come to the emergency room complaining of shortness of breath.

When I saw him the morning after his admission, his sister was just getting up from the recliner by his bed. She was alluring, two tones darker than her brother, with the same thick hair. Her nose, where it met her brow, was flattened, unrefined, and yet somehow attractive. I sensed she was proud of her nose, like a boxer is of his.

Enrique looked tired behind the oxygen mask, his breathing worse than the last time I had seen him. Still, he seemed more peaceful, or perhaps only more accepting.

He asked me about my holidays, even though the words came out muffled by the oxygen mask. His face glowed when he spoke of his vacation in Monterrey. "My friends . . . most fabulous Christmas for me. They did . . . everything," he said, making a sweeping gesture with his arm, suggesting a Christmas that would never be matched.

I eased his mask off only to find that his tip-of-the-nose Kaposi's lesion had blossomed into a bulbous, pitted mass that overhung his nostrils.

"When I was coming back. Across the border," he said. "The customs man. Put his head in the car and . . ." He gulped for air. "He asked me. If I was going to. A fancy dress ball!" Enrique and his sister laughed at this recollection.

His lungs had fine crackles in both bases. The friction rub I had heard over his heart, and which had disappeared with the chemotherapy, was back. On his chest X ray, the masses that I had assumed were Kaposi's were a little bigger than before. But now he also had a diffuse haziness to both lungs that I thought was a pneumonia. I didn't think it was *Pneumocystis* because I had put him on Bactrim as a prophylaxis against that disease months before. Still, I would start empiric treatment for *Pneumocystis* while we tried to make a specific diagnosis.

"Have you had breakfast?" He shook his head. "Good, don't eat anything. I'd like to do a bronchoscopy this afternoon." It was, I explained, a procedure where I would go down with a fiberoptic instrument into his trachea and bronchi, take biopsies if need be, wash out small segments of his lung to try to find the infectious agent causing his problem.

He shrugged his shoulders, as if he were resigned to whatever I had to do.

"Anything else I can do for you, to make you more comfortable?" I asked.

"Can you prescribe time pills?"

"I'm sorry? What are . . ."

"A joke," he said, smiling mischievously. "More time on earth." Then he sighed. "My mom will be here in an hour or so."

"Does she know what's going on now?"

"We never talk about it . . . ," he said, looking at his sister.

She brushed his hair back from his forehead. "She knows," she said to me with assurance. "My mother has known from the time he was a little boy . . . that he was really her little girl." She stroked his brow and smiled as she said this, showing strong, even teeth. Her English was accented, but good. Spanish was clearly her first language. "When he was young, he would tell Mama how much he loved her, how pretty she looked. There's nothing she does not know."

Enrique looked at his sister tenderly. I found it difficult to keep my eyes off her face.

○

Enrique was emblematic of the new style of AIDS care in the nineties. AIDSology, I called it. I had given him chemotherapy for his Kaposi's sarcoma because I was as familiar with the chemotherapy for these tumors as the oncologist. I would perform his bron-choscopy and therefore didn't have to enlist the help of a pul-monary physician. I had done a skin biopsy on him. In the clinic, we did bone-marrow biopsies and other procedures as the need arose. I had even pulled a tooth or two.

In the early days of AIDS, it had not always been easy to get con-sultants from other disciplines to see HIV-infected patients, or treat them as promptly or as courteously as we wanted. It had been frus-trating, paralyzing. As a result, HIV specialists had learned to become jacks-of-all-trades.

Now, twelve years after the epidemic had begun, eight years after HIV had been discovered, the climate of AIDS care in America had changed. My present medical students had heard about this disease in junior high school. It was rare for physicians to express distaste for taking care of persons with AIDS, or to make off-color remarks about a patient's sexuality, something that had been common in the early days. Oh, we still had our full complement of homophobes, but the power balance had swung the other way. One senior resi-dent had made a prejudicial comment to my physician's assistant, Della Nabhan, about "those homos" and she had been merciless, hounding him, telling him and everyone within earshot that this was a reflection of his own sexual immaturity. It had served as a potent warning.

○

The endoscopy suite where Enrique awaited his bronchoscopy was primarily used by the gastroenterologists. Dr. Zuckerman and his colleagues were well published, intellectually curious, and always willing to do endoscopies of the stomach or colon, or perform liver biopsies on our AIDS patients when the need arose.

David was there, waiting too. When he had free time from his rotations, he would seek me out, tag along. I tried to let him know of interesting patients or procedures I thought he should see. We waited for Linda, the endoscopy nurse, to finish what she was doing and join us with Enrique.

To my surprise, I saw Raju, the Indian intern who had been on the ward rotation with David and me, lying on a gurney. He was, he told me quietly, volunteering for a study in which they would place a tiny gastric tube via his nose into his stomach and monitor his gastric juice pH for twenty-four hours. Prior to inserting the tube, Linda gave Raju some Versed intravenously, a Valium-like drug that would ease passage of the tube. As David and I watched, Raju's eyelids fluttered and in a few minutes he seemed to be in deep meditation, his fingers clasped together and resting on his belly. Linda put K-Y jelly on the tube.

"Dr. Raju?" she said to him. "Which nostril would you like me to put this in?"

His eyelids opened slowly, and a dreamy expression came to his face. "Whichever nostril you think is more beautiful, Linda," he said with an angelic smile and then closed his eyes again.

O

Enrique's nose and pharynx had been anesthetized with xylocaine. He was lying in the darkened bronchoscopy room with the head of the bed raised slightly. I gave him two milligrams of Versed. The dose was small but strong, so he could respond to commands but later have no memory of the procedure. A pulse oximeter displayed his oxygen saturation. Even with supplemental oxygen he was saturating at 85 to 89 percent, not ideal. "Enrique! *Como esta?*" He flashed a thumbs-up sign at me. Two other students and a resident came and stood beside us.

I slid the bronchoscope, an instrument slightly thicker than a pencil, up Enrique's left nostril and then watched my progress on the TV monitor in front of me. The bronchoscope was flexible, like a hose, and had a control that I worked with my right hand, which allowed me to bend its tip up or down. My left hand was farther down the shaft of the scope, near where it entered his nostril, and this was the hand with which I fed the scope in or pulled back or applied gentle torque. On the screen, the back of Enrique's tongue came into view, and then his epiglottis and now his vocal cords, which quivered with his every breath. I squirted some xylocaine directly past his cords into his trachea and, after giving this a chance to work, I eased the scope down, working its tip so that it slid down between the vocal cords without traumatizing them.

"Imagine," I said to the students, "that you are in a spacecraft going headfirst into the trachea. The only way to orient yourself, left and right, up and down, is to think of your eye being at the end of the scope, the image on the monitor like the view out the windshield."

The trachea resembled a tunnel we were passing through, a tunnel with a pink, shiny lining, and supported by C-shaped rings of cartilage whose outline was visible through the mucous membrane. I could see the students were transfixed as we came to the carina, the place where the trachea divided into left and right mainstem bronchi.

"A fork in the road," I said.

Just above the carina we could see vivid purple to cherry-red patches, as if someone had smeared jelly on the mucosal surface. "These are the Kaposi's sarcoma lesions," I pointed out. There were more as I went down further into both the left and right bronchus and explored their subdivisions. "Picture?" I said, and Linda reached around my hand and snapped a switch, taking a Polaroid image. I took a few more shots.

"How do you know where you are, Dr. Verghese?" David asked.

"The only way to know where you are is by where you have just been." It sounded like an aphorism for life, not just for bronchoscopy. "If I'm in doubt, I just pull back to the bifurcation of the trachea, to the carina, and then start again from there."

Linda pointed at Enrique's oxygen saturation: It had dropped to 80 percent. We roused him, asked him to take a few deep breaths, which helped, but not much. I slid the bronchoscope into the lung segment that on his chest X ray seemed the most involved. I wedged the bronchoscope as far as it would go. Now, working rapidly, Linda pushed several syringefuls of normal saline through a port on the side of the scope, for a total of about 150 milliliters. Then, by depressing a button, I sucked back as much of this fluid as I could through the suction port into a sputum trap. "This is what we call bronchoalveolar lavage, a method to sample millions of alveoli, and, with any luck, to find the organism—if there is one—that has taken advantage of Enrique's weak immune system."

I was done. "David, you want to drive out?" I passed the scope over to David, positioned his hands in the right manner, and told him to gently pull out, using the toggle to keep the scope in the center of the trachea. He hadn't expected this, and was nervous. The other students looked envious. I put my fingers over David's, and guided him. We pulled back to the vocal cords, then went down one more time to the carina, and then I let him pull out on his own.

I wrote orders for Enrique to go to the recovery room for an hour. I filled out the lab slips and the procedure note. Enrique was fast asleep.

"Thanks," David said when we were alone.

○

In the waiting room, we found Enrique's mother and sister. They stood up as they saw us. I introduced David, then showed them the Polaroids of the Kaposi's inside Enrique's trachea. I had brought his chest X ray with me, and I held it up against the ceiling lights and showed them the Kaposi's but also the new infiltrate at the periphery that looked like an infection. Things might worsen before they got better, I said. If they got better.

His mother, stoic till then, brushed tears from her face. She said something rapidly in Spanish. The sister explained, "He loved Christmas. My mother says she's glad he had a wonderful Christmas. She thinks it's as though he is ready to go."

I didn't know what to say. Then the mother touched my hand and said, "*Gracias,* Doctor." The sister came forward, her face inches from mine, and hugged me, and said thank you. I could smell her hair, her body, a crisp, unadorned scent. I didn't want her to let go.

○

The day after the bronchoscopy, David and I went to see Enrique's alveolar fluid. Under the microscope I thought we would find *Pneumocystis,* but instead we discovered an organism I had been long expecting to see in El Paso: *Coccidioides immitis.* I had to move the slide around to find it, but every few fields, scattered among the alveolar macrophages and the neutrophils, the thick-walled spherules of *Coccidioides immitis* sat like huge land mines. I pointed them out to David. Each spherule was a hundred times the size of the adjacent white blood cells. "You see those tennis ball–like structures within the thick outer wall of the spherule? Those are endospores, each of which can become a spherule."

"Christ!"

"Amazing this, don't you think? That a fungus can exist in the soil in a form similar to the furry mold on bread, nothing like what we're seeing under microscope—"

"A hyphal form?"

"Exactly. And then we breathe it in when we're walking through the desert. Enrique probably got it when he was a child stirring up soil near a creosote bush. Then, in his body, the fungus morphed into a different form: From mold in the soil it became these bomb-shaped baskets, collared by white blood cells, unable to do anything but sit there. Then, when he got HIV . . ."

"His lymphocyte count dropped, his cellular immunity waned . . ."

"Right. And the fungus came alive: The spherule ruptured. Out came hundreds of endospores, each of which grew to form a spherule with hundreds of endospores within, each of which . . ."

"And you and I can get this?"

"You and I probably have it by now. It's endemic here. But if your immune system is intact, usually nothing happens."

We walked back from the lab to the hospital.

"The full expression of this fungus's dimorphic life cycle means death for the host," I said. "Makes you wonder whether we are dimorphic too. One form on earth, and another on some other host, a form that we can't imagine . . ."

"And therefore came up with terms like heaven?" David said.

"Or hell."

O

Outside Enrique's room a nurse crossed our path and exchanged a significant look with David.

"Wow!" I said, when she was out of earshot. "I felt those sparks from twelve feet away."

He shook his head, as if such forces were beyond his control, but he smiled secretively.

"By the way," I said, "did you enjoy the rodeo?"

That stopped him in his tracks. "*You* put her up to that?"

"No," I said, giving him a gentle prod on the sternum, "*you* put her up to that. Walking around with your helpless-babe-in-the-woods-don't-know-shit-about-America con."

I pushed open the door to Enrique's room before David could

reply. The television was turned off, and only the sound of oxygen bubbling through water could be heard. His mother and sister were on either side of him, stroking his arms, their faces sorrowful, tearful. His eyelids were half closed, the eyeballs drifting up. The rapid fogging and unfogging of his face mask revealed his respiratory distress. He was much worse off than the day of the bronchoscopy.

We had a diagnosis, I explained to Enrique, and to his sister and mother. We would use a drug called Amphotericin B, given by vein, in high doses against this fungus. With luck, the drug would work quickly to make him feel better. As for chemotherapy, we would hold off for now. The fungal infection was the more pressing problem.

News that a specific infection has been identified was usually cause for celebration, for hope, but they seemed to know that it was too late.

Before I could ask, his sister told me that they had talked about it and decided that if his breathing got worse, he did not want to be on a ventilator. He would sign a "do not resuscitate" order.

Enrique did not utter a word during all this, opening his eyes only occasionally. I told them that I would prescribe a very small dose of morphine, which had the effect of "cutting off the lungs from the brain, so he doesn't get anxious about his breathing," words that I had trotted out often to students and to patients. If his breathing became worse, they were to let us know.

He lifted his fingers once off the bedsheet as I made to leave, a wave that was thank you and good-bye. His sister too glanced at me, a look both concerned and tender, as if in her grief she had enough heart to worry about me, about my reliving this scene again and again, a little piece of me chipping off each time.

○

I stayed in the hospital late that evening. On a television in the house-staff lounge I caught a press conference in midtown Manhattan. Arthur Ashe, looking wan and pale, announced that he was suffering from AIDS. He had probably been infected for a decade or more. By some miracle, his wife and child were uninfected.

Earlier that year, during the Australian Open (which Jim Courier won, and in celebration of his victory had jumped into the Yarra

River), I had noticed the strange discoloration of Ashe's skin, remembered the bypass surgeries he had had in 1979 and 1983. The thought of AIDS had crossed my mind. But then I'd pushed it away. It seemed inconceivable that anyone that famous would be able to keep a disease like AIDS a secret.

Heartbreaking now to watch the news conference, to see Ashe poised, collected, pushing his glasses back on his nose, a Wimbledon champion, speaking in the measured voice of a scholar (the author of a three-volume book on the black athlete), showing the dignity of a statesman and the composure that had been his trademark on the court.

Composed, that is, until he mentioned his daughter's name, Camera. Then he lost his composure, fought back tears. I could not hold mine back.

I checked on Enrique before I left the hospital. He appeared unchanged. I thought there was a good chance that he would survive a few more days, perhaps even turn the corner. The family did not think so, and there were other members there. His friends from Monterrey would arrive shortly, his sister said. I paged the resident on call, a sensitive South American lady who was *simpática* as far as AIDS went, a favorite of our HIV patients. Yes, she'd be delighted to attend to Enrique and the family through the night. I encouraged her to use morphine judiciously if he seemed to be struggling.

○

Back at my apartment, there was a message from David. "Did you hear about Ashe? Bummer. Call me if you haven't heard. Oh, and by the way, one of the radiology technicians told me the other day that you looked like Julio Iglesias. That you were so polite and this-and-that. I said Julio Iglesias had more hair . . ." I laughed aloud hearing this. I picked up the phone to call him, then remembered that at this hour I might wake his landlady or the other boarders.

I must have fallen asleep in the recliner. Sometime during the night, the resident telephoned to tell me that Enrique had died. My first thought, to my annoyance, was that I must tell David, but I could not since he had no phone in his room.

And then I was awake, alert.

"Dr. Verghese?" she said, unsure that I had heard her.

"What time is it?

"Three-fifteen."

"Was it . . . hard?"

"He was alert. I gave him the morphine twice, the last time an hour before he died. His breathing was worse. The family was taking it well. They declined an autopsy. They told me to tell you thanks, and that they would be in touch."

21

July 5, 1975, center court, men's finals, Wimbledon: This is the picture that lingers: Arthur Ashe sitting in a chair during the changeover, eyes focused on his hands, his posture that of a Buddhist in prayer. Later I learn he is not meditating. He is staring at notes that he hides in his palms.

○

The night before the match Ashe talked to Roscoe Tanner, the hard-hitting serve and volleyer whom Jimmy Connors had decimated in the semifinal. The harder Tanner had hit, the better Connors had played, feeding off the pace. Tanner had served out of his mind and still won only eight games. Ashe also consulted with Donald Dell and Dennis Ralston, his Davis Cup captain, trying to come up with a game plan to defeat Connors.

Ashe's game is tailor-made, on paper, for Connors. Despite the dissimilarity in their temperaments, their games are strikingly similar. Ashe's countenance may be impassive, composed, but on the court, he is normally not one to temporize. He hits freely, attacks, and goes for winners.

But no one in the world that year is better at hitting out, attacking, going for winners, using pace than Jimmy Connors. If Ashe's face masks his emotions, Connors's is a window to his soul. In his eyes, his grin, his snarls, you see brashness, arrogance, lewdness, pixieish charm, and, of course, utter self-confidence. When perturbed, Jimmy will stick a racket between his legs and simulate masturbation. Ashe, at most, will square his shoulders, tighten his lips, push his glasses back up the bridge of his nose, and hunker down for the next point.

O

The bookies have Connors as a three-to-twenty favorite. Ashe, at thirty-two, is no longer the same player who, in 1968, was ranked number one in the United States. He is perhaps a half-step slower, his game not quite as intimidating as before, certainly not intimidating to Connors.

Just before Wimbledon, Connors filed a libel suit against Ashe for three million dollars, because Ashe had said to the media that it was "unpatriotic" for Connors not to play the Davis Cup. The pros have banded together to form the ATP—Association of Tennis Professionals—of which Arthur is the president. The only holdout is Connors, who has sued the ATP for twenty million dollars for barring him from their events.

This is Ashe's last chance to win Wimbledon. He beat Borg to get here—Borg who, incredibly, will go on to win the next five Wimbledons, a feat that no one in attendance that year can possibly imagine.

O

Ashe has not commented on Jimmy's lawsuit, but he shows up on court wearing a USA Davis Cup warm-up jacket. It is the only hint of gamesmanship we see from Ashe for the rest of the day.

His tactics become apparent when the match starts. He eschews his usual hard, flat serve and instead hits the heavy slice, the can opener into the deuce court, dragging Jimmy off the court. Connors has the best return of serve in the game ever, but this angled serve that lands halfway up the service sideline and hooks out to where the stockade of photographers are clicking away is one that even Connors, particularly with his two-handed backhand, can barely get a racket on. When he does get it back, Ashe is at the net and hits an easy volley to the open court.

During the rallies, Ashe gives Jimmy no pace, slow-balling him, hitting dinks, chips, and underspin shots that hardly carry and that land short in midcourt, shading to Jimmy's forehand. Because of Jimmy's unorthodox grip on the forehand—it resembles a Western grip, and yet the ball is hit flat—he has difficulty with the short low ball on this side. He tends to rush the shot, runs through it as he hits it. Many of his shots hit the tape, fall exasperatingly back. He has none of the clearance that topspin would give him. When Jimmy succeeds in getting this tricky forehand over the net and in the court, he is looking for Ashe to try to blast the ball past him. Instead, Ashe lobs over his backhand. Time and again he brings Jimmy in with short balls and then lobs him. Ashe keeps most of his ground strokes and approach shots down the middle, taking away Jimmy's angles. Jimmy is famous for hitting angled winners on the dead run from the deep corners of the court. But on this day Ashe does not give him that opportunity.

Ashe wins the first two sets 6–1 and 6–1. The crowd is in shock. The crowd is decidedly in favor of Ashe. But they appear unprepared for the underdog to prevail. Connors looks, according to Peter Ustinov, who is commenting on the match, "like a Scotsman who has mislaid his kilt." His twitches and his tugs on his shirtsleeves become more pronounced. He blows on his hand again and again, as if trying to thaw it from a deep freeze. His face shows anxiety and even fear behind the bluster.

○

By sheer determination, Connors claws back in the third set. At a few crucial points, he lures Ashe into hard-hitting duels. Connors wins the set 7–5.

Jimmy is up in the fourth, 3–0. The crowd is numb, sensing they are going to be disappointed by Ashe, feeling sheepish about having so vocally backed the underdog. Ashe's failure is their failure.

○

The changeover.

Ashe in Buddha posture, face motionless, eyes focused on his hands, sitting on his chair, his back to the umpire. He understands how much the crowd wants him to prevail. He is worried. His temptation, as he sees the momentum swing back to Jimmy, is to retreat to his natural game, to go to autopilot, to slash and smash, to hit out and then let the chips fall where they may.

That is the easiest thing to do, no cognition or effort of will is required.

Many thoughts must pass through his mind: Perhaps he thinks of his father, newly widowed, returning from the hospital when Arthur is seven, clutching his boys to him, weeping, saying again and again, "This is all I got left." Perhaps he thinks of Richmond and the solitude of his tennis, hours against the backboard. Perhaps he recalls that it is an act of will, of faith, that took him from that backboard to becoming a junior champion, to playing for UCLA, to winning the U.S. Open title, to winning the Davis Cup. Or perhaps he thinks none of these things, only of the match and where he is playing it.

He has come this close to the most coveted title in tennis. And, once again, it is not merely his hopes, but the hopes, strangely, of the English crowd as well as the hopes of blacks everywhere that rest on him.

Yes, what is required of him now is not a physical act so much as an act of faith. He must stick with the strategy that befuddled Connors and won him the first two sets. He cannot retreat to autopilot.

He glances at his notes.

He takes a deep breath.

He must exert his will, play this unconventional off-speed style if he is to win.

He rises from the chair. The crowd does not realize that the greatest battle is already over.

It happened in Arthur's head.

22

I arrived at the hospital parking lot just as David pulled in. His hair was still wet. His short-sleeved blue shirt was, as always, rumpled, and badly in need of ironing. He reached to the backseat for his mustard-colored tie, already knotted. He was about to slip the noose over his head when I took it away from him.

"Here," I said, and handed him a paisley red-and-green tie I had brought in my bag, also knotted, ready to wear.

"That was nice of you!"

"Couldn't stand the sight of this thing anymore. Diarrhea yellow gets old after a few months. And have you heard of such a thing as an iron?"

"Watch," he said, putting on the tie and then pulling on his white coat. "See? No one notices."

"You need to get your own phone line. I would have called you back last night."

"Can't afford one," he said glumly. "Soon, though. I'll be done paying off one of my loans." I told him about Enrique's death.

We walked toward the glass doors of the Texas Tech building. Through the glass I could see an obstetrics senior resident coming toward us, and I held the door open for her. She said, "Hi, Dr. Verghese," but pointedly ignored David, almost shouldering him aside. He stood back, head lowered.

"What was that about?"

He shook his head, as if it were not worth discussing.

"She used to be my classmate. She and I and another guy used to study together, cook together . . . She's pissed. Ah, well . . ."

"Pissed about what?" I was indignant that anyone should treat him this way.

"I don't know exactly. It was during my bad times, before Gloria shipped me off to Australia . . ."

"And?"

"I don't remember everything I did. I see their faces and how they react to me and I know that it must have been something bad. I know she tried to help. Sat with me in the ER till the wee hours when I came in for bleeding ulcers. It was all that aspirin I used to take. She'd drive me home, bring me food. She lent me money . . . She cared. She was a friend, and I let her down is the bottom line."

○

He came into my office with me. While I tugged on my white coat, David deposited his backpack in the corner. I had told him to feel free to use my office when I was rounding, that it was unlocked. He hadn't thus far except to keep his backpack there. The lockers were in the student lounge where his classmates hung out. I sensed he wasn't comfortable there.

"Mind if I tag along?" he said. "Don't have to be in the nursery for a while yet."

"If you help me dig out a folder in radiology."

The file room clerks in radiology seemed to know him well. From behind the counter, I heard one of them tease him about his new tie and then look at me and giggle.

We walked the folder over to one of the radiologists, who sat in the glow of a view box. I put up the chest film of one of my patients with HIV infection. The chest X ray flaunted a new, rounded mass at the edge, a new whodunit to be solved. David stood deferentially in the background as I gave the radiologist a synopsis of the problem, and what I thought it might be.

The radiologist, seeing David, pointed out for his benefit the clue that the mass in the left side of the patient's chest was outside the pleural space, not intrapleural. "That's Felson's extrapleural sign," the radiologist said to David. Then, turning back to me, he said, "I can do him this afternoon, if you want to schedule it with CT?"

We went to book CT time, so that we could pass a needle into the mass under the guidance of the CT scan.

"He has a nice pleural rub. Have you ever heard one before?"

David shook his head. "Well, then, come and listen. It's a precious physical finding."

Before we returned the film, David said, "I wasn't entirely clear on that extrapleural business back there . . ."

I put the film on another viewer and went over it with him.

"Got it," David said.

"By the way, how can you tell whether this is a man or a woman?" I asked David.

"Breast shadows?"

"I can take you to two bars in El Paso where, if you use breast shadows to determine gender, you'll go home with a boy."

"Don't know, then."

"See here, see where the cartilage at the end of the rib is calcified? See how it forms a cup-shaped depression? In a woman it would be the opposite, a prong, a phallic projection. Felson—the same Felson the radiologist was quoting—called it 'radiologic penile envy.'"

David looked disbelieving, so we scanned the other films on the view box until I found a chest X ray of a woman.

"See that?" He nodded. "I have Felson's book on chest X rays. It's a slim volume. I'll lend it to you. You can read it in a night."

"Yeah, right!"

We returned the X ray to the file room ladies. It was my turn to stand back while David talked to them. As we were ready to leave, one of them called out to me, "Bye, Dr. Verghese," and gave me a smile that was more in the eyes than the lips.

"That's the one who said you look like Julio Iglesias."

"Oh God."

"And I told her you said she looked like Gloria Estefan."

"Get out of here!"

Just then his beeper went off. When he looked down and saw the number displayed, the expression on his face, till then amused and roguish, changed to disgust.

"I was looking forward to seeing the patient, but I can't." I was puzzled. "Got to go to pathology for a urine drug screen. When they call, I have to drop what I'm doing and be there in fifteen minutes." He glanced down the hallway. "Got to drink some water. I'm bone-dry." And then he added, "I shouldn't complain. The pathologist who supervises the test is a real decent guy. Somehow we manage to chat about everything from cricket to politics, and all the while he's watching the urine go from my dick to the cup . . ."

○

That evening, the boys and I bought a television and a VCR. Ostensibly I was buying this for their sakes. But, in truth, my desire not to miss the summer tennis bonanza—the French Open, Wimbledon, and the U.S. Open—had inspired the purchase.

At the apartment, the boys chanted, "*Blues Brothers*! *Blues Brothers!*" I had introduced them to the movie and it was one of their favorites, perhaps because it had as many songs in it as a Hindi movie from Bollywood. With each number, whether it was Aretha asking for some R.E.S.P.E.C.T., or Belushi and Aykroyd doing "Stand by Your Man," we got up off the floor to dance. Pizza from Domino's was on its way.

The phone rang and I could barely hear David's voice above the music.

"Didn't realize you were busy . . ."

It was a night that he should have been at an AA meeting on the west side.

"I'm watching *The Blues Brothers* with the boys. Are you at your meeting?"

"I got busy in the neonatal ICU. That's why I missed the biopsy. Missed the meeting. I just got home."

"Something wrong?"

"Naw . . . I'm kind of at loose ends, that's why I called."

"Come over? Pizza's on its way." I knew David's evening meal was often plain spaghetti, which he ate straight out of the pot. No sauce, no cheese.

"Umm . . . No. It's too late. Sorry to bother you. Get back to Steven and Jacob. Tell them I said hi. We'll talk tomorrow."

○

Late that night, after the boys were asleep, I went through the rest of my collection of videotapes. I turned the screen to face the corner where I sat, away from the sleeping bags so the flickering image would not disturb them.

I put on the 1981 Borg-McEnroe Wimbledon final where McEnroe finally prevailed, effectively sending Borg into retirement. I hadn't seen this tape in years, and already it looked dated, as if the tape had been slowed. I was used to seeing a different game on television: nineties players were bigger, taller, more powerful, and brought serving speeds up to 120 miles per hour.

I switched to a tape a friend in Tennessee had sent me, but which I had not as yet watched. It was Borg's comeback attempt in 1991 in Monte Carlo, after a layoff of almost ten years. The thought of his return to tennis had excited me—his off-court life after retiring had been a disaster: leaving Marianna for Jannike Björling with whom he had a son; leaving her for Loredana Berte, a faded Italian singer best known for "Non Sono una Signora" (and indeed there was nothing ladylike about her); the stomach-pumping overdose/suicide episode in Milan; the terrible business deals.

For his comeback Borg insisted on playing with his old Donnay wood racket. Though Borg looked fit and moved well, his shots had no sting to them, and his game, which was so perfectly matched against McEnroe a decade before, looked pedestrian against his journeyman opponent, Jordi Arrese.

It was sad to see the man I had so admired, the man who had been the best tennis player in the world, look so . . . ordinary. It was pitiful to see him get pushed around by a lesser player. An idol from the past, now revealed to be hollow.

I would have loved to watch this tape with David. It would have interested him for the same reasons it did me. I wished that he had come over.

I was as familiar with the rhythm of David's life as I was my own. I had the pulse of our friendship, and this call on a Friday evening felt like an irregular beat.

I lost interest in the match after a few games, probably because I knew that Borg had lost, 6–2, 6–3. I stopped the tape and crawled in with the boys.

○

It rained all Saturday morning, a steady drizzle with occasional thunder that made the telephone line crackle. I dropped the kids back at their mother's, early. They were going to a birthday party.

When I returned to the apartment, I stood at the door, looking in.

The sleeping bags were in the middle of the carpet. An empty pizza carton sat on the counter; the last two slices constituted the kids' breakfast. And in the corner on top of the new TV were five empty Beck's beer bottles. I had almost killed a six-pack. There was the sound of water pouring out of a drainpipe next to my balcony and hitting the ground below. The sky outside was the same color as the gray carpet. Without the boys, the place seemed forlorn.

I called David but his line was busy.

I called my cousin in India. She and her husband had just broken up; he had turned out to be an alcoholic. He had left, and she was cleaning up the house, preparing to sell it. She said she had found bottles hidden all over the house: in the flush tank above the toilet, in a flowerpot on the veranda. When she was emptying the bedroom, she found on a storage shelf just below the ceiling "ten dozen empty quarter bottles of rum." Her husband (someone I was once very close to and fond of) would come home from work with the bottle concealed in his briefcase or on his person. He had the energy and imagination to sneak the bottle in, but once he had drunk it, he was incapable of the effort required to take it out. "He stood on a chair, put the empty up on that ledge, pushed it out of sight with a stick that he kept up there. Just imagine!" She said she had to haul away carton after carton of empty bottles.

○

This story depressed me even further. And the talk of empties prompted me to pick up my own, and to fold the sleeping bags, clean the apartment.

I was tempted to go for a drive, but where would I go in the rain? Other than David, there was no one in El Paso whom I met with socially. I had imposed this isolation on myself, feeling shame in my domestic situation. I had told no one about my separation.

I dialed David's number again. Perhaps I'd suggest a movie or that we go out and eat. The phone was busy for a long while, and I was getting annoyed.

"It's about time you got off the phone," I said when I got through. "How are you?"

"Fair . . . I was talking to Gloria. My telephone bill is unbelievable. It's the biggest item on my monthly budget."

"*Amor de lejos, amor de pendejos,*" I said. Love from afar, love for idiots.

His laugh was pained. "Yeah, I am a *pendejo*, sitting here and try-ing to keep the flame burning in New Jersey." But he shied away from revealing more. "I got back late yesterday evening. It took me forever to finish up at the newborn nursery," he said. "The car wouldn't start. I didn't try to fool with it. Waited for the bus, and it was ages before I got home."

"Maybe the rain shorted something in the ignition?" I offered. If the Isuzu did nothing else, it provided a safe topic for conversation. If I were to rib him about the car, I was sure he would come up with a spirited defense. But I sensed that this wasn't a day to pick on the Isuzu. The man was down.

"Were you okay last night? The boys and I were dancing away . . . And I got a VCR. I was watching old tennis tapes. You'd have enjoyed it."

"If my car had been running, I might have come over. I was pretty down." Then he said, "For a fraction of a second, the thought of using again crossed my mind. They say don't even debate it, don't let it stay in your head—call someone right away. That's why I called."

"Jeez, you should have said something!"

"The thought . . . that's scary enough. And to call you, to call my sponsor, to say a prayer grounds me, helps remind me of where I am . . . you know? And then I wrote in my journal for an hour or so. Felt strong again."

Interesting. He kept a journal too. I wondered if it was like mine, a tennis journal. And how long had he had this habit?

"What are your plans?"

"I'll probably go read in the library. Finish some notes in the nurs-ery. It was hectic there yesterday. If a preemie sneezes or any of its functions change—which happens to at least two or three of them every day—you draw blood, get a chest X ray, and start treatment for sepsis. You don't ask why, you just do it. That much I have learned."

"I know what you mean. Parents see them as very unique, but at that age, they all look the same." A contrast to my work with HIV, where there were so many different *stories* one heard.

"It is. It's formulaic. But, I'm getting the hang of it. It's taxing physically on the one hand, but when you learn to be efficient, it feels good. I think I'm doing okay compared to the intern who gets reamed every day by the attending. His problem is he's trying to *think* when he should just do."

I offered to help him start the car.

"Thanks. Don't want to even think about the bloody thing today. I want to go to a meeting. Mickie is going to take me later."

"Mickie?"

"My landlady."

o

The next day was gorgeous, sunny and bright. Saturday seemed like a hallucination. The Sunday *New York Times*, fat and turgid in its plastic sheath, was propped up against the front door. An enterprising young man had started a delivery service. It didn't matter that it was costing me a small fortune. I had learned my lesson driving around on Sundays looking for the *Times*. Only a few select groceries ever had it. Everyone, including the young man who delivered it, depended on one distributor who flew the paper in from Dallas or Houston. If it didn't come by eleven o'clock, it wasn't coming at all—as if El Paso were an island in the South Pacific served by a fickle air service.

Since David's car was out of commission, I didn't think our regular tennis game was on. I sat on the porch with a cup of coffee and read the paper, every bit of it, including the classifieds. This, I said to myself, is normal, healthy: A man sits in his apartment on a Sunday reading the *Times*. The birds are singing, the neighbor is vacuuming . . . but when David telephoned at ten and said, "I got the car working. You want to play at the usual time?" I took off as if I had been offered a parole.

o

The bright green leaves of the ocotillos in the front yards of houses I passed now displayed flamelike clusters of flowers, evidence of the rain. Mesa Street was vibrant, alive, the parking lot of the Village Inn crowded with people in their Sunday best.

When I met David on the courts, my mood was the opposite of what it had been the previous day.

"Blue sky, no cloud in sight, the air still, the tennis courts beckoning . . ."

David's face, his T-shirt, and even his socks drooped. He had been on the phone all morning with Gloria. He had even missed church. It may have been paradise outdoors, but he was still in the dog-house.

"What did she say when you told her you had thought of using?"

"I hate to rock the boat." He shook his head, as if the boat was already in danger of tipping over. "Didn't tell her. She's holding on by a fragile thread because of everything we've been through . . . I want her to be confident, to believe that it will all work out. But, you know, she makes it tough."

From the start, David's shots were mechanical. Instead of dictat-ing the pace, he was content to be my foil, to let me be aggressive and inventive. Without his even being aware of it, the force of my shots pushed him farther and farther back, and as I hit inside-out forehands deeper into his backhand corner, his slice returns were falling shorter. And yet he wasn't playing tennis reluctantly or to accommodate me. I sensed that he reached for the tennis the way I did, looked forward to our twice-a-week dates. This kind of tennis was healing, the rhythm of our to-and-fro drill perhaps as salutary as the church service he had missed. Still, if I could have tied musi-cal notes to his strokes, the tune that emerged would have been a lament.

And suddenly, while we were at the net, picking up balls, his mood changed. He began to cackle. His eyes, which had seemed gray a little earlier, were now clear blue, and his tongue sat on his lower teeth, thick and lewd, peering out through his grin. "To get so crazy because of one woman—it's pathetic, isn't it?"

Sure, I'd go along with that if it improved his mood.

"I need to put her into perspective. Maybe I should start seeing someone else, huh?"

"There's always the rodeo . . ."

He spat on his palm and worked it into the handle. "Women! I tell you . . . ," he said.

I chuckled in agreement and he strutted back to the baseline, looking eager, bouncing on his feet. Now it was my turn to be pushed back from the baseline, to be rushed, to stab at balls and try to block them back.

The barometer of his moods, I realized, depended on Gloria and how their most recent conversation had gone. While playing tennis, he had been carrying on an internal dialogue with her. He was trying on different skins, trying to clothe his soul to allow him to either be with her, or be rid of her. To my embarrassment, I realized that my facial expression and tone of voice had changed to match his: When he'd spouted commitment, marriage, family values, it had made me pensive. When he'd lumped her in the general category of "Women!", I'd slipped into a preadolescent frame of mind, the common bond of young boys—the dislike of girls.

The last ten minutes of our tennis was pure magic, a free-flowing battle, hard and ferocious, like the first round of the Hagler-Hearns fight, swinging each other from side to side, painting the lines, hitting on the rise. I found out that when I could generate tremendous pace and depth, we were, at least for a short exchange, almost equals.

"Steven and Jacob say they 'hate' girls—one thing they both agree on," I said as we packed up to leave. "They will never kiss a girl, they claim. When I told them kissing was the easy part, they thought I was making fun of them. They got so mad they were choking on their pizza. I pointed out that their mother was a girl. Steven said, 'She's not a girl. She's a mommy. That's different.'"

David laughed at this. "Maybe they're smart enough to know that women can torture them," he said. "How come we lose this wisdom when we grow older?"

"Beats me."

I asked David if he wanted to see a movie in the evening.

"No thanks, I . . . I guess I'll try to raise Gloria on the phone." As he pronounced her name, a dour expression came back to his face.

○

I sang along with Ian Anderson on the radio, belting out the lyrics, drumming on the steering wheel, bopping in my seat as the traffic flowed up Mesa Street. Speed up, slow down for the lights, speed up, peer into the cars moving in formation with me, study the occupants . . . Perhaps because of the music, vintage Jethro Tull, I felt as I had as a teen when, after years of pining, then begging, I got to drive, taking sensual pleasure in motion, in mastery of a stick shift, completely conscious of the asphalt unfurling before me, and the signals it sent back through the steering wheel.

The day stretched ahead of me, full of possibilities. I'd pick up the kids, perhaps go to the park, then the video arcade, eat out, take a drive. In the evening I'd curl up again with Gabriel García Márquez and the enchanted world that spun out of the pages of *Love in the Time of Cholera.*

Only imaginary women populated my world.

Well that's all right by me.

23

David knew of a wonderful bicycle ride that he said we must *take. We* would follow Route 28, pass through La Union, Chamberino, La Mesa, and eventually reach La Mesilla in New Mexico, a quaint but touristy town, a miniature Santa Fe, a stop on the Camino Real.

There was a bike at Mickie's place he could borrow, and if I could find one we'd be all set. He and Gloria had taken this trail, and along the way they had seen a beautiful house—his dream house—which he wanted to show me.

I'd promised David we'd go, but I kept putting it off. Why revisit a trail he'd explored with Gloria? Why not blaze a new trail that would be our very own? Besides, cycling seemed so much more cumbersome than when I was a kid on my Hercules: the oafish helmet, the shades, the cleated shoes, and the spandex—I couldn't see it. Sixty miles on those narrow saddles? What if I got blisters? What if we had a flat? What if . . .

It was silly to fret so, but I couldn't stop thinking about it. I was both excited and fearful about this bike ride, as if it were some kind of test.

On an impulse, I visited a bicycle showroom. The salesman had not an ounce of body fat on him, his calves were bigger than my thighs, and he greeted me as if I were a true aficionado, a believer—he knew no one who wasn't. Dangling from the ceiling and laid out in shiny rows were racing bikes, mountain bikes, trail bikes, downhill bikes, tandem bikes, touring bikes, BMX machines, tricycles, but nothing so simple as a bicycle. My Luddite streak was aroused. Would that I could wave a wand and bring back a simple pedal bike, bring back wooden rackets, bring back doctors who didn't need batteries of blood tests to diagnose conditions that were staring them in the face, bring back . . .

I came out of the shop with a mountain bike—because I liked the straight handlebars—but I had the salesman replace the knobby tires with narrow street tires, and a saddle from one of the geriatric tricycles. I lied and said I already had the helmet and the rest of the necessary paraphernalia and a wardrobe full of spandex. By this time the salesman was dubious.

I mentioned none of these anxieties to David. I did tell him that I now had a bike.

○

The morning of our ride, David came over early and we watched the French Open semifinals between Courier and Agassi. I had asked him to stop by a west-side deli and pick up two baguettes, Brie, croissants, ham, and juice. I had coffee ready.

We padded around the apartment barefoot, grabbing the edibles during the changeovers. I noticed that David's feet were high and arched—no wonder he frequently complained of foot pain—and there were hard calluses on his toes from a lifetime of tennis.

We lay on the carpet, pillows against the wall, transported to Stade Roland Garros and the red clay. Agassi had, at the prematch press conference, made a remark about Courier: "I don't think he has a lot of natural ability to fall back on."

"The nerve!" David said. "He should shut it and play tennis."

We yelled instructions to Courier, cheered when Agassi made a mistake, used body English to try to influence a ball that was an ocean away. After watching a point where Jim Courier banged a serve, forced a short return, ran around his backhand, and hit a powerful forehand from no-man's-land into the corner for a winner, David said, "Boom. That's it right there. The modern game. Forget about the volley. The only time these guys go to net is to shake hands."

When Courier won 6–3, 6–2, 6–2, we stood and exchanged a stinging high five.

"There are many different talents besides hitting a tennis ball," Courier said after the match. "Having guts on the court is a talent; having desire is a talent; having the courage to go for a shot when you are love-forty down is a talent . . ."

○

The Upper Valley was on the western edge of El Paso. Here the Rio Grande bled into irrigation canals with names like Montoya Main and Three Saints and from which a lacework of smaller arteries shot south and north, branching into arterioles, capillaries budding off to cover every property in the Upper Valley, feeding pecan groves, fruit orchards, fields of cotton, or, simply, a front lawn. The ditches were dry during winter, dark scars running behind the house and grounds. But in late March they filled with water and formed a silvery hem that paralleled alley and fence. Following a published schedule, the *alcalde*—once a very powerful person in the life of a Spanish colony—unlocked the ditch box, after which property owners opened their sluice gates, and then opened successively smaller gates in their fields or lawns or orchards until they had their fill of water. In this part of town, a vacant lot did not sit covered by blow sand that neither weed nor creosote bush could hold. Instead, it disappeared in an overgrowth of cottonwood and trumpet vines and chinaberry and willow—a testament to how water could transform the desert.

We parked my car near Country Club Road and unloaded the bikes. We wore T-shirts, shorts, and sneakers—our tennis uniform. Off we went, turning onto Country Club Road where the giant cottonwoods on either side of the road formed a shady canopy and littered the ground with their seeds. The leaves had a mirrored texture that made them shimmer and give off a dry, ringing sound with the wind.

After a mile of experimenting with the gears, I found a setting that seemed close to what my old Hercules had been like. I didn't touch the levers again.

Looking back over my shoulder in the direction of my apartment, I saw a different view of the Franklins. The mountains were farther away than I was used to seeing them, and grander because my eye could take in the entire ridge, see the deep grooves, as if made with the tines of a giant fork, on its side. The land this close to the river (which, in the Upper Valley, no one called "the river," but instead, "the levy" or "the canal") was flat and a thousand feet closer to sea level than where I lived. I found this extraordinary: that in the same city your house could be in the desert with roadrunners and rattlesnakes as neighbors, or on a mountainous volcanic rock perch with hawks and coyotes for company, or here in a verdant valley where even as the suck and splash of water reached your ears a mosquito found the juiciest part of your earlobe.

David turned off into a residential area and we rode parallel to a canal, on a raised dirt path from which we could see into the backyards of houses. I smelled what I thought was jasmine but turned out to be honeysuckle spilling over the back wall of a corner home that we were approaching.

"This is it," David said, stopping and leaning on the wall with a proprietorial air. Through the sycamores and through the branches of a weeping willow sat a grand old hacienda with pink adobe walls and a tiled roof. The trees and the walls afforded privacy, a shady enclosure, and the house too had gathered itself to face inward, all its rooms opening to a large central patio. The entrance presented to the outside was a tall archway hung with heavy wooden doors that led not into the house but into a courtyard paved with alternating saltillo and decorative tiles, almost an Islamic motif. Somewhere behind this courtyard was the front door. A rough-hewn bench sat in the courtyard, red clay pots with petunias, African daisies, and sweet alyssum all around it. Bougainvillea spilled off a trellis.

This was a house that had been reproduced in oil and watercolor paintings in the kitsch galleries of Santa Fe and La Mesilla, an image so commonplace, the postcard embodiment of the Southwest, that it had become a place-mat motif, a spoon-holder image, almost a caricature. David looked at me, to see if I was as awed by this as he was.

"It's gorgeous," I said, and it was, but it didn't do for me what it did for him.

"If I won the lottery . . ."

"You don't have to win the lottery. There's no reason you can't aspire to it."

He looked doubtful.

"You're going to be a doctor, not a stable hand. If you go into practice, you can afford this."

"I guess," he said, a bit deflated, as if he preferred the house when he thought it was unattainable. To suggest he might one day own it robbed it of some of its charm.

On the corner of the property was a stable and a horse run. Two horses watched us indifferently. The horses' origins were similar to the architecture of the house: brought by the Moors to Spain, and by Cortés to New Spain or Mexico, and finally by Oñate to New Mexico.

The long sigh, and I knew what was coming. "Been a while since I've come this way," David said. "Gloria showed me this route. We stumbled on to this house. To see her in this setting, against this fence, made me see her in a different light. You know what I mean? All this history and the river . . . till then she was a girl I met in the hospital."

Had their last interaction been pleasant? So far he was in a good mood.

We set off, back on Route 28. A pickup truck coming in the opposite direction passed dangerously close, the driver giving us a look that suggested he didn't think anything without a motor had rights to paved road. I swiveled my neck to give the man the finger. He saw me in his rearview mirror and reciprocated.

David hadn't even noticed.

"If you could have seen her then. She was a patient's aide, I was a third-year student, fresh from Lubbock. Those huge eyes . . . her hair . . . Every time I passed her, I'd say hi. Very much aware of each other, you know? Then me and an attending physician were at a bedside and she came to take the patient somewhere. I was flustered. My attending asked me what kind of diet we should order for the patient, and I said, 'Regular diet.' It was a trick question—the patient had a nasogastric tube in place, connected to wall suction. He was NPO." (Nothing by mouth.) "The attending thought this was hilarious and I could see Gloria trying not to laugh. I was mortified."

His laugh sputtered like a lawn-mower engine that had not yet caught, but his face colored at the memory. Listening to him, I no longer focused on my bicycle. I was gliding along effortlessly, feeling foolish for having worried so much about the trip.

"I began to think about her a lot, you know? That delicious and utterly painless way that you daydream about someone?"

"Oh yes . . ."

"Of course, I hoped she was daydreaming about me too. I asked for a date but she made an excuse."

"I don't blame her. She saw through your charms."

"It only made me more interested. If that was her plan, it worked."

We pedaled in sync, riding abreast of each other. This story of their meeting had the quality of a fable that was at the core of their relationship. It was all too familiar.

"You heard Rajani's version when you came over for dinner. What she didn't say was how much she resisted me. The same thing—a frostiness, refusing to take me seriously. We had met once. And when I ran into her two years later, I offered her a ride back to the YWCA where she lived. On the way she agreed to stop for an ice cream. Out of nowhere—probably 'cause I knew I wouldn't have another chance—I said to her that I thought she was fascinating, and that I wanted to pursue a serious relationship—"

"You actually used that word? 'Relationship'?"

"It clunked in my mouth even as it came out. She laughed so hard she almost choked on her ice cream."

David was sniggering. My turn to flush at this memory, to recall how she had looked around the ice cream parlor, as if it might reveal evidence that I had used this come-on before. Her eyes told me she saw me as frivolous and immature—not ready for marriage. Not the way I saw myself. Perhaps she had been right. Perhaps now she regretted not going with her first instinct. But, even as I thought that, I was sure neither of us could imagine a world without our boys.

"When I won her over," I said to David, "months after that meeting, it made me feel that I had in hand something of infinite value. Of more value perhaps than if we had simply agreed over ice cream to proceed further."

"So it was all her fault for playing hard to get?" David said, trying to keep a straight face.

We pedaled in silence for a long while after that. We rode through acres of pecan plantations, then cotton, riding through La Union, Chamberino, La Mesa.

"If Gloria had succumbed to my charms right away," David said, "would I have decided that she wasn't worthy of me? As if the only woman good enough for me is the one who can resist my charms?"

"Bingo," I said.

He let out a strangled sound, meant to be a laugh.

I had been talking about a relationship that had ended, dissecting out the seeds of its failure. But his was a relationship for which he still had great hopes.

"I do know," David said, "that when things start to go well is when I get restless, find myself sabotaging it. Not just with Gloria, but with others in the past."

If he brought about the phone fights with Gloria because of a transgression of his, was he motivated by the need to reenact her capture?

"When I relapsed about a year into it, she didn't walk away. She saw me in all my ugliness. I told her to leave me, that I was no good for her. But she wouldn't. Her loyalty during that period . . . it's something I can never dismiss. Do you see? There isn't a doubt in my mind that I love her."

But it wasn't me he needed to convince. More than ever I sensed his ambivalence. "Love" was such a poor word to describe the tempestuous, tortured, raging, ecstatic tsunami of emotions that threatened to undo him.

I understood now that *he* could never be the one to end it. For him to renounce her or to lose her was to renounce himself, his dream house, his dream. And if she renounced him, it would take away the last vestige of self-esteem, a self-esteem that I could see was not formed by his talents as a tennis player, or the fact that he was a doctor-to-be, but mainly by the fact that he had attained Gloria.

The woman in his life was like a mirror with the power of magnifying his figure to twice its size, or shrinking it to the size of an ant, and he kept morphing between the two forms.

24

I saw David late one afternoon when he came to my office to pick up his backpack. He told me that Gloria was coming into town the next day. "She'll be here for two weeks."

"Great!" I said, but what popped into my head was whether she would take away our Wednesday and Sunday routine.

He didn't call for a week. I thought that he was probably staying over at Gloria's parents' house, and so I didn't call him. The weekend came and went. By the middle of the following week, I still hadn't heard from him. I knew his schedule as precisely as my own—he was in obstetrics and gynecology: clinics in the morning, lectures at midday, operating room twice a week. Occasionally I spotted his backpack in my office, but it would be gone by five o'clock when I came back from rounds. I searched my desk to see if he had left me a note, but there wasn't one. The thought even crossed my mind of peeking into his backpack for clues to what he was up to. Gloria had simply swallowed him up, eliminated him from my life.

While I shaved on Friday morning, I had an imaginary conversation with David in which I chastised him for his fickleness. And then I had a conversation with myself asking why I was acting this way. I had come to rely on our tennis dates, they were the central ritual of my fractured existence—his too I assumed. Did he not feel the itch to meet, to play?

That evening I stopped by Rajani's house to pick up the kids. Every time I visited, I saw Rajani blossoming, as if in my absence the roots she had put out had finally broken through rock and found rich, loamy soil. She had dug up a large oval patch of lawn and planted rosebushes. The bushes were already thick with tight, colorful buds, standing tall and proud and ready to prick flesh. Her mother had an identical garden.

A beat-up pickup truck with Chihuahua plates was parked outside and two men were laying a sprinkler feed and putting brick edging around the rose bed.

The carpet had been torn off the bedroom floor and a wooden floor laid. She had invested in a sleigh bed, a rich, polished work of art. Did I want the platform bed? Otherwise she was going to throw it away. The wood paneling in the living room had been painted white. She was taking piano lessons and an upright piano sat in the corner. Her eyes had lost their murkiness and sparkled; there was a lightness in her step, a cheeriness.

How could I not think that my presence had inhibited this blooming? I was like a blight that had been eradicated. In my apartment, I woke to piles of books around me, more books with bookmarks in them in the bathroom, coffee cups on the tops of books, and clothes tossed on the floor, as if in that disorder I found the same satisfaction she seemed to find in order.

○

On Saturday morning, two weeks after Gloria's arrival, David called.

"Abraham!" he said, his pitch rising on the last syllable.

"David!" I said, forgiving him at once.

Yes, Gloria was still in town. Yes, it was going well. She was leaving on Sunday. Did I want to play tennis that morning? Gloria had other plans and he was free.

I agreed readily. When I hung up, I felt ashamed for being so cross with him. And yet, if Gloria didn't have other plans, would he have called me? Still, I needed to play.

We met at the courts at nine-thirty in the morning. Gloria was to pick him up at ten-thirty. He wore a watch, hers I presumed, and he glanced at it frequently.

I was bouncing on my feet, anxious to test the engine and see if it still worked after the layoff. So sweet to hear the ball come off his racket, to meet it squarely in the center of mine, to find in just a few strokes a comfortable depth. Yes, my shots were still there, even sharper than before. And David played with his usual grace. But a rhythm, a mantra to build on, eluded us. I blamed Gloria for that—

the strange sight of a watch on David's wrist was the mark of her presence.

We played a few service points. For the first time since we'd met, I could read his serve. From the placement of his ball toss, I could anticipate that can opener that would swing me out wide. I hit two of them back for winners. This didn't escape him, and he made an adjustment. The American twist serve, the slice, the flat cannonball, the in-swinger into-the-body now came from almost the same ball toss.

We stopped not because we were bushed, but because the watch spoke. I went out with him to the parking lot.

To my surprise, Gloria was already there, seated in her car, the engine turned off. She was writing something on a piece of paper on her lap. Her long hair fell forward, hiding her face. When she looked up, I felt a quickening within me: It wasn't just that she was beautiful, it was the reserve and strength in her gaze that startled me. I had a sudden insane fantasy of whisking her away.

She stepped out of the car on seeing me and we were reintroduced. I was reminded of something I completely forgot in David's presence: that others saw me as David's boss, his mentor, a senior doctor who had befriended his medical student. If he and I thought of ourselves as equals, Gloria saw it quite differently.

"I was getting ready to leave you a note that I'd meet you at my mother's," she said to David. How she expected him to make it there was unclear, as she had dropped him off in her car. David glanced at the watch, made as if to say something but didn't. He looked at me apologetically. I knew I should excuse myself but I didn't want to.

"How are your studies going in New Jersey?"

"Very well, thank you," she said. "Hope to be done by the end of the year."

She stood there, her arms clasped behind her back, rocking on her heels, pleasant and polite.

"Well, it was nice to see you again," I said and shook her hand once more, tapped David on the shoulder, and walked off, feeling as if their eyes were on me.

From my car, I watched them pull away, Gloria driving. Her features had hardened, the smile she had for me was gone. She gripped the wheel with both hands. David's body was turned toward her, and he sat rigid in the passenger seat, one hand braced on the dashboard, his eyes on her face. She looked straight ahead, her lips moving rapidly, jerking her head forward once as if to emphasize a word.

In that image, that last head movement, having no idea what she said, I knew that all these months she had been measuring him, that she was unsure about whether she wanted to continue with him. And he didn't know this as yet.

○

I wasn't ready to leave the club. I called the boys and asked them if they wanted to play. So far they had shown little interest in the game, but I could hear Rajani in the background encouraging them to say yes.

I stood them on the service line with their junior rackets and had them imitate me as we hit a forehand. "Stand sideways, point with your left hand, keep the racket back, and after the ball bounces, step, and swing at the ball."

Then, I stood by the net, and bounced balls just in front of them. By the second hamper of balls they were timing their step and swing, making decent contact with the ball. I could see the thrill in their faces when every so often they struck the ball in the racket's sweet spot and saw it spring off the face, charged with energy. I gave them a good target: me. They tried to nail me, and in the process their shots were clearing the net.

We stopped with just that forehand lesson, before their interest flagged.

○

On Monday, the day after Gloria left, I gave David a ride home from the hospital. The Isuzu was in the shop.

"Oh, it was great!" he said about Gloria's visit, but his face didn't quite match the voice. "On Saturday, we walked on Rim Road. You know, near the tennis club? And we saw this house for sale. A cute little house, like a doll's house. It was an open house and the realtor was right there. She went over how we might buy it, using her calculator to figure out payments and so on. You have to see it. Old, adobe, exposed beams, cozy, just perfect . . . a city version of that house in the Upper Valley. Much smaller, of course. Seeing the house and then sitting down with pencil and paper and thinking how we might buy it was . . . exciting. I mean . . . it showed me that we were serious."

"And?"

"We'll have to see. On my intern's salary and what she'd make when she starts working . . . we might just do it."

I saw Gloria walking through the house, David chattering behind her. I could see her eyeing the rooms, imagining how she would refurnish them, seeing herself lying on a bed, or sitting on the sofa, but unable to see David with her in that picture.

○

We arrived on the street where David lived, the house where he rented a room from Mickie. David had met his landlady at an AA meeting when he'd come to El Paso after his year-long hiatus. He had heard she took in boarders, people in recovery. She welcomed him to her house.

He had not encouraged me to visit before, opting instead to come to my place or Dolce Vita. Perhaps because of the stereo having been stolen from David's car, I had formed a vision of a seedy neighborhood, a ramshackle dwelling on a street crowded with cars, *cholos* hanging out on the streets. Instead, what I found was a pleasant side street of neat, modest, one-story brick houses. The front yards were well tended; some of them were fenced in. The windows were barred on most of the houses, and the mulberry trees and the maples suggested a neighborhood that was twenty or more years old. We pulled into the driveway behind a small sedan with a metal harness on the trunk to which was strapped a motorized wheelchair. I remarked to David that it was not what I had pictured.

"It's a different place at night, believe me," he said. "The coyotes rule."

We entered through the front door, into a hallway. A lady was coming toward us from the living room, pushing a walker ahead of her.

"This is Mickie," David said.

Mickie was a short, chunky woman. David bent over to kiss her on the cheek. The moon face and acne were telltale clues to the fact that she was on cortisone and had been on it for a long time. Mickie clutched my hand in both hers and held on, smiling broadly.

"I'm dee-lighted to meet the man David calls his 'mate.' I thought maybe he made you up. An imaginary friend. David has no other friends." Her voice was so high-pitched it scraped the ceiling.

David looked embarrassed. "Except you," he said.

"Of course me. Did you park behind my car, honey? I have to go to a meeting in the northeast in an hour . . ."

I told her I had brought him and that I wasn't staying long.

"Stay as long as you like. Come on in, mate," she said, putting one hand on my arm possessively. "Oh, before I forget, David, you had a call from Gloria," Mickie said. "She says it's urgent you call back."

David went off to make the call and I followed behind Mickie's walker. We went into a dark, paneled living room, cluttered with piles of magazines, tables big and small, all stacked with papers. There was a path between these obstacles just wide enough for her walker. I guessed Mickie was in her late fifties, but the years of hard living had taken their toll. Perhaps for this reason I felt she had no time for pleasantries or posturing, and couldn't give a shit what you thought of her or her house. She accepted you and, by God, you accepted her if you wanted to—she wasn't going to lose sleep over that.

"Don't know if David told you," she said as she groaned and eased herself down onto the sofa, "but I have angina, insulin-dependent diabetes, hypertension, collapse of my vertebrae from osteoporosis, bleeding gastric ulcers, and polymyalgia rheumatica, and . . . oh . . . aseptic necrosis of the hips."

She cackled after rattling off this list, as if she had arrived at the point where illness had transmuted itself into absurdity. A multitude of medications were lined up on the coffee table in front of her. There were framed needlepoints and macrame on the wall and an unfinished macrame on the sofa. She picked this up and began to work on it, talking to me as if we were picking up a conversation we had started a while back:

"Oh, yes, we do spend a lot of time here. Just David and me. Yeah, he keeps me company—sits right there where you're sitting. He loves to hear the story of all my illnesses, how they started, what the symptoms were, how they were diagnosed. What medications I take for them. He says he's learned more medicine from me than from any textbook! He sits there and looks up the things I tell him in the textbook you gave him, and he says, 'Classic, Mickie, bloody classic!'" She burst into bright laughter again.

I could faintly hear David's voice from behind the door during the lull in our conversation. He sounded as if he were pleading. Mickie leaned over and lowered her voice to say, "That girl is driving him nuts."

"Women!" I offered.

She wrinkled her nose. "No. It's *men*. There's not a woman worth all that. Trust me, I know."

We both were quiet now, eavesdropping. David seemed to be doing more listening than talking. Mickie shook her head. The genial expression on her face hardened.

"The other day when they hung up, he took the receiver and beat himself on the head with it." I must have looked incredulous, so she demonstrated with an imaginary telephone, as if to a deaf-mute. "Whacking himself! There was blood above his ear. I had to go over there and pull the phone away from him. I said, 'David, why are you doing this?' 'Because I'm *bad*, Mickie, Gloria says I'm bad.'"

She leaned back, as if she had unburdened herself, and it was now for me to pick up the load.

"Why?" I finally said. "Why does he think he's bad? The drugs?" I asked.

She shrugged her shoulders and her eyebrows almost disappeared over her scalp. "Could be." We were silent for a few moments, until we heard David's voice again, beseeching. "I think it's because he can't stay true to her. You know David. He's a helpless womanizer. And because of his guilt, he tells Gloria or she catches him in a lie."

Helpless womanizer? I had the illusion that I knew everything David was up to. There were a lot of women who were attracted to him, ready to give him a come-on, but I assumed that nothing came of this, that it was just banter, and that he was loyal to Gloria. It was an assumption that suited me, suited my sense of order. But now I could see the face of the ICU nurse who wanted to take him to the rodeo; I remembered the nurse on the sixth floor . . . and a woman in the lab . . . and one of the clinic secretaries. Every one of those encounters could be and perhaps had been sexual. Perhaps he rationalized his quick dalliances as different from and not endangering the sacred bond he had with Gloria.

Mickie went on. "It's part of the twelve steps, you know. Admitting your wrongs—it's step number five: 'We admitted to God, to ourselves and to another human being the exact nature of our wrongs.'" Here she stopped, the better to make an AA teaching point: "But, you see, I think she's not the human being that he's supposed to confess to. And I have to remind him that part of making amends—which is step nine—is to make direct amends 'except when to do so would injure others.'"

She smiled with the satisfaction of the pedagogue who had mastered her material.

We heard David's door open. He came out of the room, carrying the telephone, and our conversation ceased. He appeared excessively cheerful—it didn't ring true. He set the phone down on a little side table in the hallway. Before he could say anything, another door opened and two hands lifted the telephone and pulled it out of sight. It was so sudden that we laughed.

"My fellow boarder," David said to me, tossing his head in the direction of the hallway. "Mickie," he said, sitting down next to her, almost leaning on her, their faces inches from each other.

"Mickie, I'm broke. Can I wash your car? Run errands? Or mow the grass?"

"Don'na, mate," she said, imitating him perfectly.

"I'll do anything, Mickie," he said, his tone pleading.

"Anything?" she said, rolling her eyes.

"Almost anything."

"All right, David," she said, sighing, pinching his cheek, holding on to it and shaking his head like a little boy. "All right. Go ahead, mow the lawn."

25

One evening after a late admission, I gave Della Nabhan a ride home. We headed west on the freeway, and then she directed me up a steep road that seemed aimed at the very top of the Franklin Mountains. Abruptly, the road veered right and ended in front of a pillbox from which a security guard eyed me warily. Despite seeing Della in the car, he took down my license plate number, peered into the car, and then retreated into his dark booth. The barrier did not go up at once.

"Right after the second set of buildings . . . downhill here . . . past the pool . . . pull in here." The condos were brick with black, sloped roofs. They were each positioned on the edge of the property for great views. Some were large duplexes, while others were flats not unlike mine. "They used to call this Queen Hill," Della said. "In fact, I bought this condo from two of our former patients. They died before you came."

○

On the way back out, I spotted a clearing off to the right at the edge of the property, abutting the mountain. Had I been looking the other way I might never have seen it. A pool perhaps? But no, the pool was next to the clubhouse. On a hunch, I turned the car in that direction, following a circular road.

The condos formed a perfect ring around the property, but for this gap, in which sat a tennis court. Even before I got out of the car, I could see this was no ordinary court, but a court set in its own rock amphitheater. It extended almost to the very edge of a canyon. Across a narrow chasm, a concave rock face rose several hundred feet into the air, leaning back over the court, dark and foreboding, as if a caped shaman were holding back the mountain, keeping it from tumbling onto the court. The other side of the court opened to a sweeping view of the plains below, and a huge horizon. I had to sit down on the bench to take this in.

The sun had just set and its afterburn colored the giant canvas with splashes of red, yellow, orange, magenta, fuchsia before conceding to ink blue on which backdrop the stars appeared, as bright as a porch light turned on in the middle of a dark prairie.

Beneath that old canopy of stars, perhaps two thousand feet below me, El Paso and Juárez came alive to the night. The white, sober streetlights of El Paso gave way to the shimmering green lights of Juárez, a tropical and brazen green that seemed to throb and surge, that seemed to say, *Ni modo*—anything goes. As I gazed at those lights I could almost imagine the notes of a *corrida* and hear a haunting male countertenor voice, a sound so natural to both Mexican and bebop music, but so foreign to Anglo music. The lights ended abruptly to the south, where the ancient Chihuahuan desert began, the terra incognita that Oñate crossed so long ago.

26

The following Sunday, late in the afternoon, David met me at the bottom of the hill leading up to the condo. He locked the Isuzu and jumped into my car, because his yet-to-be-rebuilt transmission was suspect. At the gate, I blithely invoked Della's name. Again the scrutiny, that, minus the dogs, was reminiscent of crossing back from Juárez to El Paso. After a while, the barrier went up.

David shook his head, amused by all this.

"Trust me," I said. "It's something to see."

The gate to the court was unlocked. I heard David mutter under his breath as he stood in the center of the court and looked across the canyon. The sun was still up and the rock face looked even more imposing than when I had first seen it, pressing down on us, tempting a step back. And when he turned and looked the other way, his eyes had nowhere to stop: What seemed like the entire desert Southwest was laid out before him.

All he could say was, "Christ!"

"What'd I tell you!"

The court surface, when I dragged a toe over it, was as smooth as a blackboard. Not a crack or bubble or scuff mark. I bent down to peek at the service line: Not a single fiber from the nap of a tennis ball was visible.

David came to the same realization. "Bugger me dead. It was waiting for us."

I put away my old can of balls and popped two fresh ones. Tentatively, we took up our positions. No stretching, and for the first time ever in our playing partnership, no dink'em warm-up. David held up a ball, rotated it like a jeweler displaying a gem, and then, with a flourish, put it into play.

The sound of the ball being struck splintered the silence and then reverberated as if it were coming from the mountain. It echoed as if we were hitting not one ball, but three successive balls. We played for one hour, without saying a word, pausing only for me to find the switch box and turn on the lights when the sun sank beneath the horizon. The rhythm of our play seemed to find its natural meter here. From David's silence, I knew that in all his travels, he had never played in a setting as charged as this.

I understood now that *this* was why I had dragged David here. If our tennis partnership was special, different, sacred, like a marriage, we had finally found a setting to match.

○

A flip of the switch and the court was back in darkness. Way below us, a river of headlights flowed on I-10, and beyond that a smaller stream on the Border Highway. To our left, on what was called Crazy Cat Mountain, houses built on concrete stilts glowed like spaceships in the dark.

David had his feet on the bench and was hugging his knees to his chest. I felt I had been part of a ceremony and we were now savoring the afterglow. It was a while before either of us felt inclined to speak.

"When I was down there, using," he said softly, pointing with his chin in the direction of the freeway and the river, "I remember sitting along the canal and looking up this way. Looking at the houses on Crazy Cat and being envious. Regular people, having dinner, then reading before bed, sleeping under sheets—not driven to shoot up. And the junkie who was with me, a laborer from Juárez said, 'Those poor bastards'—*pobrecitos*—'who live up on the mountain. They have to carry their water all the way up there.'" David cackled at this thought. "The guy had no concept of running water!"

He was silent after that, but I could feel his mood darken with this memory.

"You know, I never look in the mirror when I shave? I do it by feel. In the shower. I can't stand to look at myself too closely. What I see in the mirror . . . makes me dislike myself."

I said nothing. This was David talking to David, David hearing himself. In the after-tennis quiet, when the body was worn, achy, but still, the mind lifted its veil, slipped through its everyday pretenses.

"Once, in the middle of a three- or four-day coke binge—at home, not on the street—I barricaded my door. I could see shadow people, kept hearing voices. I imagined that somehow somebody had sneaked in and was in the bathroom. I could hear his breathing in there. I worked up the courage to kick open the bathroom door—like in the movies—and stood to one side, out of the way of bullets. Then I charged in."

He stopped here, as if that was all he had to say. "It was you, right? Your reflection?" I finally said.

"No . . . it was a frightening, evil-looking . . . stranger. He had my face. But he had lost so much weight. He hadn't shaved, his eyes were red and sunken. He was a loathsome creature . . ."

He turned to me and in the dark I thought his face was contorted with shame. "I checked myself into detox that very day. It didn't last. I ran away and was back to using. But that's the image I still see when I am shaving . . ."

27

Most of David's classmates had left town, completing their senior electives in some other city, or else interviewing for internships. When you did see them, they had their noses buried in the "green book"—a book that listed all the internships in America—studying it with more diligence than any textbook. They were preoccupied with "the match."

Each senior student submitted a wish list of his or her choice of internships; hospitals made a similarly ranked list of the students they wanted as interns. And until match day, students worried whether fate would give them their first choice or their seventh choice, worried whether it was chutzpah to put down Harvard or Stanford when they suspected they were, at best, Baylor material.

I never saw the green book in David's hands, nor did I see him in the library, queuing up to use one of the manual typewriters to fill out application forms. Other students had come to me for letters of recommendation, but not David

"Why bother?" he said when I asked. We were sitting across from each other in my office. "The dean's letter is sure to have 'chemical dependency' or 'rehabilitation' in it. I can't picture too many internship directors reading past that to see what my grades are, or that I've been clean this long."

He was probably right. His application would go to the same stack as those from foreign medical graduates (FMGs). The better hospitals, or the more lucrative specialties (surgery, obstetrics, emergency medicine) at lesser hospitals would never need to dip into that pile.

"You can't practice without an internship."

"I'll take my chances with the scramble. Don't have a choice."

In the twenty-four-hour period after the match, hospitals that didn't fill their positions, and students who weren't picked, scrambled, like spurned lovers on the rebound, for a mate. Most FMGs found their positions during the scramble, typically at inner-city hospitals, and particularly in internal medicine, pediatrics, or family practice programs—less lucrative specialties not in demand by American medical graduates.

"It's a relief not to have to fool with the interview process," David said, but I knew it hurt him to see his peers sitting in the lounge like debutantes before a ball, comparing dance cards. It was perhaps why he had started to use my office as more than just a repository for his backpack. I'd find him there writing up his case histories, or reading the *Harrison's* I had given him, a book that, despite its heft, he carried everywhere. He occupied a tiny piece of real estate on my desk, and immediately gathered up his papers and offered to leave when I arrived, but I'd wave at him to stay seated. If someone came in to talk to me, David would discreetly slip away.

"I'd like to travel, get away for a while," David said, looking out of the window wistfully. "I thought of going up to see Gloria if she's not too busy . . . But money is terribly tight."

"How's she doing?"

"Oh great, great . . . She's taking a heavy load this summer. She'll probably be busy studying . . ."

"I've been thinking about this research project," I said, surprising myself at how readily I came up with an alternative that would keep him around. "I'd like to do a chart review on pneumonia—" I said, making up the project as I went along, "—a retrospective survey on severe pneumonias here in El Paso. We've had quite a few patients like Mr. Rocha—more than I remember in my other jobs."

The interest that showed on his face spurred me on. "Hard work, of course. But I have a little research money that I can pay you— you'd be helping me greatly."

"I'd love it! I had a job lined up at a psych center in Santa Teresa to do admission histories and physicals for one of the doctors. It's a couple of hours in the evenings and some weekends . . ."

"You can still do that. The hours for this project can be flexible."

"If you're sure that's okay . . . I'm desperate for money."

"You know you can ask me if it's that bad. Man can't live on spaghetti alone."

His self-conscious laugh told me this was no joke.

"I did a retrospective study with Jack Peacock two summers ago," he said, changing the subject. "We looked at the Thomason experience with cardiac contusion after car wrecks. Published it in the *Southern Medical Journal* . . ." He smiled shyly, proud of this. Not many students at Texas Tech had the gumption to take on a research project, much less see it through to completion. It made me feel that he would have been my first choice as a summer research assistant . . .

On the other hand, I'd thought up the project specifically for him. I didn't want him going to New Jersey, didn't think it would be healthy. But maybe even this was too noble a thought. I just wanted him around, I didn't want an interruption in our tennis ritual, and I didn't want to share him with Gloria.

o

The next morning when I got to work, David's car was already in the parking lot and I found him seated in my office, sipping on coffee, with another steaming cup awaiting me on my side of the desk. He had certain favorites in his wardrobe that he never tired of: khaki slacks, polyester black pants that were shiny in the seat, a short-sleeved blue shirt, a mauve shirt with epaulets. But this day he was wearing the paisley tie with his most formal shirt—a white long-sleeved one. He had even made an attempt to iron it, though the cloth was reluctant to let go of its wrinkles. A yellow legal pad sat in front of him. His face broke into a puckish grin. He was pleased to be in my office in a capacity other than that of visitor.

We went first to see the administrator, to fill out forms, so he could be paid. I took him next to the office my secretary shared with three others and explained to her what he would be doing for the next month or so. "No introductions needed," Sandy said.

Back in my office, I gave him a reading list and extracted a number of relevant papers from my files for him to review. I suggested he go to the library and do a literature search before we began.

"This is what I have in mind: We'll create a form that you will then use to review each patient's chart. We'll have to decide what to include on the form: demographics; the tests done to isolate a causative agent; the chest X ray findings; the progression and regression of the pneumonia; risk factors such as HIV, or steroid use . . .

Eventually, when we have a stack of forms, we'll begin analyzing the data, looking for trends."

David stood up, scooped up the papers, parked his pen behind his ear, ready to hit the library. "Was there anything else?" he asked. He stood in the doorway, looking at me inquiringly.

There were, I thought, so many different Davids: the retiring Aussie, the stylish tennis player, the downcast lover, the thoughtful friend, the mischievous Lothario, the recovering addict, the plodding medical student. But the David of that moment—attentive, cheerful, animated, a happy amalgam of all his personas—was the David I found the most engaging. If he could only keep that recipe, draw it up on demand, it would serve him well.

"No," I said. "That's all."

28

A week after David started on his research project with me, Dr. Lou Binder came through for David. He offered him a position as an intern at Texas Tech.

Lou, who was the associate dean of students, had seen David through his string of relapses. It was Lou who, after Gloria had shipped David off to Australia, gave him a mandate: Go through rehab at Timberlawn in Dallas, stay clean for a year, and Tech would take him back. Many other medical schools might not have been so patient. Now, two years later, Lou's faith in David seemed to have been justified: David had done superbly in his fourth year, and would soon graduate.

David accepted a position as one of four transitional interns. Unlike a "straight" internship in medicine, surgery, pediatrics, or obstetrics and gynecology, David would spend three months in each discipline. It would allow him a chance to add one more clean year to his record, this time as a doctor. A transitional year was a prerequisite for some specialties such as radiology, ophthalmology, and even emergency medicine.

David was ecstatic. His future was more certain now than that of his classmates who were still waiting for match day. He called me the night he found out to tell me the good news. When I saw him at work the next day, he was in my office, bent over a form, a pen clasped in his peculiar chopstick grip, his left index finger keeping his place in the chart. A good half of my table was now his. When I came back from rounds at lunchtime, he was not there, but forms sat neatly in a pile, on top of an accordion folder in which he had organized all the background papers pertaining to the study. He had left one form on my part of the desk with yellow Post-it notes on the pages where he had questions. In the late afternoon, when I returned to my office once more, he was hard at work, the pile of forms visibly larger. I was the one treading quietly, trying not to disturb him. But he pushed his chair back, closed the chart, and put his papers and the folder into his backpack, which was so full now that he ported his *Harrison's* in his hand.

"Can I ask a favor, Abraham? Can I come by the flat and make a phone call to Australia? To my parents? I'll pay you for the charges. They've disconnected the bloody phone at Mickie's place because my housemate hasn't paid his share of the bill." In all this time, he had never named his housemate, as if this was not a person worthy of that courtesy. I had never seen the man, only heard his gruff voice on the phone, and seen his hands emerge to grab the instrument on the one occasion when I had visited David.

I knew that David's father was a mathematician trained at Oxford and MIT, an academic who taught in a university. I remembered David telling me that he called his parents when he learned he had been accepted to medical school. His father's comment was, "So you decided not to pursue *real* science." David had been a graduate student in biochemistry at the time. That comment had made me think of his father as distant and remote, but still someone whose approval David wanted. When his parents had visited in David's third year of medical school, David told me, their failure to respond the way David thought they would to Gloria had triggered his relapse.

○

I let David into my apartment and I went out to the communal mailbox. When I returned, David had opened the fridge and helped himself to a Coke and a slice of pizza, leaving one slice for me. He was on the balcony, his shoes were off, and he massaged his instep. I made myself some tea and went out and sat with him.

After a while, David fished out a bulky address book from his backpack and went back inside. It occurred to me that I should leave the apartment and let him be alone. But he had already started dialing. The sliding door of the balcony was half open. I could see that he had taken the phone to my recliner. He sat on its edge, his free hand picking at a loose thread on his trousers. The ease and fluidity of movement that I associated with him on and off the court was gone. An adolescent awkwardness had replaced it.

The moment the phone was answered so many thousands of miles away, his body became still. "Hello, Mother," he said, his pitch rising on the word "mother," which made it seem as if he were asking a question.

A few how-are-yous and I'm-fines were traded, and then there was talk of the weather. No lightness. No laughter. Instead it sounded like a play-by-play from a Miss Manners book on overseas calls to pater and mater. David was now hunched over, a mask of politeness frozen on his face.

I heard him ask his mother if he could "speak to Father?" Not "Daddy," or "Dad." But "Father." When his father came on the line, the same preliminaries were exchanged and then David said, "Father, I hate to ask this and I know you may not have the money, but I've had some repairs on the car, and some more work I have to do on it. Do you think you could lend me a thousand six hundred dollars?" Evidently his father thought it was too much. There was a silence and then David said, "Well, could you lend me a thousand two, then?" which, after a while, it appeared Father agreed to wire to him. I sensed David had more to say, but the telephone call was over, wound down at the other end. If he said good-bye, I missed it. I had assumed he was calling to tell them the good news about his internship, his imminent graduation, but it never came up.

He put his finger on the switch-hook, then ever so gently replaced the receiver on the cradle, and sat back on the recliner, pulling his feet into him.

I felt terribly sorry to see him, still sitting there, clutching the phone to his chest, as if he were loath to let go of the physical connection with the instrument that had brought his parents' voices to him. In a fetal position, he looked so forlorn and forsaken. Surely, if his parents could have seen him, they would have swept him into their arms and comforted him, no matter that he was no longer a child but a doctor-to-be. He had left Australia right after school, an all-boys grammar school. And his problems since then perhaps made it impossible for his parents to see him as a child any longer, made them forget the boy-child who had left Australia to chase his tennis dream.

He was unaware of me. As I studied his face, what I saw on it was unadulterated shame. He had felt shame before he made the call, and more shame now that the call was over. His parents must have been deeply disappointed, shocked by their son's entering a world so foreign to them: cocaine, needles, detox, rehab. And nothing he had done in the last two years of rebuilding had diminished his shame.

Now David got up, returning the phone to my desk. "Ah, well," he said cheerily, coming out to the balcony and easing into his loafers. "That's that, then." He pulled a twenty-dollar bill out of his shirt pocket and showed it to me. I waved it off. He placed it under my teacup on the little table on the balcony.

"I have to go. I don't want the engine to get too cold. It might not start."

I made to give him back the twenty-dollar bill, to say something. But as I moved toward him, I could see that his eyes were glistening and that he shrank from my approach.

He was at the door now. To even shake hands would have upset his tenuous state.

I let him walk away.

29

On Sunday morning, I called David before he left for church.

"Do you mind if I bring the kids to the court? I've been trying to give them tennis lessons. They have about a twenty-minute attention span at the most, after which I'll send them to the pool and you and I can play."

David watched us for a while. I had the kids demonstrate their forehand form, make a few mock swings, and then we tried the real thing. David called out encouragement and they took lusty swings. Perhaps because they were self-conscious in his presence, they had a hard time hitting the ball, either stepping in too late or swinging too early.

"Let me teach you the backhand, now," David said to them. "The backhand is the more natural stroke," he said to me. "The motion of drawing the arm across the body is intuitive. It's why we tend to fling a Frisbee in a backhand motion."

This was a revelation to me. I thought of the forehand as the first stroke, certainly the key shot in my arsenal, as fundamental to my game as the Green Bay sweep with pulling guards was for Lombardi. But for David, that backhand slice of his was at the core of his game. It was an effective stroke, and the harder you attacked it, the earlier he took the ball, knifing it back almost before you finished your follow-through. It was the perfect counterpunch, low and penetrating, but David's backhand was at its heart a defensive shot.

Though neither of us hit a two-handed backhand, this is what we taught the boys, and in just ten minutes, they were making decent contact with the ball and, moreover, hitting with more control than they had shown on the forehand.

But their minds were elsewhere. I took them to the pool where they would stay under the watchful eye of a lifeguard and the parents who took turns keeping tabs on the kids.

○

When I came back from the pool, two men, one in his sixties with gray hair, and another, younger and athletic looking, were chatting with David.

"We've been challenged to some doubles," David said, introducing me around. As he and I walked over to our side, David said, under his breath, "The older man played at Wimbledon."

"Good god!"

"Yeah, but don't forget that that was some forty years ago."

It was the first time in a long while that I had played competitively. Our opponents were excellent doubles players, the older man crafty and consistent, the younger man quick and powerful. It was easy to tell they had played together before. I was nervous, made many unforced errors, lost my serve twice, and felt that I was letting David down. David was relaxed, enjoying himself, while with each game I felt the pressure on me rise. I wished David hadn't agreed to this. We had a tennis ritual that was well defined, the boundaries clear. Why did we have to try to change it? Doubles made me look inept, like a pretender.

They won the first set handily. As we changed sides, David said, "Go for your shots. I'll back you up. Trust me, just go for it."

Go for it I did. I took my time with my first serve, remembering to sway first forward and then back before leaning into the serve. I hit an ace. David, turned so that our opponents could not see his face, grinned and waggled his eyebrows. As we put together a few more points to hold serve, I realized that I had been playing as if the match depended on my game, not *our* game. I hadn't taken advantage of my partner's skills or created opportunities for him. Now, when David received serve, I stood at the net, confident of not being nailed, as I knew David would deliver the ball to the server's shoelaces. I teed off on the return of serve. I hit a forehand whenever I could run around the backhand.

My first serve seemed so much more effective than it really was because David was at the net, ready to put away any loose returns. Even if I had to spin a second serve in, David's net play put the percentages on our side. The second set was close and we lost in a tie break that could have gone either way.

When our opponents left, David said, "We did great! That's the thing about doubles. One plus one sometimes equals three. The closest I came to succeeding on the tour was in doubles. Had a big old South African partner, as strong as a mallee bull. He used to slam that ball."

"Like me?"

"Not as good as you."

○

We sat poolside, watching the boys.

The previous day, an invitation to be a guest of Dr. David Smith at his graduation from medical school had arrived at my apartment.

Dr. David Smith. Such vindication and pride for me to see those words centered on the page. I had never been as invested in a medical student as I was in David. Almost a year had passed since we'd first met. It had taken me a while to realize how fragile his hold on the doctor dream had been, how many times the needle had brought him close to losing it. To his father, he would never be a *real* scientist, but in my book, he had the potential to become something better, a caring and careful physician.

Unfortunately, the graduation ceremony in Lubbock fell on a date when I would be speaking at a meeting elsewhere. I couldn't cancel. I hesitated to tell David this.

"Got the invitation for your graduation yesterday," I said.

"Neat, huh?"

"I am so very, very proud of you." And then, to my surprise, I couldn't speak. We could talk candidly about so many things. But to bring the lens to bear so directly on the friendship made us self-conscious. And perhaps that was why I was tongue-tied.

"Abraham," David said, bailing me out when the silence had become quite uncomfortable, "all I can say is thank *you*."

I found a voice after some throat clearing. I told him about my dilemma with the date.

"I can't imagine anyone taking the trouble to fly to Lubbock," he said. "Don't give it a second thought."

I asked him if Gloria was going. Were his parents coming from Australia?

"No. But Mickie wants to go. Can't stop her. And I'm honored that you'd want to come. But really, Abraham, the ceremony itself isn't significant. It's . . . the journey that counts. I'm finally done."

His original classmates, the class he had started with, were long gone. Some of them, like the obstetrics resident who now shunned him, were finishing up their training. Others were already in practice. David would be capped and gowned with a medical school class who at one time was three years behind him; most of them were much younger than he. They were running around planning the graduation dinner, anticipating match day, snapping photos to use in roasting the faculty, getting nostalgic, and, interestingly, a little cocky, as if they already had the degree. There were parties to go to every night. Relatives to be received. A few private receptions at the Sheraton, the Hilton, the country club . . . For David, there would be none of this. For a moment, I toyed with the idea of throwing him a party at the apartment. But who would I invite? And where would they sit?

I did sense a burgeoning confidence, a diminution of the self-effacement that I remembered from when I'd first met him. He said that he and Gloria had been "at it" on the phone that morning, but even this didn't seem to affect him. (What did they find to argue about when they were so far away from each other?)

"When you look in a mirror, can you . . . are you happier with what you see now?"

He let out a sharp whoosh of air, and shook his head. "Maybe it's my curse. When I achieve something . . . I diminish it. As if I'm saying to myself, 'If *you* could do it, it can't have been that big a deal.'"

I made as if to cuff him on the back of his head, and he ducked.

"Honestly. I'm already thinking about a residency. Where do I go? What specialty do I want to go into?"

I had assumed that his carrying *Harrison's* around all the time, the way he had devoured Felson's radiology text, and all the hours of tagging along with me in the hospital meant he wanted to be in internal medicine, a vain assumption on my part.

He must have read my mind, because he said, "I don't mind internal medicine. But honestly, I find its loose-endedness unsettling. I mean, the patients in our pneumonia study . . . it's not clear what many of them had. And Mr. Rocha, for example. We don't know what he had—"

"Did you see him when he came to the clinic?"

"Yeah. I saw him."

"And how was he?"

"Fine."

"Fine?"

"Okay, he was great. Said it was all like a bad dream for him . . . doesn't remember much."

"Forget about him. Did it do something to you? To see him normal? Alive?"

Was David simply being difficult? Did he not see the triumph in the survival of a man whose lungs had been unable to oxygenate his blood, a man whose kidneys had failed, a man who just two or three decades before might have died? Mr. Rocha's being able to walk into David's clinic like Lazarus had done nothing for David.

"But I don't know if it was anything *I* did. Some other team wound up getting him off the respirator and sending him home. He's better, but we don't know what happened . . ."

I looked away in irritation. Wasn't that the very essence of medicine, to make people better, to help nature along? Scientific inquiry had its stimulus in patients like Mr. Rocha, who presented with something unknown.

"I think I like things black or white . . . ," David said, his tone wheedling, as if trying to coax me back. "The *in between* is killing me."

"Are you talking about you and Gloria, or about Mr. Rocha?"

His laugh was strangled. How accurately my arrow could strike when its tip was whetted with anger.

"It could be both," he said.

"Internal medicine is like that. Lots of chronic diseases that don't get better, or, patients like Mr. Rocha who defy labels."

I was trying to defend my specialty. Despite the frustrations, there were challenges, diagnostic puzzles that needed solving. I liked the fact that the field was vast, almost limitless. And if you specialized in a subspecialty of internal medicine (such as cardiology or infectious diseases), there was still the need to keep up with advances in the rest of the field. It made one a perpetual student, a posture that I respected more than the posture of absolute mastery. Obstetrics, for example, which I had enjoyed as a student, felt as if it were a field that one could master in a short time. There were a certain number of fixed paradigms and predictable responses: uterine contractions weaken?—start the pitocin drip; baby's heart rate drops, and labor doesn't progress?—cesarean section. Great skill and judgment were required. But my bias was that it lacked the intellectual challenge of internal medicine.

"Temperamentally, I think I'm more suited to, say, something like surgery or emergency medicine."

So *that* was where he was leaning.

"I'm able to make a clean disposition with the patient, you know? Trauma comes in. Cannulate the airway. Stick in a couple of chest tubes. Pop in a central line in the neck. Stabilize the patient and then ship them off to surgery. Or wherever."

The way he said this annoyed me, as if he had, after all, picked up the "five-tubes-and-you-are-dead" lingo. *The House of God* by Samuel Shem was written as a brilliant satire, but it was amazing how many students had taken it as a literal text, bought into the "gomer" (get-out-of-my-emergency-room) lingo.

As a student I had enjoyed working with my hands. I had found surgery particularly exciting, almost a sexual release. Many students went with those first feelings, the immediate sense of worthiness that came from *doing*. Among male students, it was predictable which ones would react that way, feel empowered by "shoving in a couple of chest tubes" and decide that the titillation *they* felt (never mind what the patient felt) meant they had received their calling.

"I suppose I'm looking for what's most comfortable for me, what suits my temperament—it sounds selfish."

I bit my tongue. Perhaps he was looking at himself more realistically than I was. Temperament had so much to do with our choices. I had moonlighted in ERs for years during training and I enjoyed (if one can use the word "enjoy" in such a terrible context) the adrenaline rush of dealing with trauma. But I missed the sense of continuity of care. I missed watching a disease unfold, witnessing the outcome, good or bad. To see Mr. Rocha for the one hour of his transit through the ER wouldn't have satisfied me. It would have been like seeing the beginning of a movie and leaving.

Temperament explained why the nicest, friendliest folks seemed to go into pediatrics. It explained why ER docs were adrenaline junkies who were into rock climbing and bungee jumping.

But what served the patient the best? The surgeons I admired the most at Tech—like Jack or Ed Saltzstein, the chief of surgery—were those who seemed to have transcended the knife-wielding bravado and become thoughtful, caring craftsmen who did see the big picture. But perhaps what got them in the field in the first place was the "stick in a couple of chest tubes" mentality that David was espousing. Who was I to pass judgment?

30

David began his internship on July first. His first rotation was in family practice, and he thought it would be relatively easy. Still, until he found out what his schedule would be, which nights he would be on call, our tennis was on hold.

He now had a locker along with the other house staff in the call room of the hospital. I looked for him when I got to work, but there was little reason for him to be in the Tech building and nothing of his remained in my office except for the pile of forms from our study. He had almost finished with the chart-review phase; what remained was to analyze the data.

I did see him on his first day as an intern, though not in the hospital. I had gone to the Sunland Park mall with the boys. We went first to a bookstore where the boys promptly sat crosslegged under the comics rack and read. We were on our way to the next stop, the video arcade, when I looked down and saw David on the lower level. I was so surprised to see him—it was an evening when he was usually at an NA meeting downtown—that I didn't at once notice the woman he was with.

David was nodding, listening intently, his eyes smiling, his mouth half open, anticipating the punch line. She was using both her hands, elbows angled away from her shoulders, slender fingers circling each other as if to indicate a shape. I could see them clearly, and if they so much as tilted their heads they would see me. I stepped behind a pillar. She was taller than he, all vertical lines, straight hair framing a slender nose, pipe-stem jeans that ended in pixie boots.

David put his head back and the decrescendo guffaw followed, but still he didn't see me. He had three shopping bags in one hand, buoyant in her wake, completely attentive to her yet not servile. A couple pushing a baby carriage and, with eyes only for the shop windows, collided with them, a bump that startled all four of them into an awareness of where they were. David, his hand at her elbow, smiled his apologies, looked down at the baby, and steered them clear.

"There's David," Steven said, looking down at them, and then at me, realizing at once that I was hiding.

"Who's that with him?" Jacob asked.

"Shhhh . . ." Steven said, pulling Jacob behind the pillar with us. "Probably his girlfriend," Steven said in disapproval.

○

I looked for David the next day. Midmorning, I was standing waiting for the elevator, my mind elsewhere, when he emerged. My eyes were drawn first to his shirt collar, a virginal white collar, not wrinkled, not flopping out onto the lapel of his white coat, instead sweeping down to frame a tie that was not in his usual repertoire of ties. I looked up at the face again, to make sure it was him.

"Don't say a word, Abraham."

Black slacks and shiny new shoes completed the outfit. Perhaps this was what I had seen in the shopping bags.

"Dr. Smith!" I said, fingering his silk tie, though there were interns and students with me.

"Dr. Verghese!" He was squirming and bashful, flushing at this attention. "Had to bring some new life to my wardrobe."

"Indeed, I'd say you succeeded." I used an expression he had once used to describe a Texas Tech secretary who had a penchant for dressing like a debutante, as if her goal in life was to top her previous day's ensemble with a more striking one, a process that would surely culminate in her sitting behind her typewriter in a tiara and evening gown. "You look done up like an organ grinder's monkey."

David, for once, didn't blush. My team was on the elevator now, holding the door for me. David backed away, as if to spare himself further assault. "Call you later, Dr. Verghese?" he said.

The transformation was startling. Just a few weeks before he had sat in my office in a dull, checked shirt, with those dreadful khaki pants, counting on his white coat for concealment when he stepped out. I had watched him hunched over the table, painfully balancing his checkbook, using my office calculator. There were three monthly checks that went to pay off his medical-student loans. And two other debts from the past he'd said. I'd watched as he had addressed the envelopes, copying from the bulky address book. He'd shown it to me, laughing as he said, "My life is so compressed that my first girlfriend, my two wives, and now Gloria are all in here!"

○

That evening David called and asked me if I wanted to play tennis late, under the lights, at our secret court. "I'm not far away. I'll pick you up outside," he said.

I was listening for the bronchitic rattle of David's car coming down the hill when a shiny car silently pulled up next to me. It was the Isuzu. A new muffler and a wax job made it, but for the slight yaw as it approached, almost unrecognizable. There was a regular driver's-side window in place of the cardboard.

"Well, well," I said as I slid in. The upholstery was spotless, the dash gleamed from Armor All, and the interior smelled of a pine forest. I nodded in appreciation at the new stereo deck playing "American Woman," David's favorite song. He pulled away smartly, marching through the gears, glancing at me to see if I noticed. "It goes like buggery when you put the foot down," he said. And indeed, it made it up the hill to the condo effortlessly.

He was coasting in the internship, he said, finding the workload of family practice easy, spending a lot of his time helping the other interns. "And," he said proudly, with a sidelong glance at me, "teaching the third-year students. I remember how much of the basics I was taught by interns. Attendings often take it for granted that you know. Takes an intern to really appreciate their level of ignorance."

The security guard at the condo waved us in. But on the gate to the court was a massive padlock.

"The German lady, I bet," David said. When we had played at the condo last, a woman had come by and asked whether it was necessary to use the lights when the sun was not as yet down. David had turned on his charm, explaining to her in the thickest Aussie accent he could manage that it eliminated shadows, made the transition from sunlight to floodlights smoother. She had resisted him completely, asked him which unit we lived in. We invoked Della's name, but the woman was dubious. She left us both feeling like schoolboys who were about to be reported.

We got back in his car and drove off to the club.

"My AA and NA meetings . . . are getting to be a pain, to be honest. How am I supposed to find time now? My sponsor thinks I have an attitude problem." He normally spoke of his sponsor with reverence. "He won't let me cut back on the meetings. And Tech, of course, requires me to do what he says, not enough I pee on demand for them twice a week . . .

"I went to jail today," he said, turning to grin at me. "To run a meeting. It's supposed to keep me humble. They look at me—a doctor. It's supposed to impress the shit out of them."

"Does it?"

He shrugged. "Naw. They're not shocked to think a doctor has been where they are. They have no trouble imagining that. You know, funny though. I think I can look at them and tell who will succeed and who won't. It's like I have a nose—"

"I saw you in the mall the other day," I interrupted. David's mouth fell open. As if I had chopped his legs off. "You looked like you were having fun. Wasn't Gloria, was it?"

He retracted his head between his shoulders, said, "Oops," and then laughed. "No. That was Emily. I've been meaning to tell you about her," he said, shaking his head, as if she were a weather pattern that had blown into his life, a phenomenon over which he had no control. Something that had just *happened*.

Emily was a regular at the AA meetings at the Arid Club on Douglas Street. "Her drug of choice was food!" he said as if it still amazed him. "She still *has* to consume her drug every day. She can never avoid it. It's not cut and dry like it is for the rest of us—use: relapse. Don't use: sobriety. She has to restrain herself from taking too much."

"Aren't there rules about your . . . dating someone within the program?"

He grimaced. "That's part of what my sponsor is annoyed about, can you believe it?" he said, as though I was sure to see the absurdity in this. "Anyway, when I'm doing well, my fridge has at least milk in it. When I was using, there was nothing in there but the ice trays. For Emily," he said, laughing, intrigued by the observation he was about to make, "a full fridge is an invitation to disaster!"

We pulled into the club parking lot.

"I'd like you to meet her sometime."

"What about Gloria?"

David didn't seem embarrassed by this question. "I don'na, mate. I honestly wasn't looking. There was some chemistry between us that I could feel for some time."

"Uh-oh. Chemistry."

"Seriously!"

At the club, David's game was playful, effortless, teasing me with angles and drop shots. I hit a vicious backspin drop shot. He ran from behind the baseline to dig it out just before it touched the ground a second time, in the process losing his balance, almost falling over, dropping his racket. I had come to the net too, and the ball sat up for me; I popped it right at his belly. He caught it with both hands. After a beat, he yelled, "Howz-at," and tossed the ball up and caught it again as if this were cricket. We doubled over laughing, leaning on the net cord.

"Chemistry, my ass," I said.

"It's not the way you think."

The way David explained it, a weekend AA jamboree had put Emily and David in the same small lunch group. David took the plunge and told her he was attracted—the chemistry—and that he could sense she felt the same way. He did tell her that at that point in his life he needed *not* to get into a relationship—his sponsor's instructions. (Which made me wonder why he approached her at all.) But chemistry compelled him to say what he said. Then, a few weeks later, David called her to see a movie and on the day they were supposed to go, he canceled because he felt guilty, knew it would be more trouble, and that he still had "issues" with the other "relationship."

I wanted to say something sarcastic about the AA-speak, the vocabulary that was meant to be revealing but instead cloaked real emotions from their owner. After having resented Gloria all this time, I felt a peculiar impulse to come to her defense.

"We decided not to date but we fell into the habit of going to the

Coronado park after the meetings, and sitting there and watching the sunset and talking. For hours. Not a date."

"Not a date?"

"No. Not a date."

These not-a-dates were on the same evenings when the boys and I had had pizza. How long had this been going on?

"I was candid," David said, his expression earnest, as if he had not only come clean with her, but with me. "Told her about the marriages, the coke, the relapses, the year in New Jersey with Gloria."

But what he wasn't candid about, what he didn't mention to Emily, what he had adroitly sidestepped with me and most of all with himself, was what *Gloria's* expectations were. He most definitely had not come clean with Gloria.

O

Just a few days later, I saw David eating lunch in the cafeteria with a woman who had to be Emily. At close quarters, I could see why David was attracted to her: Her blue eyes made you want to come clean.

I felt as if I were intruding, even though David waved me over, stood up, and pulled out a chair for me. In that movement of sitting down with them, once again I breathed my own isolation, felt the shallowness, the seclusion of my world, how it was populated only with my children and David. Even as I sat down and unloaded my tray, I resolved to not be so reliant on David, to widen my own circle.

The two of them were eating off one tray. "You get free food as an intern," David said. "Just wave your badge at the cashier. I think I've already put on a few pounds."

"No more spaghetti?"

He made a dismissive sweep with his hand, as if those days were behind him. "I come by here evenings before I leave. I eat dinner and then go through the line and fill a Styrofoam container to take home. For Mickie."

David had abandoned his half-eaten entrée and was working on the first of two yogurt bars. Emily picked at a salad. Neither Emily nor I seemed willing to open our mouths and say much in front of the other.

"Abraham," David said, "I've decided to try to get into an emergency medicine residency after the internship."

I was surprised at how acutely disappointed I was to hear him say that. I thought it was the wrong choice for him, given his past problems with cocaine. ER work was hectic, stressful, quick highs, lengthy lows—not unlike cocaine. It was a field with a significant burnout rate. But it was vain for me to want to shape him in my mold. Perhaps this was the moment when I needed to step back and let him grow.

"They liked my work when I rotated in the ER as a student. They have reservations, of course. They were burned by Julius." Julius, a former Tech star student, had begun the residency and was then forced to drop out because of drug use. "But I've been encouraged to apply . . . Would you mind writing a letter, Abraham?"

"No problem," I said, but my throat was dry and the words seemed to stick there.

David went off to answer a page, leaving Emily and me sitting together, both of us nervous. It had been a while since I had been around a good-looking woman and I was self-conscious, taking small bites of my food so as not to be caught with my mouth full. Emily was no more at ease than I was. Still, neither of us spoke, and then the awkwardness made us look at each other and laugh. Her mouth was wide, with strong teeth.

"David's been telling me about the research paper you guys are doing," Emily said, taking the plunge. "Sounds as if you are almost done."

I nodded. "It's all his work. He's got an aptitude for research."

"He's very grateful to you, you know. He looks up to you," she said. I was pleased to hear this, but surprised that our friendship had already been discussed. "Outside of the support groups, I think you're the only true friend he has."

David returned. "I've got to run up to the ward," he said, as if that were a distraction, his main business being in the cafeteria.

"I'll be fine," she said. Had I not been there they might have kissed.

"David's quite taken with you," I said softly, once he was gone.

She smiled most naturally, as if she knew this to be true and was happy about it. And then she blushed.

"My first time seeing him in this environment. So different from the AA meetings. Have you ever been to a meeting, Dr. Verghese? Oops! Not to imply you were addicted. Sorry—"

"I've never been. And please call me Abraham."

"What I was going to say is I wish you could see him at a meeting. People 'share' at these meetings. But David . . . Well, David is painfully honest. Taking big risks and putting it all on the table, sharing straight from the heart. Stuff we can all relate to even if we don't have the courage to say it . . ."

David had talked about being bored with meetings, while Emily was presenting him as the savior of the meetings. His "painful honesty" hadn't kept him from getting into this date-but-not-a-date situation, one that Gloria was bound to object to. For a man who liked things cut and dry, black or white, he was letting the boundaries get very blurry.

"But I kind of wanted to, I don't know, almost laugh at him. Like he was trying to make me laugh? His clothes, the car—the first time he tried to give me a ride in the car it broke down." She giggled, a sound so pleasant that I wanted to hear it again. "And living at Mickie's . . . It made me feel sorry for him, you know what I mean?"

I did indeed.

○

David was no longer alone. When we met on Sunday, even though Della had given me a key to play at the condo court, David opted for the club. That way Emily could go for her walk up Rim Road and Scenic Drive and when she returned she could wait for us in the shade, in the clubhouse. At one point we saw her silhouetted against the sky, a loping yet rapidly moving figure whose arms were held high and pumping.

"I'd rather play tennis," David said, "than go with her on those killer walks. Did it once and I was sore in places I didn't know I had muscles."

When we went for coffee to Dolce Vita, Emily was with us. I had been prepared to resent her, for the jealousy I had felt the moment I first saw her to build. But to my surprise, as I sat across from her at a table, not on the bar stools, I found myself enjoying her company, delighting in her laugh. I kept waiting for her to give me a reason to be annoyed with her, but it didn't come.

With her around, David was cast in a new light. His speech and the topics we strayed to in Dolce Vita were necessarily different now that she was present. He kept coming back to AA and NA, to recovery. His emotional barometer, which, even during the course of one hour could be unstable and tend toward pessimism, fluctuated less around her. He was more upbeat.

"The best part about recovery," Emily said, "is not having to lie again, or to live a lie." When she was ill with bulimia, she said she had lied to her mother about her vomiting. As her weight continued to drop, her mother had insisted on listening outside the door every time she went to the bathroom, and so Emily had resorted to throwing up only when she was in the shower, the noise of the water drowning out the sound of her retching. That was all she said, and I thought of her then as a stalwart, a backbencher who didn't proselytize, but whose testimony when she chose to speak was powerful, perhaps more powerful than David's. Recovery was a quiet component of her character. It had given her a peace and equanimity, a generous and optimistic outlook on life that showed in her eyes, that didn't disappear when you scratched the surface.

Yes, this mutual investment in recovery and the lack of too many illusions about the other's past was a novel way for David to begin a relationship. Emily quietly but rigidly controlled those elements of her life she could control, and there was much David could learn from this. She acknowledged, when I asked, that she jogged or walked every day—sometimes twice a day—and I imagined she kept track of the mileage and the time expended. I had seen several pairs of track shoes and a warm-up suit in the backseat of her car. David, as if showing her off, asked her how many calories and fat grams were in the muffin I was eating, and she said, "Roughly three hundred, and . . . about ten fat grams." I imagined she kept a running total of her caloric intake and energy expenditure. If she went past her caloric limits, she made up for it with exercise. If she exercised too much, she ate sufficiently more to compensate, though that day at Dolce Vita she didn't eat anything. She just had water.

○

As we sat there, I thought that perhaps we could, after all, go from being a duo to a comfortable trio.

But there was one name that had not been uttered at the table: Gloria. It would have been churlish for me to bring her up. She may have been absent, but she lingered in my mind, a powerful figure placed there by all that David had said about her.

She would not look benevolently at this scene in Dolce Vita.

David may not have been fearful, but I was.

31

It is three in the morning. The coach is awake and cold and shivering. He has heard a sharp sound, like the report of a rifle.

He knows what it is: one of the thirty Donnay rackets he carries for his player and that are stacked in the clothes closet has imploded, collapsed in on itself from the tremendous tension of the strings. It is a familiar sound, but still, each time it startles him, makes his heart race, more so when it wakes him from sleep. He looks around the room, as if the sound still echoes in the corners.

He had asked other coaches whether this ever happened to them and they had looked at him strangely. It is only his boy—he still thinks of him as a boy—who wants his rackets strung at such an extraordinary tension, twice that of McEnroe. Ninety pounds means they are dancing on the edge of the tolerance of the wooden frame. It is difficult to find a stringer willing to work with such tension, to risk having it explode, sending projectiles of wood splinters and gut in his face. There is only one man in Sweden whom they trust.

Ninety pounds of tension makes the racket feel as stiff as a skillet, but it is what the boy wants. It suits his big, looping ground strokes, gives him a control and precision that no one in the world can match.

On several occasions, the rifle-crack sound has shattered the calm of a first-class cabin at thirty thousand feet, causing flight attendants to scream, drinks to be spilled, looks of panic to come over the faces of passengers. The boy never flinches or blinks when this happens. He sits, observing quietly, while the coach explains, pacifies, pulls out the frame from the bag and cuts out *the strings before they warp the frame. If the frame is warped, they give it away as a souvenir.*

Once the implosion happened in the customs lounge in Milan and instantly the machine-gun-bearing carabinieri surrounded them, muzzles raised. And the previous year in Britain, just before they stepped out of the locker room for a quarterfinal, the coach was double-checking the tension, holding the racket in one hand and slapping the heel of his other hand against the strings. The racket shattered and gut and wood wrapped around his wrist like a handcuff. "It must have been more than ninety pounds," the boy said, walking away, even as the coach tried to free himself.

○

He lies still, knowing he must get up, open the bag, and cut out the strings. The rackets are stacked on top of each other, like a fine china service in green chamois. He idly wonders if it is possible for one racket to snap and set off a chain reaction with the others inside the giant duffel bag. He tries to imagine that sound.

He searches the suite for the thermostat and, finding it, turns off the air conditioner.

He listens at the door that separates his room from the boy's; he thinks he hears something. The door opens softly and she stands there. He is embarrassed to be seen there in nothing but boxer shorts, as if he were eavesdropping. She too was awakened by the sound, has come to the door, and now looks at him as if he has some answer for her. He shrugs. She smiles, sadness in her smile. They both turn to look at the boy: He sleeps, facedown, his arms spanning the width of the bed, his head buried in the pillow, his blond hair tangled and covering his shoulder blades, his spine rising and falling slowly. Surely in sleep his heart beats even more slowly than its usual sixty or so a minute. Once in the press it was reported that his heart pulsed at thirty-six beats a minute. It has become perpetuated as a truism, quoted so much that no one would believe him if he disputed it. Thirty-six is an aberration. Perhaps it gets that slow in sleep.

"Do you think he hears the sound in his dreams?" he whispers.

She thinks about this. She leans to his ear. "When he dreams, he concentrates on what he is dreaming about and ignores everything else."

It is the seriousness of her reply that makes him laugh, reach out and touch her on the shoulder, gently. Their communication is usually wordless, and their topic is almost always the boy. His touch tells her to go back to bed, to try to sleep. His communication with the boy is like that too. After years of traveling together they speak only when one of them is moved to. The girl has been with the boy for a few years—they are married now—and she has slipped into an orbit much like that of the coach. They are two satellites around the boy, the star. She and the coach have been sucked up, consumed by his needs. She has let her own career lapse, stopped competing on the women's tour. She had given up her ambitions in order to further his. It is perfectly reasonable, she is a talented player, but compared to him . . .

She closes the door and he thinks he hears the creak of the bed as she climbs back in with the boy.

○

He finds the racket and cuts out the strings. He checks the exact order of the rackets. The previous night he and the boy had held their "harpsichord recital"—her name for the ritual that goes like this: They lay out fifty rackets on the floor of the coach's room. The boy, a racket in each hand, taps the strings of one racket with the frame of the other. They both lean forward and listen intently. If necessary, he pings it again. Based on the pitch, he places the racket on one of two piles. When they are done, they go through the rackets that have made the cut, the ones whose sound resonates with some inner standard both coach and boy have memorized. They now rank the rackets: The first six will be used in that order and the order is never changed. If, during a match, a string breaks, the boy will walk to his bag and pick up the next one without a second thought. The racket whose string just snapped is the fourth racket. Tomorrow they will have to go through the remaining twenty-four rackets and pick a sixth.

He replaces the rackets and contemplates going back to bed, but he knows he will just toss and turn there. As he grows older, he sleeps less and less. It is, the doctor told him, tension. How many pounds? he wanted to ask. He declined pills because, for the most part, he wasn't tired from lack of sleep. But he misses the escape into sleep, he envies the way the boy rises from a chair, says good night, and falls on his face on the bed into deep sleep for ten hours. More and more he thinks of the boy as a perfectly balanced creature, put on earth for only one reason, to play tennis. Everything they do, from the vigorous massage the coach administers, to the meticulous watching of the boy's weight, is designed not to interfere with the symmetry of the body that allows it to play tennis the way it does. A few ounces too many or too few might change the balance, alter the delicate levers around the joints that allow him to hit the ball just so.

○

He slides open the door to the balcony and steps out of the icy room and leans against the railing. He almost chokes as the Florida air clogs his nose and throat, like a hot, wet rag. He can feel sea spray in the wind. His sweat glands are jarred awake. When he looks at his forearm, he can see a fine sheen of sweat forming underneath the hairs.

He sits without moving for three hours. The sea on this half-moon night is full of sound, like a creature that is awake and playfully trying to rouse the world. Nights like this, awake, he plays in his head with his invention, what has now become his obsession. He is consumed with an idea for a racket. He has a name for it already: the Protagon. The racket is strung in such a way that the main strings descend to a focal point within the shaft. Within the handle is a camshaft that allows the player to adjust the tension by turning a knob in the base of the handle. Once he mentioned this idea to the boy, who listened with detachment and mild curiosity, as though to say, Why do you even think of such things? Surely your life with me as my coach is a full life, yes?

Yes. His life as the boy's coach is a full life. Or, rather, he has no life of his own. He took up this life willingly. In the process, he has become part of one of the greatest records in tennis his-

tory: *five Wimbledon titles, six French Open titles. But he knows that the life is winding down. The boy's game isn't erratic or fading, but the boy, who can be out there all day and night, getting the ball back one more time till he wins, is bored. And then there is McEnroe. Thus far the boy has imposed his baseline game on others, like Connors, and even on McEnroe when he first appeared on the scene. The coach has ideas, ways to counter an ascendant McEnroe. The boy probably knows already what he needs to do. The coach can tell the boy is trying to decide simply if he wants to change his game, not if he can.*

The coach isn't reluctant to give up the travel and the luxurious but stupefyingly monotonous hotels. It is a sybaritic existence that can fascinate only people who have just enough money to experience it occasionally. To live in such places year-round is to long for an uncarpeted floor, for a kitchen, for an overstuffed, worn armchair, for the familiar creak of a shed door. He will willingly unload the burden of making travel arrangements, scheduling practice time, lining up partners, timing meals before matches, enduring press conferences, meeting with sponsors, planning the calendar a year or two ahead. But, for the first time in their partnership, he has greater ambition for the boy than the boy has for himself. The U.S. Open title eludes them, as does the Australian Open. He does not want the boy to finish his career without winning all four Grand Slams at least once. But, he can sense that the boy is winding down. The other life— whatever is out there after tennis—is beckoning him. And when that moment comes, the coach will be silent, help him make his exit, stifle the arguments against retirement that even now he rehearses in his mind.

But the Protagon will be the coach's own legacy. It will be a record of his own, some tangible way in which his name will survive independently of that of his ward, be spoken separately from the boy's. A coach, in the sense of someone telling the boy how to play, had always been superfluous. There was nothing to tinker with in his game. His powers of concentration were awesome, and of his own creation. In an interview once the boy had said, "I try to reduce the game to its simplest level: I try to get the ball back over the net one more time than my opponent."

The adjustments the boy made for the grass of Wimbledon—a surface on which no one thought he could be dominant—he had made himself: He had worked on his serve; he had developed the backhand slice approach specifically to hit to Connors's forehand; he had worked on the drop volley, a shot that still looked so awkward when he executed it, but one that caused the ball to drop over the net and die, unanswerable. The coach was in reality a gofer, a valet, a masseur, a connoisseur of the boy's body.

The Protagon will not be a racket for a touring pro. Instead, he pictures someone out there, a club player, a man with some other profession—a doctor or a lawyer—who will benefit from this racket. He pictures this man going out to hit, and finding that nothing is going quite right. That his baseline tactics are not working. At this point the player can simply twist the grip on the racket, drop the tension five or ten pounds, and have the ball come off the racket like a trampoline, use it to serve and volley, use it to block service returns, dispense with much backswing on the ground strokes. The player could, in other words, emulate McEnroe.

Or, on a hot, muggy day, if the ground strokes seem to be working well, the owner of the racket can crank up the tension, convert it into a stiffer wand, use it to camp behind the baseline and take huge swings at the ball, give it topspin and loft, control, and, like the boy, pin his opponent behind the baseline—

He hears someone open the door between the two rooms. He hears the sound of a toilet flushing.

He gets up, stiff from sitting outside for so long.

He must look for the room-service menu.

It is time to order breakfast. And to pick another racket.

32

When I met David on the tennis court at the condo the following Sunday, he was pale and there were dark circles under his eyes. I knew what had happened even before the words were out of his mouth. There was only so much entropy a system could tolerate before a correction came about.

"It's over with Gloria," he said, as if he were passing news on to me that would fell me, and so needed to watch me carefully. I didn't flinch.

"Emily and I drove out to Mesilla yesterday," he said in a leaden monotone, "along the route you and I went, cycling."

Also the route that he and Gloria had cycled. I could see him in my mind's eye, standing Emily at the wall of his dream house, presenting it to her just as he had to me.

"We were having a good time, walking through the crafts shops. We ate dinner. Then, in the *Placita*, we ran into Gloria's brother."

The brother had been strolling with *his* girlfriend. Introductions were made and the two couples parted pleasantly.

But the telephone wires had hummed so that by the time David got home after dropping Emily off, Mickie had a message for him: Call Gloria, ASAP.

He had delayed, agonized, but finally his fingers had tapped out the touch-tone refrain that meant New Jersey. Gloria snatched up the phone on its first ring and lashed into him, shamed him for his deceit, trotted out all his previous betrayals, summed them up and closed the case and their relationship "once and for all," David said.

"She refused to hear my explanations,"—what explanations could he offer?—"and hung up on me." I pictured him still holding the phone, words of explanation stacked up on his tongue, tumbling back into his pharynx, all jumbled together now.

After reciting this tale, David stood there, his face sagging like a wet canvas, waiting for sympathy from me, waiting for me to commiserate with him.

Did he really think that his seeing other people was all right with Gloria? Did he not know that there would be a price to pay if she found out? Perhaps it was bad luck that he was spotted, but had he taken pains to hide the relationship if his intent was to keep it from Gloria?

I held my tongue, didn't even cluck it, because I saw the canvas twitch. He was on the verge of losing all control, bawling perhaps. I stepped closer to him, and he shook his head as if to say he was okay.

For a moment, I wondered if he was putting me on. For weeks now, he and Emily had been a couple. But here he was speaking as if he didn't see that losing Gloria had any connection with his dating Emily. No, the great love of his life had been felled by a freak lightning bolt, but he would be brave and struggle on.

I knew him to be intelligent. I had to probe his reasoning, though gently. I had to see if he understood he was responsible, that he must have wanted it to end, that consciously or not he brought it about. I wasn't passing judgment on what he did—men did it to women all the time, and the other way around. But I was curious as to whether he understood the concept of consequence.

"David . . . it was coming, wasn't it?"

He looked perplexed.

"She was bound to find out? And you knew she'd go apeshit when she did?"

He chewed on this as if it had never occurred to him. Then he shook his head, as if I had misunderstood, he hadn't explained it to me well enough.

"You see, Abraham, in my mind . . . I never broke my bond with Gloria. I was trying to explain that that hadn't changed . . . she wouldn't listen."

Where did Emily sit in all this?

I was surprised he hadn't canceled our tennis date. We stood at the net, but the last thing on his mind was tennis. As an afterthought now, he picked the tennis balls out of my hand—no stretching—and we began to rally from the baseline. I felt as if I were hitting against a machine that delivered the ball at a precise length, but couldn't care less what I did with it.

Later, when we came to the net to gather balls, he stood there, disinclined to resume playing. But I found out what had given him the motivation to get out of bed that morning and come to the court.

"I'm going to move out of Mickie's place. Emily and I decided yesterday, before all this happened, to move in together. I can finally afford an apartment." A trace of excitement crept back into his voice. "There's this place, the ground floor of a house in Sunset Heights that we have an appointment to go see. It's supposed to be sunny, spacious, beautiful—"

My expression stopped him.

"You were making plans to move in with Emily yesterday?"

"Yeah, but—"

"That meant it was over with Gloria before she called?" My saying the name made him wince. "And what does it mean to Emily that you are moving in with her? It means you are in love with her, right?"

"I *am* in love with Emily. She's wonderful, wonderful . . ."

Again he looked at me as if I just didn't get it. I was utterly confused by what I was hearing.

We went back to playing, but my concentration was gone. A steadier partner would have been hard to find. But the tennis was not the same.

As we gathered up the balls and I packed my racket bag, David came out with the thought that had been brewing in him for the last few minutes. An explanation. For me.

"You see, Abraham . . . Gloria . . . there is something about her that I can never completely let go of—"

"Then why . . . ?"

"If she were to call in the next five minutes and tell me to come back to her, I would. That doesn't take anything away from Emily—"

"Yes it does. Does Emily know that?"

"No."

I drove away perturbed, my usual post-tennis euphoria tainted. Silly me: When Mickie had called David "a helpless womanizer"

I'd thought she meant he was unable to resist sexual temptation. But perhaps I had underestimated Mickie. She had in mind what I was now witnessing: the overflowing of the chemistry, David's inability to separate his loves.

○

When I called David the next evening, he was chirpy. The house in Sunset Heights had been everything he imagined it would be. He had signed the lease. His sponsor—with whom he had to clear this sort of thing—had reluctantly given him the green light, and he would move the next day. The momentum, the flow, the rapid changes had pushed Gloria and his discomfort to the recesses of his mind. He didn't mention her and I didn't bring it up.

I offered to help. But he said he had so little that he could do it in one trip. And they were getting a pickup truck for Emily's stuff. I wished him well. Since he didn't mention a tennis date, I didn't bring it up either.

The two events—the breakup with Gloria and the move to a new apartment with Emily—were connected in David's mind, but not the way they should have been. He acted now as if the breakup with Gloria had *resulted* in his moving in with Emily. As if it were true, true and related.

But at this point, the logic involved was of interest only to me, important only that I keep clear in my head what had happened.

33

Now that David and Emily were living together, I saw even less of him.
He had a new phone number. The blithe voice on his new answering machine was part Yank yuppie, part Croc Dundee—"Hoi! Emily
and I aren't in at the moah-ment but . . ." It made me picture them
in a sun-drenched room with all the windows open. Different from
when it was just the two of us, reaching out from our dark lairs on
either side of the mountain. Still, David made it a point to call me
every three or four days—his tone was that of the big brother, the
settled one, checking up on his younger ward, but I thought he was
really calling to show me that my misgivings were unwarranted, and
that he was all right.

A week after he moved in, he called to tell me that Dr. Walsh and
Dr. Nelson, the directors of the emergency medicine residency at
Texas Tech, had interviewed him. They had concerns, given his past
and their own experience with problem residents. "But they said if I
did well in the transitional internship, I'm in!"

"Good for you."

"Of course, it's provisional. I have to keep up with the meetings,
get good sponsor reports, keep clean urines . . ."

○

I called to set up a match two weekends after he moved. He had me
hold, and then, after a muffled discussion, he came back on the
line to say he would have to pass, because he and Emily were going
to a couple of west-side garage sales and then to visit the consign-
ment stores in the Upper Valley. What had been inviolate in our
friendship, the tennis, was now relegated to a lesser place. It
depended very much on their schedule as a couple. It was not para-

mount in his life, the way it had once been with us, the way it still was with me.

The two of them were buying furniture and decorating—playing house. He was feathering his nest, while my pleasure came from the very lack of furniture, from living largely at floor level.

They swung by my apartment after one of these excursions. I could see surprise register on Emily's face when she walked in, though she gamely took off her shoes and sat on the floor. I think she felt sorry for me. David understood that there wasn't a stick of furniture that could have made me happier. The U-Haul box that the boys and I used as a dining table was now rich with pizza stains and wax trails down the sides from the night we had lit red and purple candles. I had reinforced its corners several times with packing tape. It sat in the middle of the room, an art object.

○

A month went by without our playing tennis. I gave the kids more lessons, went riding on my bicycle, exploring the town. Late at night I got in my car to roam even farther afield. But I still longed for the resumption of our ritual.

Finally, on a Sunday, we met for tennis at the club. It was a glorious hour of tennis, so much so that when Emily showed up toward the end of the hour, I was resentful of her, reminded acutely of what had been taken away.

We went together for lunch to a Greek restaurant off Mesa. The conversation turned to Julius, the former Texas Tech ER resident who had been dropped from the program because of drug use, and who had recently died in another city of an overdose.

"He is why the ER people were so wary of me," David said, his mouth full of food, but a malignant expression coming to his face. "What a stupid fuck! He was never, ever, truly in recovery."

I stopped eating to look at him. David had known Julius fairly well. Their paths had crossed in NA meetings. It was an uncharacteristically vicious thing to say.

"Julius was the consummate smooth operator," David said, as if to explain Julius to me. "I don't think he ever intended to quit. He just didn't get it. He didn't get it."

○

After lunch David and Emily insisted I come by and see their place. It wasn't far from where we were, and though I really had no desire to see their love nest, it would have been rude to refuse.

I followed them to the Sunset Heights neighborhood, a part of town I had explored with the boys and alone in my late-night meanderings. It was one of the oldest residential parts of town and one of the first planned neighborhoods in Texas, the brainchild of a New Yorker, J. Fisher Satterthwaite. El Paso had laughed when the project began in 1885, because the land was so unpromising, full of igneous rock and with little soil. Satterthwaite was undaunted, spending huge amounts of money to tear down hills and create a system of graded streets. A flowing traffic pattern was in place—before the advent of the automobile. Gas and water lines were put in and the lots landscaped. A central park was built, with a trolley station that ran down to the business district. *Paseños* stopped laughing. Satterthwaite's quote that "no city in the country ever grew downhill" had become El Paso's theme song. By the nineties, developers had pushed so far up the slopes of the Franklins that the houses on Crazy Cat seemed only a few hundred feet from reaching the top.

Sunset Heights offered wonderful views of the river and of Juárez. It was the choice area from which El Pasoans with binoculars watched the exciting May 1911 revolution across the river, as Orozco and Villa and Madero attempted to overthrow the thirty-year rule of the dictator Porfirio Díaz. The battle for Juárez was a spectacle of artillery, firearms, and, finally, hand-to-hand combat. The wealthy Mexicans—*Porfiristas*—who fled the revolution that ousted Porfirio Díaz came to El Paso and bought and lived in the mansions of Sunset Heights.

I followed David and Emily past the Trost House. Henry Trost, a colleague and admirer of Frank Lloyd Wright, had designed many of the houses in Sunset Heights, as well as the major downtown buildings. I parked behind David's car. To look around any street in Sunset Heights was to see a catalog of architectural styles: Classic Revival, English Tudor, Mission Revival, California Bungalow.

It was still a romantic subdivision, a throwback to another era, with a view that justified its name. But the freeway had come up just below it, and the winter smog from inversion was centered squarely on Sunset Heights. Many of the mansions were boarded up, with gang graffiti visible. Some of the old scions of El Paso still lived here. But others had cleared out, partitioning their homes and renting them out as apartments. As an island of gentrification, it was suffering severe erosion.

David and Emily occupied the ground floor of a two-story home that was at least a hundred years old. Broad brick stairs led to a veranda. From a foyer we entered a huge living room and dining room with polished wood floors, even more spacious than I would have guessed from the outside. Facing the street was a sunroom where Emily had petunias and daisies sitting in pots. The furniture in the living room was of the heavy, wood variety, decorated with oversized pillows and throw rugs. A folio-size photography book sat on the glass coffee table. I saw David's *Harrison's* on a shelf together with a set of bound books—perhaps an encyclopedia. A buffet table held trinkets and small portraits. Philodendrons, and spider plants in hanging pots, soaked up the light streaming in from the tall windows in the dining room. I was embarrassed now to think of how Emily had sat on the floor of my flat, her back against the wall, drinking soda out of a can.

I remembered the moment David had first walked into my new apartment, how much he had liked it, how it had been so much more than what he had at Mickie's. Now it was my turn to express admiration. The appearance of the house belied the short time they had been together. At any moment I expected two toddlers and a golden retriever to emerge from the bedroom.

If I did envy anything, it was not David's new place but what he now had with Emily. There were nights when I longed for company, a woman to hold hands with on the balcony, a woman to read to, and later to make love to and fall asleep with, limbs twined around each other under the sheets. The trouble was, I wanted this on only some nights. Most nights I was loath to give up my solitude.

Emily played the gracious hostess and fixed iced tea for us, complete with a twist of lemon and a sprig of mint. She brought this out on a tray.

I looked at David as we sat together in the sunroom; he appeared distracted, proud to show me the place, but embarrassed, like a new groom, by his domesticity. It was more than that, however: He looked trapped, just as I probably had when he'd come to dinner.

We were talking shop, he and I. I was telling him about the AIDS clinic, how central it was to my workweek. What frustrated me though was that there came a point with each patient where AZT or DDI or DDC did nothing. I told him how I had taken one patient off AZT because he was clearly dying, and the drug was giving him side effects. His family came to me in great alarm, asking, "Why did you take him off the medication?" My explanations didn't seem to satisfy them, and to take him off AZT meant to them that I had given up all hope. I put him back on a lower dose, and when he died a few weeks later, the family took this in stride.

There were new strains of HIV showing up in Africa and even in America. I waxed eloquent about the ingenuity of this virus, its ability to mutate, and now, its ability to show that it had cousins and relatives—new strains—also capable of causing AIDS. "God knows what other viruses are lurking out there, sitting in the blood supply, waiting to be discovered," I said.

I realized that both David and Emily had become very still. His face was twitching.

"My HIV test has been negative," David finally said. "I took one just a while back, when Emily and I got together. We use protection, of course. I thought I had nothing more to worry about." He smiled wryly. "I hadn't thought of *other* viruses till just now."

Emily looked at me steadily.

David continued: "When I was using, I put myself in all kinds of situations. I can't even remember half of them. It's a miracle I've been spared; I *hope* I've been spared."

I had frightened the two of them with shoptalk.

"Listen," I said to David, "I'm sorry I alarmed you. The regular HIV test detects most variants of the HIV virus. You needn't worry." When I saw that this didn't really reassure them, I said, "If you're concerned, we can do the test again, but really, if I were in your shoes, I wouldn't worry."

"Okay. If you say so," David said, and sat back in his chair, but I felt as if I had thrown a damper on the works. Soon after that I took leave of them. I shook David's hand. I hugged Emily.

○

The feel of the house, its richness of objects, lingered with me after I left. David's recovery, his return to "normal" society, seemed physically complete. He had graduated, begun an internship, had secured a coveted residency in emergency medicine, had a home, a girlfriend . . . and yet he had looked cornered.

The humility that I had associated with David was missing; an arrogance had shown itself momentarily in his comment about Julius's death. But why begrudge him his confidence, his right to be opinionated? Perhaps it was my fault, my wish—society's wish—to impose humility on all addicts. When he lived his pathetic existence at Mickie's, when he had nothing, when he was remorseful, self-flagellating, he was an easy target for my pity and my noblesse. Was *my* discomfort with the visit because he had broken out of that mold? Outgrown me?

No, there was more to this than my envy. David seemed ahead of himself: This appearance of the long-married couple was out of step with where he was emotionally.

Emily was not naive. If I had seen a blind spot in the way David had closed his chapter with Gloria, and begun this new one with her, she had seen it too. There was a jarring, pricking, exposed edge to David that I could not explain.

○

I went directly from their house to see Mickie, stopping only long enough to telephone her, feeling sadness as my fingers tapped out David's former number. I had a good reason to visit: For some time now I'd had in my car samples of some of the medications she used every day. Her insurance didn't cover all her needs and Medicaid had not kicked in yet.

I told her I wanted to drop off these samples. But what I was really after was enlightenment. Perhaps Mickie understood what was happening with David.

I looked for the telephone cord trailing under the door as I walked in.

"Where's the guy who used to room here?"

"Oh, he skipped out. Still owes me rent. I wish he didn't exist."

I followed Mickie into the house. She moved even more slowly than before, leaning heavily on the walker. The piles of paper on tables had grown logarithmically since I'd last been here. Mickie told me she was trying to get all her medical bills and payments sorted out, and to have everything within arm's reach. It was too much effort for her to bend down and retrieve things from boxes. I put the bag of medicines on top of a pile of papers. An elaborate crochet piece on the sofa was almost complete: It was an Egyptian theme with a central sphinx and profiles of pharaohs around it. On the coffee table was an orange diabetic syringe, a bottle of insulin, and an alcohol swab half out of its cover.

I noticed for the first time the bookcases behind the sofa. I walked over and saw that the shelves were filled with hardcover books. Some novels, but mostly volumes that had to do with recovery. I remembered that at one time Mickie had worked as a counselor.

"David been by?"

"Hell, no. He's called, though, I'll give him that." She smiled now. "I miss him, I tell you. I miss the way he'd walk in and say, 'Hi, it's Daaiy-vid,'" she said, imitating him and then laughing her bosomy, raspy laugh. "I love that boy, liked him from the moment I met him. He was such good company. I worry about him. David's so vulnerable, so innocent."

"He isn't exactly innocent, Mickie," I said. "You know that, don't you?"

"Ah, but he is, Abraham. He isn't innocent about the world. In fact, he knows too much about the world. *Yet he knows nothing about himself.*"

This was an astute observation. But it could be said about a lot of people.

"He's ignorant about who David is," she went on, "and what David needs. He's like a little baby. Between you and me, I didn't really care for the idea of his moving out."

"Me either. You know he broke up with Gloria?" I said, fishing.

"Gloria, Emily—it's all the same thing."

"But don't you think he should have—"

"He wasn't ready for any of it. He still has so much recovery work to do. Ah, well," she said, loading the syringe, pulling up her skirt to jab the orange syringe into her thigh as casually as if she were crocheting. She pulled it out, and tossed it onto the table.

"Do you know he was fascinated by these syringes? Every evening when he came in he'd ask me if I'd taken my insulin. If I hadn't, he'd help me. Sometimes, he'd handle the syringes, look at them kind of wistfully. And then he'd say, 'They are too small for me, Mickie!' He got off on the injecting. When he was out of drugs, he'd take water in a syringe and inject it into himself."

I thought it ironic that David had worked as a phlebotomist during his year away from Texas Tech, when he lived with Gloria in New Jersey.

"One night he came home and said, 'Mickie, it's still there!' And I said, 'What's there?' He said, 'Under the bridge, all those users, they're still there. I happened to drive past and they were there sitting and injecting.' I said, 'David, you didn't think for a moment that when *you* stopped using that everyone else would just give up?' It's one of the fallacies in AA. The alcoholic thinks that once he stops drinking, his neighborhood bar is going to close. He can't imagine their going on without him."

I was curious about "under the bridge." Which bridge?

"Well, it's more an expression, at least the way I use the term," she said. "To me, it means rock bottom. It means you panhandle by the traffic lights at the I-10 feeder roads. And then you crawl under the ramps for the night and use."

"But David mentioned a particular locale he drove by," I said. "Where was it?"

"Oh, I don't remember. It doesn't really matter. I think he was referring to the spaghetti bowl near Texas Tech, or maybe the bridge near Paisano."

"And he must have . . . slept there? Lived there at one time?"

"I'm sure he did. And when you reach that stage, then anything goes: sharing needles, sex with whoever, male or female. It's a very dangerous place. You can get robbed or killed." She didn't seem as interested in the bridge as I was.

I left feeling that instead of learning more about David, he had become even more mysterious to me.

34

An invitation on short notice to speak at a medical meeting in Stockholm took me out of town. From Stockholm, I added a side trip to India. I was away for almost three weeks. When my plane was about to land in El Paso, I felt a quickening, not just at being back and seeing the boys, but because where my fellow passengers saw a dry, dusty cityscape below, the flares of the Chevron refinery and the smokestacks of the Asarco smelting plant sticking out from the haze, I saw the mountains, picked out the highway running through town like a central artery, and felt a voice within me say that I was home.

I went to work my second day back. Late in the afternoon, I saw David from a distance. He was in a green scrub suit, sitting with the rest of his surgical team in the cafeteria.

There were two surgical teams, one run by a thoughtful and skilled chief resident, the other by an equally skilled but obnoxious one. David was with the latter team. He was slumped in a chair, his feet casually draped over another chair, his mask over his throat and his surgical cap pushed back on his head. He held a cup of ice in his hand and chewed on ice chips. There was an insouciance, a laxness to his posture that I thought was atypical of David. He had subtly adopted the cowpoke, swaggering manner of the team leader. Even the female medical students who had been elegant and graceful on the internal medicine service now looked slouchy and insolent.

This wasn't terribly surprising. I knew they made rounds as a group at five in the morning, then again at six in the morning with the surgical attending, then went off to the operating theater or to clinics, and ended the day with rounds at seven at night—if they weren't on call. This would go on for three months. The manner-

isms and societal rules had to rub off on him. I didn't try to
approach David. He did not see me.

I left a message for him on his machine that evening and for a few
days we played telephone tag, setting up a date for a match without
having spoken directly to each other. When I was about to leave for
the court, my beeper displayed 0-6, and then a hospital extension. I
didn't call the number—I assumed he had been unable to break
away.

It was a week before I saw him again. He was in scrubs with a
stethoscope around his neck, and two beepers on his belt. No coat. I
was about to go home but he was on call and had dashed down to
see if I was in my office. I put down my briefcase. He sat in his chair,
and looked pleased to see that I had not touched the pile of papers
from his pneumonia study.

"A few days of concentrated work and I'll be done with this lot,"
he said, running his hand over the pile.

"It's waiting for you."

He asked about India and Stockholm. I had brought something
for him and Emily, for their house. I promised to bring it in to work.
He said he had seen Jacob and Steven in the mall with their mother
and had waved at them and they had waved shyly back.

"So?" he said. "Has the woman of your dreams shown up yet?"

"In my dreams, she has."

"She's out of school now, working at the pro shop in the tennis
club," David said when I asked after Emily.

"And you two are doing well together? Do you have a dog yet? A
fish tank? A camper? Two-point-two kids?"

"We're . . . not doing that well."

Uh-oh.

The lopsided smile that appeared on his face was eerie, out of
place, pain and pride mixed together, as if he were an arsonist
watching his own house go up in flames.

"Emily read my journals. When I was here on call."

His journal writing had begun as part of the therapy for his recovery, but it had become a habit as compulsive as mine. In his journals, he poured out his fears and fantasies. The relative calm of his
outer world capped a turbulent inner world, and his notebooks
were straight from that dark place.

"The journals are the most . . . honest part of my recovery. There's stuff in there that I wouldn't admit to anybody. Not in therapy, not to my sponsor . . ."

Not to me. I wished I could see the journals. I understood perfectly what Emily had done.

David's smile had vanished now, and his face was stiff with anger, the pitch of his voice rising. "Emily should bloody well have not read it. She should have known that what she found in there would be guaranteed to disturb her."

Was he culpable in letting it lie around so she could read it?

"Where were the journals?"

"In the back of a drawer."

"Why do you think you wanted her to find them?" I said, sounding like a therapist.

He shrugged. "I didn't see any need for her to look at them."

His blind spot was getting larger. He didn't see his role in her finding the journal.

"So what happened?"

"It was painful for her. There was stuff in there about Gloria. Now she's hurt. But I tried to tell her that it was meant to be a private journal."

The fault lay with Emily.

I opened my mouth to say something, but then decided against it.

"How's surgery?" I asked.

"Brutal," he said, and then, remembering himself, remembering the creed of the tribe he now belonged to, he squared his shoulders and said, "but lots of chances to cut."

35

On the last day of November, El Paso turned gray, wet, and bitterly cold.
This was not the towering summer thundercloud amassing far away,
shaped like Lucifer, flashing and glowing within itself, approaching
all day and so wide that it cast a shadow over New Mexico from
Albuquerque to Las Cruces. Instead, the gray was there when I
awoke. What looked like thick smoke showed over the top of the
Franklins, oozing over its crest. And then, as if it were too heavy to
float, it seeped like icing down the side of a cake into the canyons
and arroyos. When I looked again just before leaving for work, the
mountains had disappeared. In their place was a rampart of clouds.

The moisture left splotches on the pale stucco of houses, darkened the rock walls so that they looked black. Such grayness over the
city as I drove, a gray the windshield wiper could not clear. Then it
dawned on me: I was *in* cloud. The whole city was in cloud, and
instead of rain it was as if a wet rag lay over it.

Disease was once thought to come from noxious odors—mias-
mas—that rose up from cracks in the earth. If so, then a pestilence
had found The Pass of the North. The Asarco smelting plant and its
fecal smell, and later, the Chevron refinery's rotten-egg smell, came
through the car vents as I went east down the freeway. I drove, mut-
tering to myself, "The dark November of my soul."

My knee throbbed and a heaviness descended on me. I did not
welcome the rain, even though it was vital to the city to renew the
water base in the Hueco and Mesilla bolsons. What I liked most of
all about El Paso was the sun, the light, and the mountain, and now
all three were gone.

○

In my office, I took off my raincoat and shook out my umbrella. David walked in. I turned to him like a drowning sailor.

"My mother's very ill. She's in an ICU in Sydney. Don't think she'll make it."

"God! How—?"

"My sister called. They want me there." He said this in a monotone, as if he resented the news, resented its timing, and resented the demand that he come home.

I made him sit down in his chair. I was animated now, the weather forgotten. I could see the fatigue on his face—he'd been on call—and how this visit to me was an entreaty of sorts.

His mother had been traveling with his father when she developed heart failure. The doctors in Sydney found a damaged aortic valve and she had emergency surgery to replace it. But then her kidneys had failed and the prosthetic valve had become infected. Then she had thrown a blood clot to her lung. It sounded bad.

"Okay. So when's your plane?"

He stirred in his chair.

"I don't know what to do. My sister says I must go."

His manner was surly, irritable, his face dark and brooding. As if it was his sister's mandate to him that he resented.

"You didn't book a flight?"

"I don't have the money. I can't go."

"I'll lend you money."

What he heard he didn't like, because he slumped deeper in the chair, holding on to its arms, as if he might be pried loose and put on a plane. I looked at his pupils, his bare arms—they looked normal.

"It's a terrible time for me to take off—"

"Nonsense. This takes precedence."

"I'm not sure I can achieve anything . . . what purpose—"

"Come on, David. Your *mother*! . . . I'll lend you the money."

He sighed, as if he wished I hadn't offered this. He was in my office, he had sought me out because he knew I would tell him what to do, he trusted me to tell him that.

The surgical chief resident, he said, had been less than sympathetic and had grumbled about how the other interns would have to take extra call to cover him. The not-so-subtle message he'd received was that his patients in the ICU needed him. His mother had her own doctors in another ICU across the world to take care of her.

This infuriated me, and I didn't let him go on. "It's not *their* mother."

By that afternoon, he was on a plane to Australia.

○

Just a few days later, the low-pressure system that had come up from the Sierra Madres was still hovering over El Paso. The weather channel said it would push north, perhaps by the end of the day. Yes, rain was good for the city, but surely there was such a thing as too much rain.

I walked into my office and found David sitting there, in a scrub suit, in his chair, sipping coffee, another cup waiting for me.

"David! Did you not go?"

"I got back last night . . ."

"What?"

"They gave me grief here about being gone."

"Your mother?"

"Still alive."

I thought it lunacy to fly halfway across the world to a dying parent, be gone three days and four nights—half of that in the air—all because of a sense of loyalty to a residency. I sat down, my raincoat still on.

"There was no point in staying. She's an ICU nightmare. Cardiac surgery, then a cascade of catastrophes. Kidneys shutting down,"—he was retreating to the nouns and verbs we used to distance other people's tragedies—"cerebral anoxia, ARDS, on a ventilator, on PEEP, a hopeless case—"

"The kind you transfer to internal medicine?"

He was ready to laugh at this, until he realized I had not said this in humor, but to reflect his words back at him.

"She never knew I was there, Abraham!"

He spat this out. I had tapped into a wellspring of anger. What I couldn't understand was what the anger was about. It wasn't his mother's fault that she had gotten ill. And it was natural that his family would summon him home. He had become a prisoner of the internship—a Stockholm syndrome—so much so that he saw our hospital's need as greater than his family's need. I wanted to lean forward and ask, "Why do you hate her?" But he was shifting in his chair now, his manner that of a schoolboy who was in a teacher's office under duress.

I sat back, folded my arms, and stared him down.

"I came to give you this check," he said, dropping his eyes. "It's not much, but I'll pay off the ticket in monthly installments. I'm afraid it will take a while. I'm grateful to you for lending me the money."

When I wouldn't reach for it, he placed it under my coffee cup and walked away, closing the door behind him.

○

I called that evening. Emily picked up the phone. They had slapped David with night call his first day back.

"He *is* angry with her," Emily said when I told her about his strange reaction to his mother. "And he either doesn't know why or he won't tell me."

She said that David sat by his mother's bed, looking at her but unable to feel anything. He couldn't connect with her or feel sorry for her or cry. He told Emily he just sat there. Every now and then he would ask the nurses what medications were going in—being medically curious. But as far as interacting with her, he couldn't. He was numb—as if she were his patient.

"That's how he is now. Numb," Emily said.

"But why anger?"

"Oh . . . something about how his sister seemed to give him no credit for who he was now. Sober. An intern. She dealt with him as if he was still the same David who was sent back to Australia, a scrawny skeleton, barely alive."

All these reasons on the surface, but they failed to connect.

"And you, Emily, how are you?"

There was a long silence.

"Did he tell you about my reading his journal?"

My turn to keep quiet, which she took to be an answer in itself.

"*Don't* tell me I shouldn't have, Abe. I did it because I felt he was restless. Something was brewing. You know what was in there? It broke my heart. He was still fantasizing about Gloria. Explicit . . . intimate stuff."

She paused and her pain was palpable.

"Did you know that he still felt that way about her?" she asked.

What I had always known was that Gloria would not be that easily erased from his mind. Again Emily spared me the need to reply.

"He is the man I love. It's painful to read this . . ." I could tell from her breathing that she was crying now, finding words in between her silent sobs. "I confronted him. 'What the hell is going on in your head?' I said. 'How you act on the outside is not how things seem to be going on the inside.' . . . Do you know what he did?"

This time I could truthfully say no.

"He hit himself on the head with his fist. I was speechless. I watched, and he did it again. He brought his hand up, made a fist, and punched himself in the temple. I'm not kidding, Abraham, he was reeling from the blow. As if it were not *his* hand, but someone else's hand . . . Here he had hurt me, and now I was trying to keep him from hurting himself. At that moment I felt as if it was all unraveling."

"So what . . . how did you resolve it?"

She laughed. "We don't resolve anything. We barely get to talk. He's so busy with the internship. And then so tired when he does come home which, since he's on call every third night, is not that often. I have to fight for his time. And then his mother got ill . . ."

○

I went by the tennis club the next day, to drop off a racket for restringing. I didn't know what to say to Emily. I was going to see her the way I had gone to see Mickie, for my own sake, to find explanations.

Emily was dealing with a customer, pulling a jacket from a hanger, rifling through the rack for another one. I sat outside and watched her, saw her smile genuinely at this man, give him her complete attention. From her face a stranger might have assumed she was happy, content, when in fact she was in pain. I was drawn to her then. She was not naive, but she was trusting. I resented David for causing her so much grief. If David's journals revealed inner turmoil that belied the surface appearance, then she was the opposite. The words that came out of her mouth with me, with him, accurately reflected how she felt on the inside. Whenever there was a dichotomy between those two states, when she had to put on a brave face, as she did now, she considered it a symptom of her disease.

The customer left and I walked in. She looked up, smiled, and came to me. Even through the smile, pain and anxiety came to her face. To see me was to think of David, for that was our connection. We hugged. The news about David's mother was the same: She was alive.

"Who are you playing with?"

"Um . . . I came to get my racket strung."

She wrote down what I wanted—Prince synthetic gut, seventeen gauge, five pounds above the recommended tension—and deposited the racket behind the counter.

"Have you had a chance to talk much with David . . . ?"

"He hasn't been home. And *I* had to call him at work and ask him about his mother today before he told me that his sister had called."

"Maybe it's the stress of the internship. He's not living a normal existence. Not sleeping normally. Sometimes, never seeing daylight for thirty-six hours. It's bound to affect other spheres of his life."

She didn't think much of this explanation. I saw that when we talked about David, a wariness came to her face, the same look I had seen in Gloria.

"After I read his journal . . . I don't trust him. I asked him if he was sure that he wanted this, did he want me? And if he did, to get Gloria out of his thoughts. But the blind trust I had in him is . . . gone."

A customer walked in. I told Emily to call me if she needed anything and if there was any word on David's mother. She gave me a hug and a smile and said, "Thanks for coming to see me."

○

The boys were the one constant in my life, my unchanging ritual. If I had thought of myself as needing to be there for them, they were, in fact, much more there for me, secure in their routine, giving me faith.

I went from the club to see them, just in time to tuck them in bed and hear them say their prayers. When they asked about David, I

told them how his mother was very ill. Is he sad? Of course, he's sad,
I said, wondering why it was necessary to lie about this.

Steven led the Our Father. Jacob, as always, squeezed his eyes
tightly shut, as if by squeezing he could add extra oomph, open up a
more direct channel to God. The effort caused his cheeks to draw
up, and his nose to wrinkle, and it was accompanied by various
motor twitches in his extremities that I loved to watch. Then Steven
said his usual "Dear God, bless Daddy, Mommy, Jacob, and me,"
adding, "and make David's mother all right, and help David not to
be so sad." He opened one eye and peeked at me and smiled,
pleased with himself, making sure I had noticed that his prayer was
so topical. "Oh yes, and keep us warm and safe in our beds," he
said. To which Jacob added, as always, "And *no* nightmares," before
they both said, "Good night, God."

○

Predictably, David's mother died a few days later. It was a day we
had arranged to play tennis, one of his rare evenings off. He didn't
cancel, punch in a 0-6. Instead, he met me on our secret court at the
condo and gave me the news there.

It was cold, my knee ached, and I scrambled to keep the ball in
play. David fussed with the handle of the racket, and when spit
wouldn't solve it, he retaped it. Then the net strap required adjusting. Later he was dissatisfied with the pressure in one ball, and he
lobbed it into the canyon. He was, I thought, wanting to find peace
in the sound of the ball, in its echo through this canyon, but peace
eluded him.

I thought of everyone I knew who had lost a mother. I remembered
my father, in his forties when his mother died in India. I thought of
Jacob and Steven's hell if they should lose their mother; they lived
with her primarily and she oversaw their schoolwork and their everyday needs. She was so much more the focal point of their world than
I was. Meanwhile, the man who *had* lost his mother was gracefully
hitting a tennis ball, yet not deriving much pleasure from it.

After the tennis, we stood around. The city lights below us were
needle-sharp in the cold air. The two cities appeared hunkered down
for winter. It was crazy to play tennis this late, in this weather. Had it
been summer we might have sat on the bench and visited. Maybe

we could go to Dolce Vita and perhaps there he would open up? But no, just when I was about to suggest that, he said, "Nice game. Thanks for coming out. I'd better head back."

"How are you feeling?" I asked, treading into that space that he wanted to keep clear.

"When I saw her, she was already gone. The news today did nothing for me."

It hadn't done much for him the day he had heard she was ill either. I wanted to shake him, shout at him: David, I'm your friend. Open up. He clearly had trouble expressing his feelings when it came to his mother. And even greater difficulty—judging by what had happened with Gloria—in identifying exactly what he was feeling.

And then he said that he and Emily had become engaged—a matter of giving her a ring. "We've tentatively set a wedding date for the end of my internship." He smiled wryly at me, as if to say, See how far I have come? But what I saw was that he had sidestepped his problems with Emily by doing an end run, coming up with an engagement ring. It was the way he had sidestepped the Gloria issue by moving in with Emily.

He reported the engagement as dispassionately as if he were telling me about sunspot activity predicted for the next year. Or the death of his mother.

36

About the time the giant strand of lights, eight stories high, in the form of a Christmas tree, was being strung up on the outside of the hospital building, I rounded a corner of the sixth floor of Thomason and ran into Gloria, almost knocking her over. We backed away, then came forward and greeted each other like long-lost acquaintances. She had finished her pharmacy degree in New Jersey. As part of her agreement with Thomason, which had paid for her training, she was returning to work for them for a year.

"Welcome back," I said, pleased to discover that I was no longer tongue-tied in her presence. In her pharmacy uniform, she looked like just another employee—albeit a very attractive one. You have no idea, I wanted to say to her, what a force you are.

I paged David, wanting to forewarn him. Instead of answering, he materialized at my door.

"I've seen her," he said, as soon as he walked in. Despite his green scrubs, the blue mask dangling on his chest, the tourniquet at his waist, he looked devastated, his bluster and bravado stolen.

It had happened on the fifth floor, perhaps an hour before I saw her. He had walked out of a patient's room and there she was, side-ways to him, working at a desk. She looked up, said hello, and that had surprised him. He had assumed that she was in the same state as when they had last talked months before, and now that he was before her, she would try to scratch his eyes or knee him in the groin.

But she was the model of composure. "Congratulations," she said, and when he stared, unsure, she added, "On being a doctor." David stammered back that he was proud that she had finished all her training. And that he was sad that things had not worked out. She heard him out, gave him a knowing smile, and turned back to her work.

Her arrival and their meeting had utterly broken his concentration. Being in her physical presence had unnerved him, reduced him to a helpless state. If she was demystified for me, she still wielded the power, still had chemistry with David.

"I dread running into her again," David said.

I hated to hear those words. The building blocks of his life—doctoring, recovery, Emily, money, tennis, house—were stacked in a manner that was dangerous and unstable. And to this tottering edifice Gloria had been added.

"How about tennis this evening?" I said, trying to salvage something of that day.

"Yeah," he said, his face brightening.

○

From the parking lot, I saw a dust storm approaching. To the west, the sky was cloudless and a deep blue, but to the east, a brown-yellow blanket was advancing, still many miles away. Once the dust storm arrived, it did not so much blow as blanket the city, at which point one was strangely unaware of the storm, it was not as threatening as when it loomed on the horizon. *Paseños* ignored dust storms, going about their business, the tennis club staying open. One tolerated the crusting in the nostrils and the gritty sensation in the eyes. And when the sun set, the dust created a spectacle that was well worth the discomfort.

When I reached the condo, there was no sign of David. The wind was kicking up and it would have been difficult, but not impossible, to play. Still, he had said he was coming. I walked to the pay phone near the clubhouse, paged him, and he called back promptly.

"Sorry! I saw the dust storm and assumed it was off," he said.

"Yeah, you're probably right."

I walked back to the courts. The sky was now blotted out, replaced by a brown-gray canopy, except to the far west where an orange, perfectly round fireball had formed, looking like light at the end of the tunnel.

37

The year 1993 started auspiciously. In January, the Cowboys won the Super Bowl.

But early in February, Arthur Ashe died. All through the previous year, I had seen glimpses of him on television, giving speeches, appearing at fund-raisers for AIDS, working on his memoir. I saw fatigue in his face, could imagine the fevers, the mouth sores, the difficulty in swallowing, the medications he took that were identical to what I prescribed for my patients in the clinic.

At work I searched faces to see if this news affected others the way it affected me. Only David called to see how I was doing. He knew how closely I had been following this story.

"I'm taking it personally," I said. To discuss Ashe with David, a topic of little interest to anyone else, was to miss David, to see how much our friendship was withering from lack of attention. We had not played tennis in almost six weeks. We blamed the weather—though the previous year it had not stopped us.

o

At the end of February, David came stumbling through the doorway of my office, looking shell-shocked and completely unnerved—so much more emotion than when he had heard his mother was ill.

I made him sit down. His beeper kept going off. I took it from him and put it on mute.

He let out a big sigh. "I saw Gloria," he said, in the tone of a man who had seen something completely outside the spectrum of human experience. It had happened in the cafeteria, just a few minutes before he'd come to see me. And though his beeper was going crazy and he had six different tasks to complete, he had gone and sat next to her. The world around him had disappeared. He was aware of only her.

"The words just came pouring out of my mouth, I couldn't help myself. I said, 'Gloria, you know I'm still in love with you. If you just say the word, I'll leave Emily tomorrow and be back with you.'"

"No!" I said, thinking of Emily, thinking of the chaos that those words must cause. "David!"

"I couldn't help myself, Abe."

And indeed, slumped in the chair, he looked powerless, a rag doll swept along by the forces that kept sucking him back into Gloria's orbit.

"Could she help herself?"

"She was biting her tongue. I couldn't tell if she was tempted to just jump back in with me again. Or if she was getting ready to tell me off. But she just smiled and said nothing—"

Gloria had declined to enter the maelstrom. That much was clear. "And?"

"Seemed like a lifetime. She just sat there, and then she shook her head. I dragged myself off the chair and left and came here. I felt like a chook with its head cut off."

I wanted to chastise him. I wanted to point out how illogical his actions were. The effect of Gloria's slow head shake on him was staggering. His face was pale but his cheeks were blotchy red, as if she had slapped him. He looked to me now for comfort, for me to reassure him, the same beseeching look I had seen when Gloria had broken up with him.

I was silent. If this was cruelty, it was the only cruelty I could bring to bear. Why try to point out the glaring flaw in his behavior, his reasoning, when I knew he wouldn't see it? It was better this way; I wanted him to register what was happening, let it sink in. If at times I functioned as the supportive listener, now I had to be the mirror that accurately reflected his actions back to him.

Eventually he dragged himself out of the chair. I handed him his beeper. He shook his head as if to bemoan fate, and I shook my head too. "This is my last week of surgery," he said. "I start internal medicine next."

With a little wave, and an attempt at a smile, he shuffled out of my office, back to the hospital to shoulder his yoke.

O

That afternoon when I got home, David called me up. It was unexpected, and when he asked if I could play tennis ("I'm going crazy," he said, sotto voce, as if Emily might be close by), I heard it once more as a plea for commiseration, empathy, not really tennis.

Yes, I'd play, I said to David. I had no more words for him, but if tennis would make him feel better, then I was game. Maybe he needed to feel the ball smack the strings and vibrate up his arm and into his chest, maybe he needed to run hard, stretch and leap and bend, maybe he needed to be dwarfed by the overhang of rock, feel the ache in his feet and thereby discover his center. Maybe insight would come in this way. His home life and his hospital life were both complicated now—the court was the only arena where he knew exactly what to do. As for me, after Ashe's death, tennis had become poignant. To play was to remember him, to give him this tribute.

"The condo, right?"

"Yes . . . there."

I had told the boys that I would be by to tuck them in that night, but now, guiltily, I talked to them on the phone and said, "I have work to do," and that I'd see them the next day instead. They didn't seem to mind. Some days I would rush over there, my guilt and my need for them peaking as I walked in, only to find them absorbed in a game, not willing to drop everything because Daddy had come. And why should they? At first this was distressing, deflating. But now I saw it as a sign of stability; they knew I was there, that I was steadfast, and so they didn't need to make a big deal of my coming or going. Only Friday nights were sacred for the three of us.

O

David was waiting for me when I got to the condo, all warmed up and stretched. The air was dry and nippy, the lights of the court displaying halos, as if we had glaucoma. David played hard, chasing down every ball, running both of us, but especially himself, ragged. His body was focused on the tennis, but his mind, I sensed, was not there at all. "Want to play a set?" I called out, for only the second time ever.

I held my serve, stayed with him. It was 3–3, then 4–4 and his turn to serve. David wasn't trying hard or being particularly aggressive, content to hold his serve, confident, I'm sure, that he could reel me in whenever he wanted to. On his serve, he missed an easy volley, then failed to chase down a ball, double-faulted, missed a half volley, and suddenly I had broken him. I was up, 5–4.

I would be serving for the set, a position I had never been in with him. At the changeover, he giggled over his run of errors. Normally, he would not have been seriously worried. Nine times out of ten, he could break my serve if he put his mind to it. But that high-pitched giggle told me that he wanted to win this set very badly, that to lose to me would make this star-crossed day much worse.

I drank water, grabbed my racket, and willed myself to prove him wrong. I thought of Ashe, and how if I played my usual game, I'd certainly lose. To win, I had to gamble. "Do or die, Abe," I muttered. "Don't get into any sort of rally with him, if you can help it. Four big serves would do it. Hit your second serves just as if they are first serves. And if you do get into a baseline rally, be patient."

I started with a great slice serve, a can opener, dragging him wide. His return caught the tape; 15–0.

Then an ace; 30–love.

Something about hitting an ace always predisposed me to a double fault the next point, and that was what I did; 30–15. David was standing well inside the baseline now, threatening to chip and charge. On the next point, Ashe guiding my arm, I hit a service winner that he could only tip with his racket. It sailed over the fence and into the canyon.

My first match point. It had to happen here.

I hit a flat serve down the middle, and he stabbed at it, miraculously got it back, a looping shot with no pace that landed near midcourt. I ran around my backhand and hit a heavy and deep topspin shot to his backhand corner. I had the offensive now. He sliced it back, carefully and with good depth, clearing the net by inches. I took it on the forehand and sent it back to the same spot. It was a crosscourt rally, like one of our drills, working the diagonal, except that instead of hitting backhand to backhand, I was standing left of center and taking the ball on my forehand. I aimed for the inside edge of the ball to add sidespin so it would pull him even wider after it bounced. If my usual topspin ball looked oblong as it traveled through the air, this ball looked like an egg on its side.

My forehands were flowing, automatic, my body weight fully into each shot. I felt I was hitting what the pros called a "heavy" ball—good pace as the ball came off the court, rather than speed in the air. I eliminated any thought of the mechanics of the stroke other than trying to hit it inside out. I stretched him wider each time. I tried to stay relaxed, not to overhit.

His backhands, even as I pressed him, were perfect. It was beautiful to watch the way he leaned into the shot, the way his cocked wrist came through ahead of the ball, the way his left arm trailed for balance, its attitude so elegant, as if it were the arm of a ballet dancer.

Pretty though it may have been, it was still fundamentally a defensive shot and he had very little margin for error. He had to take the ball early, before it reached the peak of its bounce and became an awkward shoulder-high shot. He was blocking the ball, very little backswing—more a chip than a full stroke—using my pace, generating none of his own. The ball returned to me on a laser path, rising just enough to skim over the net, a great contrast to the parabolic arc of my shots.

Back and forth we went, neither of us willing to change direction. There were a couple of times when I thought of rushing the net behind my forehand, but a voice inside me said, *"Don't!"*

I sensed a trace of desperation in his backhand, having to scramble so wide for each one, time the ball so perfectly, risk snagging it on the net cord. He had fully expected me to miss before this, or to rush the net, or to lose patience and foolishly go for a winner.

After the seventh or eighth exchange in this rally (it felt like twenty), his backhand did finally tip the net cord, but it still came over. It popped up high in the air, most of its pace gone, a "put-away" shot for me at midcourt. There was nothing scarier than a put-away ball that you were *supposed* to be able to hit for a winner.

I ran forward but made sure I did not overrun the ball. My racket was back, my feet were set. I waited as the ball bounced, reached its zenith, and started to descend. I delayed my shot until the last possible moment, forcing David to commit one way or the other. Just as I began my swing, I sensed him run to cover the open court. I hit carefully behind him, to the backhand. He could only groan, and turn and watch the seams tumble end over end, land well inside the baseline, and then leap to the back fence as if in celebration.

"Good on ya," he said, and he looked at me with the pride of a teacher whose star pupil has just given a flawless recital.

To his credit, he didn't suggest we play another set so that he could punish me 6–0 for my impudence. Instead, he trotted up to the net, stuck out his hand. "Tried everything I could to win that last game," he said. "You played that last point like a pro."

○

I sat on the bench, bursting with pride, trying to catch my breath. David stood, one foot on the bench, panting. I was dying to hear his analysis of the last game, the last point.

"Well?"

"Emily is moving her stuff out," he said.

"What . . . ?"

"She's going to stay at her dad's. She might come over on the nights when I'm not on call."

He offered no explanation. He looked at me and shook his head and laughed, as if to say, "What else can possibly go wrong today?"

All thoughts of our game were pushed away.

Emily's leaving surely was connected to his encounter with Gloria, or his mood leading up to the encounter. To me, they were true, true and related. But he hadn't reported it that way.

Had he, in the AA spirit of "making amends" told Emily about the cafeteria encounter with Gloria? Or maybe Emily was intuitive enough—and his journals had sensitized her—to pick up on his ambivalence and confusion. Perhaps she asked him, "Have you seen Gloria today?" And then he had told her. That was one of his qualities. He didn't lie to others as much as he lied to himself.

He was getting his gear together hastily now, showing no signs of wanting to linger. He clearly didn't want me to pry into why Emily was leaving. He'd never manifested jealousy before, but now he was showing me that he realized I had feelings for Emily, that I would be as concerned for her as I was for him.

I watched him drive away.

○

I wasn't ready to leave yet. The glow of my success in that last game was still with me. If I hadn't pried into his situation with Emily, it was partly because I was being magnanimous after my win. I turned off the court lights and sat on the bench.

How sad that I couldn't celebrate this little tennis victory, couldn't bring it up with the one person I would most have wanted to analyze it with: David. Just a year ago, I would have spilled out every thought that had gone through my mind during that last service game. And he would have laughed, told me how he had tried to mess me up, change where he stood to receive serve, hope that I missed a first serve. And how when we got into the rally that pitted my forehand against his backhand, the old versus the new, topspin against slice, he had been sure that he could outlast me, tempt me to either change direction or go for too much, "And then I'd have had you by the short and curlies," he might have said.

38

*The HIV clinic the following week was full of familiar faces, patients chat-*ting with each other and with the staff, as if this were a reunion. At times, one momentarily forgot that a deadly virus was what brought us all together.

I poked my head into exam rooms that were open, greeted some of the patients I knew, then lingered to visit with Elvia and her four-year-old boy. Elvia was short and petite, her wrists so slender and her waist so narrow that I thought of her as fragile, an origami construction to be sheltered from the wind. In a clinic dominated by male patients, she was in the minority, everybody's favorite. She was elegantly dressed, as always, in black jeans and a black polo blouse, and wearing a colorful vest. Elvia's heart had been stolen by a man who in a one-month spell in Los Angeles introduced her to heroin, gave her HIV, and fathered this child. She had returned to El Paso, turned her back on that fleeting madness, but the virus had given her a wake-up call five years later. Her son was uninfected, but every time I saw him, I worried about his future. His father was dead, and his mother, despite all my efforts, was dropping pounds she could ill afford to lose. A herpetic lesion on her lip a month before had taken forever to heal, remaining raw and crusted. Now, finally, it had closed and only a small scar remained.

"Stay on the acyclovir for one more week," I told her.

"Do I look all right?"

"You look as beautiful as ever." She blushed with pride. To me, that lesion on the vermillion border of her lip had been a marker for the devastation of her immune system, of how she was approaching the steep part of the inexorable downhill slope of the disease. To her, it had meant much more than that; it had stigmatized her, hurt her vanity, made her struggle to hold her head up and come to the clinic with a sore so visible on her face. She had held a handkerchief over her face for weeks, reluctant, initially, for even me to see it. "Are you eating well?"

"Oh, my mother just cooks and cooks, and I try . . ."

"Did the Marinol [THC in tablet form] help?"

"Yes. Makes me high, though—I can't take it in the morning and still handle Carlos. I get all funny."

When I was leaving, Elvia handed me a large brown paper bag that she held flat on its side. "An enchilada casserole," she said. I hugged her, exchanged high fives with Carlos, and came out to the nurses' counter.

I whispered to Della, "I think I'm in love with Elvia."

"Sure!" Della said and snorted. "Easiest thing in the world is to love a dying woman." She pushed a chart into my hand and pointed to a room where a new patient waited.

Half an hour later when I emerged from the room, I saw David at the very end of the corridor, chart in hand, leaving a room where he had just finished with a patient. He had seen me too, and I felt a thrill, an exhilaration, as in a railway station when the person one awaits materializes out of the crowd.

Already internal medicine had transformed David, invested him once again with respectability: He was rid of scrubs, and instead wore a shirt and tie and a white coat that sparkled. The prodigal son had returned from the clutches of surgery, back into my world.

I moved toward him, weaving through staff and patients, a smile on my face. David smiled back, but hesitated. As if, had I not spotted him, had we not made eye contact, he might have moved in the opposite direction.

He stood and waited for me. He looked different, and not just because of the shirt and tie. Allowing for the fluorescent light of the clinic corridor, his skin looked sallow, stretched taut over his cheekbones. He looked older, tired, as if this truly were the platform of a railway station and years, not hours, had passed since we'd last seen each other.

Above his rumpled collar, the carotids hammered a beat. My inner metronome told me the pulse was over 100. The clinician in me was alert now—the camaraderie of our clinic had not lulled me into complete inattention. I was inches from him and my senses probed and danced off his body: pupils perhaps a bit dilated, nasolabial folds asymmetric, no moistness on the tongue, a hard descent of the Adam's apple as he swallowed, a faint, almost medicinal, odor . . . and he squirmed under this scrutiny.

"Hey! You okay?"

"Hey, yourself! Fine, fine."

"You look bushed . . . different."

The buccinator muscle twitched like a horse's skin in summer, drawing up the angle of his mouth. His eyes dropped to the chart in his hand.

I felt a knot in my stomach. Softly, my words rising up from the depths of my body and reaching my mouth, I said, "David, have you used?"

He looked up now, looked me straight in the eye, hesitated for a few seconds that felt like minutes . . . "Yes."

As I was about to say something, a voice said to me, You must remember this, you must hold on to this moment, hold on to the sound of Della laughing, and a woman talking on the phone in rapid-fire Spanish, the rustle of a hand searching through the candy basket for the right piece, the way the light from the ceiling hits David's thinning crown. The observer, the journal keeper, the recorder of events had pushed aside the clinician and was looking down at this scene, saying, urgently, *You must remember this.* In the midst of everything, this inner voice kept an even pitch, maintained equanimity, saw this and every event as an augury that shaped the next.

I wasn't angry yet. Instead, I felt tremendously sorry for David. I wanted to throw up a wall around us and protect him. I knew how much it cost him to say yes, to admit using to me. How cruel that this yes should be the measure of his trust in me. Brick by brick he had built up over two years of sobriety, created some semblance of a place for himself in medical society. He had been given his one-month token, and then his one-year and two-year tokens from NA, medals for sobriety. Now they had tumbled out of his pocket and become irretrievable. He was bankrupt again.

I stumbled past him, down the corridor, needing to find a place where we would be out of earshot. It was my face I worried about now—that *I* would give it away.

I stopped at the blind end of a hallway where extra chairs and infusion couches awaiting repair were stored and where a nurses' counter sat, unoccupied. David followed me.

I spun on him, my sadness swept away by rage, a flash flood that came boiling out of me, threatening to sweep him away like loose sediment. He flinched.

"I don't know what came over me," he blurted out, perhaps to stop me from speaking. "It was Friday . . . Surgery was over . . . I had time on my hands. I knew I was going to use. And all the things I was supposed to do when I feel that way—call my sponsor, pray, call you—went out the window. My mind suspended all action and my body went and got the stuff, shot it up."

"Oh come on, that's bullshit!" It was now Monday. That meant he had shot up three days before. "Where was Emily?"

"She's out of town, she comes back tomorrow."

"You plotted this. You waited for your chance . . . Did you shoot up again?" I was hissing, trying not to raise my voice, and he was whispering back.

"I finished the last of it on Saturday, early morning."

The clinician in me was calculating the hours before his urine would be clean. But the clinician was pushed aside by the tennis partner who had been betrayed, deceived, the partnership desecrated—

"Tell me the goddamn truth. Tell me all. Don't try to color this!"

"I got more, shot up Saturday night. And the wee hours of Sunday morning. Then slept all of Sunday."

Just over twenty-four hours, the clinician figured; his urine would still be positive.

"It was stupid, just stupid," he said. "I'm dreading running into Dr. Binder, and hoping they don't call me to pathology for a urine test today. Or tomorrow."

He made a fist, and rested his head on it. His body was shaking and his eyes were moist, suppressing tears. "I hate myself, I hate what I did." Was he going to punch himself in the face? I would have let him do it, let him hurt himself.

What next? What to do with this sobbing, wretched figure? Turn him in, of course. Expose the mischief. But even as I thought of turning him in, my mind was also asking whether this lapse of his could be concealed. What if it were a one-time lapse, a momentary weakness, a slip, not a complete fall off the wagon?

"But why? David, why? . . . Why?" I said, straightening up, my hands on my hips, my feet apart, ignoring his crying.

It took him a while to stop, to look me in the eye, ready to meet his fate.

If I was ever going to turn him in, the moment for that had passed. The fact that I was debating what to do, engaging in a dialogue with him, gave me away: I had already capitulated. It was surprising now to realize that being his senior in the medical-school hierarchy really meant nothing. When the heat was on, as it was now, the role that we had both slipped into, that defined us, was that of friends, equals. His superiority on the tennis court or mine in the hospital were superfluous. It was because I was his friend that he had replied honestly when I'd asked if he had used.

○

We returned to the patient rooms. I asked him to present his patient to me. David opened the chart in his hand, but instead of reading from it, he read from an index card on which he had summarized data from the chart and from the laboratory computers. "Mr. Salazar is a thirty-two-year-old Hispanic male, well-known to this clinic, who first presented in 1989 when he was found to be HIV positive . . ."

Two students drifted over and stood by me, listening to the presentation. I looked at David as if I were studying a stranger. I saw that in the left pocket of his white coat he had a blue book identical to mine, and behind it, index cards in rubber bands. His reflex hammer—the one I had given him—was tucked behind that. He had a flashlight and a couple of tongue depressors in his breast pocket, and his stethoscope and tuning fork in his right coat pocket. He looked the model student, cast in my own image, if only . . .

"His CD4 count at the time was 550. AZT was started in September of 1990 and two months ago, when his CD4 count dropped to 140, he was switched to DDI. He has had one admission in December of last year for suspected but unproven PCP pneumonia." He put away the index card. "This is a routine follow-up, to see how he is tolerating his meds."

I looked for something to critique in his presentation, but I could not find it. The four of us entered the exam room. I took a good forty minutes with the patient, going over him thoroughly, pointing out a few minor things David had missed—a molluscum lesion near the eye, an eosinophilic folliculitis on the skin of the back and chest.

I asked one of the students to feel for the spleen and repeated my aphorism, "Let the spleen palpate your fingers, don't think of it as your fingers palpating the spleen. And don't dig, there's no gold there. Let your fingers watch and wait."

I demonstrated how to feel for radio-femoral delay. I asked David what he knew of coarctation of the aorta.

"It's a narrowing . . . usually distal to left subclavian near the insertion of ligamentum arteriosum. About seven percent of the time it's associated with congenital heart disease—"

"Which congenital heart disease?"

"Um . . . bicuspid aortic valve?"

"Go on."

"It's . . . twice as common in males . . . it's associated with Turner's syndrome, aneurysms of the circle of Willis . . ."

I was visualizing the page in *Harrison's*, and so far David seemed to be repeating it almost verbatim.

"What might you see on the chest X ray?"

"You might see a dilated subclavian vein, high on the left mediastinal border, and a widened ascending aorta. Also the 'three' sign—like the number three—along the left paramediastinal shadow . . . you might see notching of the ribs due to erosion."

The other students were slack-jawed, not knowing this was a setup, a topic that David had looked up for our team a year ago. Still, it was impressive that he remembered all this.

I had David demonstrate how to check for peripheral neuropathy by testing vibratory sense over the patient's bony prominences, and then checking the tendon reflexes. At one point, I held David's wrist as his fingers grasped his reflex hammer, and I shook his wrist, saying, "Loosen the wrist. You want to strike the tendon with a sharp, short tap that glances off. No shame in a floppy wrist in this clinic," which was good for a laugh from all present but David and me.

I spent a long time talking with the patient. If I overdid it, it was to impress on David how this alone—being a doctor—should have been enough. There was so much to learn and perfect and polish and understand in medicine. I recalled the words from the first paragraph of *Harrison's Principles of Internal Medicine*, a paragraph written by the original editors which had then disappeared for a few editions but was back in the edition I had given David:

> *No greater opportunity, responsibility, or obligation can fall to the lot of a human being than to become a physician. In the care of the suffering, he needs technical skill, scientific knowledge, and human understanding. He who uses these with courage, with humility, and with wisdom will provide a unique service for his fellow man and will build an enduring edifice of character within himself. The physician should ask of his destiny no more than this, he should be content with no less.*

Why had doctoring not been enough for David?

I left David to finish writing up his case, and to give the patient his prescriptions and send him for a blood draw. I moved on to another room. David saw two other patients, presenting one to Dr. Ho and the other to Dr. Guerra. At the end of the clinic, I asked David if he had been paged for a urine test.

"No, thank God. It's almost five, so I'm going to turn my beeper off."

o

I had David meet me on the tennis court that evening. I didn't give him a choice. Didn't ask him if he had any plans for the evening. The power and the balance had slid my way and I was wielding it. No more pussyfooting around with him. If he wanted my cooperation, my protection, by God, I would make him play to my tune. No more sitting back and watching him unravel. There were volumes I could impart to him on medicine, but there were also a couple of lessons on not fucking up that he should hear.

I didn't necessarily want to play tennis. I just needed a place away from the hospital to make sense of what had happened. What better venue than our court where, at our last meeting, he had announced, in the cryptic manner of the last few months, that he and Emily were breaking up.

David was early, waiting for me. Penitent, eager to please, anxious to decipher my emotional state.

"I know it won't happen again," he said while I set my racket bag down. "It served to remind me of why I was in recovery. It was stupid."

"It's not me you have to convince."

"You're right."

"And what, exactly, stops it from happening again?"

"It can't," he said, hearing the hollowness in that statement. He tried again, more forcefully, "It won't."

At least he didn't say "trust me." It would have been better if he had been silent. I had wanted to see him after work to extract some security, some collateral that would justify my position of keeping silent. In the hours since he'd told me, I had begun to feel morally weak, angry for now being part of this deception.

"Where did you get it?" I said, pushing his nose into it.

He had been stretching and bouncing on his feet and my question stopped him in his tracks. There was a tremulousness and a jerkiness to him, even when he was standing still, probably the effect of all his neurons firing in overdrive for two nights, fueled by cocaine, and now running on empty.

"The corner of Ochoa."

He anticipated my next question. "I'd removed a syringe from the hospital that afternoon." He lifted his arm to me, a pathetic offering, so that I could see the puncture marks in the crook of his elbow.

"You had *hours* before you actually used . . . You were in control." I was whipping him with shame, and he had no recourse but to take it.

"It's . . . the nature of the beast. It felt as though a switch had been thrown and set things into motion. Another person, another David was—"

I cut him off.

"Have you talked to your sponsor?"

If I could not be an authority figure in David's life, I knew his sponsor was. One of the terms of his being at Texas Tech, in addition to the random urine screens, was that he satisfy his sponsor.

"No! Because if I do, he'll definitely call Dr. Binder. And then it's all over." He was whining now. "I . . . really think I can control this. I really do."

I moved away from him to the baseline. I felt a twinge of remorse for raking him over the coals. Was I a fair-weather friend? Was I making up for the last few months of feeling pushed away, taking second place to Gloria, and Emily, and his house? But no, pity for him was what had allowed him to get this far.

I put a ball into play, and as I hit it, I completely lost my stomach for the tennis. I walked off and David hit the ball back to the empty court.

I sat on the bench, my head in my hands.

He collected the ball and came and sat quietly next to me.

"Does Emily know?"

He shook his head.

He was silent after that.

After a long while, I gathered my things.

"I'll call you," I said, and gave him a look that said I expected him to be nowhere but at his house.

39

The very next night a knock on the door startled me awake from my recliner. Once before I had been awakened like this, that time by the sound of a key fumbling in my lock, and someone cursing under his breath. I had shouted, "Hey," and then a voice on the other side had said, "Sorry," and unsteady footsteps clanged a retreat on the metal stairs. A neighbor, I imagined, drunk perhaps, who had absentmindedly ascended the wrong set of stairs. I had done the same thing sober.

But this knock felt purposeful, insistent. It was after midnight and I had fallen asleep with a book on my lap, a half-full beer bottle wedged between my thigh and the armrest of the recliner. David's secret had weighed heavily on me that day, made me cringe when I passed my department chairman in the Tech hallway. The knock on the door caused me to leap out of the recliner and spill the beer onto the carpet. My heart felt as if it were about to fly out of my chest. "They" had finally come to get me.

I opened the door cautiously, the chain still on.

Standing there, her eyes brimming, lips quivering, hugging herself even though it was not that cold, was Emily. She shifted weight from one foot to the other, as if standing on hot coals. She had never visited me alone before.

No sooner had I removed the chain, before I could even ask her in, than she blurted out, "David's using again."

All that day I had, like a parent, kept tabs on him. I had him come by my office morning, noon, and late afternoon, sickening of this vigil and of his contrite, tail-between-the-legs demeanor in my presence. All day he had held his breath, waiting for the summons for a urine test, a summons which, if it had come, would have ended the charade. But it did not come. When he'd said he had an AA meeting that evening, I had been relieved.

Emily sat on the edge of the recliner. I reached around her and cleared the debris. Her legs were twined together, her arms close against her body, the hands dabbing ineffectually at her face. Her eyes floated in tears, such misery in them that I wanted to reach for her, to hold her in my arms, to bodily lift her out of the wretched situation David had sucked her into. I brought her a box of tissues, then sat cross-legged in front of her.

Had she just found out what I already knew—that he'd shot up over the weekend? Or had something happened that evening? She fought for composure now. Each time she looked at me, tears came brimming out. I brought her water.

"I just came back from Austin," Emily said, finally, setting her arms down on her thighs, her eyes swollen, the tip of her nose as red as her lips. "When David picked me up at the airport . . . he smelled. He looked as if he hadn't shaved or showered, even though he had. And he'd dropped weight in just three days."

I knew the look very well.

"'What's wrong? What's wrong?' I kept saying. And he wouldn't reply. He just said, 'I'm taking you home.' I asked him again and again, 'Did you use? Did you use?' and he denied it. I asked him if there was another woman . . ."

Another woman would have been preferable.

David had dropped her at her father's house, still refusing to say why he looked strange. Emily had put her bags down and raced after him in her car, but lost him. She'd driven to David's place—their place—but he wasn't there. "I've been driving around for hours, going back there every twenty minutes or so. A little while ago his car was finally there. I knocked on the door but he wouldn't let me in. Finally he opened the door but kept the chain on. I kept screaming, 'Let me in! Let me in!' I made so much noise that he had to let me in or have the neighbors start coming out . . ."

Her blue eyes darkened as she relived the indignity of having to scream to get into the house that she had furnished with him, that they had lived in together.

"Now he was shifty, creepy to look at. I was scared. I asked him where he had been all this time. When he said 'Furr's supermarket,' my heart sank."

"Why . . . what . . . ?"

"He's writing bad checks! He buys lotion or something small for a few dollars, writes a check for thirty. If he's already bouncing checks, he must have used up all his money, our money." She began to weep again, not for him, but for herself.

I picked up the phone and dialed David's number.

"Abraham, I'm scared," Emily said, her lower lip trembling, putting her hand on mine, as if I should know this before I spoke to him. "If you see him now, he looks like a different creature, no relationship to David Smith. And he's said to me a million times that if he uses again his use escalates so quickly that it's like taking a gun to his head."

I shook my head, dismissing this. "David hurts himself, hits himself, only when he has an audience, when it serves a purpose. He doesn't do it in a vacuum."

The phone rang in Sunset Heights. I pictured it echoing off the high ceilings and wooden floors. Somewhere in that house, David, high on cocaine, heard it ring, knew it was me, and did not answer.

I was furious with David, furious at this deception that had lasted not even twenty-four hours, pained to see Emily so crushed and beaten. "How stupid! How idiotic!" I said. And in my anger, in my outrage, there was also a sense of clarity, a relief in not having to be the guardian of his secret anymore. The other shoe had dropped; no, it had crashed through the ceiling, sounded a wake-up call that would not be ignored.

I paced the floor, still holding the phone, no longer passive, a man of action. Emily had settled back into the recliner, curling her feet under her.

I asked Emily if she had the number for Jim, David's sponsor.

"It's in the phone book." She looked it up.

When he came on the line, I introduced myself, said Emily was with me, and described what had happened.

He was nonchalant, not angry with David, almost bored. A clinician discussing a familiar clinical scenario. His tone made my pacing around the apartment appear stupid.

"I'm not surprised," Jim said. "I'd seen it coming for months."

He'd seen it coming for months.

To hear that infuriated me. If he'd seen it coming and I hadn't, it made him the wise man and me the fool. And if he'd seen it coming, why didn't he do something? I was about to respond when he said, "I'll try calling David," and hung up.

Emily and I sat there looking at each other. If the relapse had been coming for months, when exactly had it begun? The moment he left Mickie's? The day his mother died? His first encounter with the resurgent Gloria?

In a few minutes, the phone rang.

"I spoke to David," Jim said. (Why had David picked up the phone for him and not for me?)

"And?"

"Oh, he was bullshitting me, in denial. So I hung up on him."

Here was a man who had no trouble putting David's behavior into perspective.

"What do we do? Should we break down the door and go get him?"

He actually laughed. "What for?"

"Because . . . he might overdose? To stop him from using?"

"David's responsible for David," he said, his tone suggesting that we were not really talking about David anymore but about me, about the annoyance he heard in my voice. "You aren't responsible for David. Don't get caught in that trap. No one can make him do anything. No one made him use. No one can stop him from using but himself."

I had no response to this.

"An addict is his own worst enemy," he said now, more gently, "and you or I can help him only when he decides to help himself. Right now, he's blown it."

○

The next morning, when I got to work, I saw David's car in the parking lot. The phone rang as I walked into my office. It was Emily.

"Did you speak to him?" I asked. "'Cause he's here."

"I know. Jim called Dr. Lou Binder. Lou summoned David to his office and asked him for a urine sample. At that point he fessed up."

"God! I wonder what Binder will do now."

"He's on a plane right now with David," Emily said, her voice catching, "heading to Atlanta, to rehab."

Part III

In these days of modern tennis a player
is as strong as his weakest stroke.

—*William T. Tilden II*

40

Carlsbad, even at midnight, is a golfer's town. The bellboy asks about my golf bag as we putter along narrow paths between manicured lawns on the way to my room. I point to the Samsonite—featherlight and rattling on his golf cart—two tennis rackets and little else in it.

"Tennis," I say, weary after a whole day of airports and planes.

I ask the bellboy whether the old man still teaches. Or is he being used as a come-on, illusory, like the spa beauty photographed on the edge of a steaming whirlpool.

"He still teaches," says the bellboy. "He's always there. Giving lessons."

The next morning at seven-thirty I call to say I want a lesson. They check his schedule and say, "Possibly." Yes, possibly even today. They will check with him when he comes in. He will call me. Fifteen minutes later, the phone rings while I sip coffee and read the calorie count printed on the breakfast menu. The old man himself is on the line. He pronounces my name carefully.

"I can take you at twelve o'clock," he says. "You want half hour?"

"One hour."

"Okay . . . You know it is a hundred dollars."

"Yes, sir," I say.

I check in early at the pro shop. I hear him talk in an office at the back. I watch some doubles on center court, and after a long time—I am very early—I sense him come out. The same voice I heard on the phone—raspy and faintly accented—asks a man sitting near me if he is waiting for a lesson.

"It's me," I say, standing and turning to face him.

He is much shorter than I imagined and absurdly pigeon-toed. After offering me a handshake, he takes off in a brisk crab walk, his trunk swaying from side to side, two rackets clutched under the crook of his arm, head held high despite the stoop of his back that robs him of more inches. He wears white cotton warm-up pants and a predominantly white tennis jacket—zipped, and upturned collar—in which he floats as if in a life vest. A floppy white cap shields his face but not the eagle eyes perched above the pointed nose. His tennis shoes are high-topped, at least two sizes too big and richly padded. The laces are very loose and yet the tongue of the shoe bulges out. I picture the varus forefoot, curled inward, scrunching the last, all the weight on the outer edge of the foot as he waddles.

"How long you been playing tennis?"

(I barely hear him, he is walking so far ahead of me.)

"Twenty years," I say. "Off and on," I add as an afterthought.

If he hears me, he gives no sign. Maybe this is something he asks without paying any attention to the answer. I imagine he gets answers like: "I just took it up last week." Or: "I have never played but I love to watch Chrissie Evert."

We are at the court.

"Show me your grips," he says, fingering his own racket.

I show him my forehand—extreme Western. He makes a sucking sound between his teeth and I think I see a grimace. The darkened sun furrows etched on his face are so close to a scowl, it is difficult to tell.

"Now show me the backhand."

Again a contortion of the face suggests he would prefer more Continental.

"The serve now."

I show him a backhand grip.

"Good. Can you slice the backhand?"

"Yes."

"Can you slice the forehand to approach the net?"

". . . Yes."

"Good." He is relieved; I am salvageable. "'Cause you can't approach the net with topspin.

"Listen to me," he says, coming up so close that I tense. *"Listen to what I am going to tell you because it is the most important thing about tennis. What's your name? Abraham? Abraham, listen to me, this is what tennis is all about:*

"The ball must be hit deep, or angled away.

"The short ball must be punished outright—or used to attack.

"The game is won at the net.

"That's it," he says.

He studies me carefully, looking perhaps for doubt, disagreement, or understanding.

I feel a sense of bewilderment. Not that any of these aphorisms—*"keep it deep," "attack the short ball," "win at the net"*—are new. Yet, at this instant, while I stand on immaculate Har-Tru no different from Har-Tru anywhere, under a pristine Carlsbad sky that could be Abu Dhabi sky, fingering a racket handle as familiar as a lover's instep under the bedsheet, a lifetime of tennis is temporarily erased and it is as if I am hearing for the first time how the game is played. The mechanical aspects of hitting the ball—head still, knees bent, eyes on the ball, the usual focus of any tennis lesson I have taken in the past—seem banal compared to the philosophy of hitting the ball.

"There is nothing else," he says, as if reading my thoughts. *"That's it."*

His scrutiny has not ceased. I am shocked at the simplicity of the explanation. It's not to be dismissed, for this is, after all, the man reputed to be the wisest strategist in tennis, the man who made Connors the potent force he is. This is the man who won three NCAA tennis championships, three Pro Singles titles, twice beating Pancho Gonzales.

I feel a warmth from him; perhaps he realizes a catharsis has occurred in the student and what follows for the teacher will be simple denouement. In the depths of the left pupil I see a hint of a cloudy-white opacity, a reminder of the passage of time.

"So now," he says, *"we will hit some balls. Some will be short. Hit them and come in. Hit deep and to the center for now."*

We begin to rally. It is a feeling akin to communion as his ball, heavy and deliberate, is met by my racket and propelled back, deep, but wobbling eccentrically, revealing a diffidence that diminishes the longer the ball is in play. He hits a short ball—deliberately. I slice a backhand approach—head down, knees bent, follow-through deep to the target—and he effortlessly lobs over my left shoulder and into the backhand corner. It is not its height that makes it unplayable—the ball is behind me before I even see it.

I go back to the baseline, rally again, approach on a short ball—and the same thing happens. He strikes my approach on the rise; a wonderfully timed half-volley lob hit with a firm wrist and careful follow-through. That lob and his killer two-handed forehand were what he was best known for when he was on the tour. The stroke begins in the misshapen feet and travels up the bowed knees and into the locked hips that are now magically fluid and supple; the completeness of the stroke fuses disparate and inconsonant parts into one synchronous thrust. The ball is struck well out in front, at the apogee of the uncoiling—as if the ball were secondary and of less import than the stroke itself. He holds the follow-through, punctuating the stroke, remaining motionless as the ball rises, spinning in the same axis as its flight, over my left shoulder and into the backhand corner that beckons.

"You need to think," he says. "That is what you need to learn. Your strokes are not bad. When you see my racket like this, you know it is a short ball—start coming in at that moment. If you anticipate, you can hit a better approach. Let us keep working on the approach."

He feeds me short balls and I approach. Unless my approach is deep enough to push him onto the back foot, he punishes it with the lob—each one identical to the one before, arching over my backhand and into the corner. I am now so intent on coming in that when he hits a high ball that lands at the baseline and kicks up, accelerating, I make an awkward high swing—more an act of self-preservation than a legitimate stroke—and I pop up a short ball. When I look up, he is two feet inside the service box, appearing out of nowhere. He slaps the ball with a hint of underspin at a sharp angle crosscourt. I hear a guttural thwump as the shot comes off his racket; his stroke epitomizes the idea of "put the ball away." I stand lead-footed, watching *the ball skid low, graze the inside of the line on its way to set the chain-link fence into song.*

"Come here!" he says, slapping the net with his racket edge.

"I knew you were going to hit short before you knew. My ball caught you flat on your heels. You had to hit short! Remember, all tennis shots are played waist-high. You should have moved back to hit that shot. Use your head."

He makes as if to return to the baseline, but thinks better of it and continues:

"If the ball is coming this high over the net, where will it bounce?"

"High and deep," I say.

"So?"

"So I must move back," I say.

"And if it comes in low over the net, like this, where will it bounce?"

"Short."

"So what will you do?"

"Slice and come in."

"Yes. Go back and let us try some more. Short ball, come in."

He walks back to the hamper, picks it up, and hooks it over his shoulder while he extracts seven balls. He sets the hamper down the same way—without flexing his back or bending at the waist. Seeing his effort, I resolve not to waste balls.

More approaches. My heart pounds behind my eyes and sweat soaks my T-shirt and forms a V on the front of my tennis shorts. If the approach is not deep, he punishes it—always with the lob. I begin to recognize the flight path of the lob; a lucent arc carved out of red Carlsbad air.

When I finally hit ten good approaches, he says:

"That is what I want! Come here."

I go to the net, grateful for a respite.

He looks around and lowers his voice: "Of all the pros, John is the best," he says. "For my money, he is the best because he knows how to read the short ball and take advantage. That, my friend, is what it is all about. That is the name of the game.

"Those baseliners—you know who I mean, the kids who just now came along—I'm not saying they cannot make money or

that they cannot beat good players. But to be a great, you have to take the short ball and come in. You have to be an attacking player. You put the pressure on the other guy. You make him make the shot."

Forty minutes have gone by and we have spent most of it on the approach shot. In the next few minutes he looks at all my other shots. He has me volley at the net. He is happy only when I hit the volley with a racket almost perpendicular to the net, angling the ball away acutely and with pace.

"That's the only kind of volley to hit," he says. "You hit your first volley from here," he says, standing two feet inside the ser-vice box. "And you angle it to where the guy is not standing. Unless the score is forty–fifteen—in which case you go behind him. If he has a weakness, then go for the weakness. Keep attacking it. Get his momentum going so it carries him off the court."

He looks at my drop volleys.

"Drop volleys are for soft balls only, and they are always hit crosscourt," he says. "Don't try it on a ball that is hit hard. Nobody can do that. Nobody.

"You can't let the ball drop too low before you hit the drop vol-ley. If you let it drop, your opponent knows you have to hit it up. And so he will be coming in. Unless he is stupid.

"If he is stupid, you will win anyway."

We practice the lob. In all the lessons I have ever had, this is the first time I have practiced the lob.

He looks at my serve, return of serve, lob, overhead, and passing shots. He makes only minor comments. I get the feeling he is uncon-cerned, given the nature of our brief lesson, about trying to correct the mechanics of a shot. It is the use of a shot that he dwells on:

"The best time to lob," he says, "is on the first volley. Because your opponent's momentum is moving forward."

I think about the lob over my backhand that he has hit at least sixteen times today.

○

When the hour is up, I help him pick up balls. He has not bro-ken a sweat under his jacket. We walk back together, me beside him, in stride, in rapture, for I feel I have been given a special insight. I think of the countless times and the many years he has done this, imparted his principles to a student; there is in it a faith and a doggedness that reminds me of the old horse-and-buggy doctor going out season after season in all kinds of weather to see the ill. When he was a top-flight player, trophies and fame were his reward, but now, in the obscurity of this court on the edge of the property, he still puts on a class act every time. I find this inspiring both as a teacher of medicine and as a student of tennis.

○

In his office, I show him an old picture of my eldest son that I happen to have in the pocket of the racket cover. My son is four and he is in a tennis hat, pointing at the camera, his dimples irresistible. I ask him if he will sign it.

I see the first smile of the day on that face and a hint of tenderness. The teeth are perfectly straight.

"What's his name?" he asks.

He writes painstakingly, laboriously, and as if nothing is more important than this, yet a felt-tipped racket would work better in those knobby hands: "To Steven: Punish the short ball. Pancho Segura."

41

A week after David left, I met Gato. Fever, chills, visible track marks, and a heart murmur were his presenting complaints. The note of the junior-most medical student had put it together: "IVDA with fever, rule out endocarditis."

I expected to see a much younger patient, not the fifty-five-year-old man shirtless on the edge of the bed, as motionless as a predator who has sensed its quarry approach. His cheekbones were puffy and prominent. Deep behind them, eyes as dark as raisins took my measure, and gave away nothing.

A comb, a toothbrush, and a razor were laid out parallel on his bedside table—not by the sink. His slippers sat neatly at the foot of his bed. He completely filled this small, confined space with his presence, as if he were at ease with being sequestered, had learned to take possession of such environments and make them his.

His ears and his brow were linked by facial musculature. When I introduced myself, his ears pulled back a good inch, and his hairline, which began almost at his eyebrows, retracted to show some forehead. I took this movement to be a hello. A half-smoked cigarette, the end pinched off, sat securely behind his left ear.

I studied him with as much interest as he did me: IVDAs of his age were a rarity. If they hadn't given it up by fifty, they were generally dead—from an overdose, infection, trauma, AIDS, or cirrhosis. Long incarceration had probably spared him.

Taut biceps, a hairless body, well-defined pectorals, and very little subcutaneous fat gave him a catlike, youthful quality. A tiger on his chest, the Virgin of Guadalupe on his left shoulder, and a devil on his right forearm were clues to the polarities in his life. Only the last, a red-and-black job, looked like the work of a tattoo gun. The rest were monochrome, dull—jailhouse art.

"When did you last shoot up?"

"Shoot up?" he said. "No, *ese*, someone's been feeding you tales. I don't shoot up."

"Save that for your probation officer. He's going to know anyway, 'cause they did a urine screen on you when you came in."

"You need my permission to do that."

"Here's your signature where you gave permission," I said, opening the chart and finding the page.

From the drawer in his bedside table, he extracted a spectacle case, unfolded his bifocals, and leaned forward, not touching the chart, to peer at the evidence. A tattoo on his flank became evident when he leaned forward. I hadn't seen it till he leaned over.

"*La Tuna?*" I said, pointing to the tattoo. *La Tuna* was a federal penitentiary twenty miles up I-10 in New Mexico. The tattoo was the head and torso of a woman, a woman as familiar to me now as if she were my own sister.

He took the bifocals off and returned them to their case and to the drawer. He gave me the prison-yard stare, clenched his fists. I held his gaze.

"Maybe you were just there visiting?" I said.

Then his face cracked and he gave me the magnanimous smile of a poker player whose bluff had been called, but who was still utterly confident that he would win in the end.

"You're pretty good, Doc," he said in a low, raspy voice, and stuck out his hand. "Gato Salazar."

"I'm pretty good with my patients—blind when it comes to my friends."

Who better to tell David's story to? How David had fooled me. How I had missed all the warning signs. Gato listened and seemed pleased to learn of a doctor in his fraternity.

"What warning signs, Doc? Don't kid yourself. It's a magnet, always out there, pulling you in. I was clean six years one time and then, just like that," he said, snapping his fingers, "I saw something orange on the ground . . ."

"A U-100 syringe?"

"God knows what it was. But yeah, that's what it made me think of. Hell, anything can trigger it. To see a roll of bills," he said, approximating it with his thumb and index finger, and smiling at the thought, "or to walk down a street where you shot up . . . Fuck, just talking about it with you makes me want to go out and get a quarter."

○

That evening a rainstorm caused a smashup on the interstate and forced me to take the Border Highway home. I drove alongside the river, my headlights on, windshield wipers squeaking prosodically, only the chicken-wire fence—the tortilla curtain—separating me from the Rio Grande. Every five hundred yards I passed a green border patrol Bronco that sat facing the river, the officers looking bored but raising their binoculars to their eyes every so often.

The Border Highway sat below the interstate, separated from it by the canal and by railway tracks. A train ran alongside me, momentarily disorienting me, making me misjudge my speed.

As I overtook the train, it struck me that this town was all parallel lines: first the long ridge of the Franklins, then Mesa Street, then Interstate 10, then the Franklin Canal, then the railway tracks, then the Border Highway, then the Rio Grande. And on the other side of the river, the parallels continued in El Paso's poorer twin: *Avenida Riberena*, and further back, *Avenida 16 de Septiembre*, then the mountains of Juárez that were mirror images of the Franklins except that in place of the thunderbird, they displayed giant man-made white letters that said, in Spanish: *LA BIBLIA ES LA VERDAD; LEELA*. The Bible is the truth; read it.

I winced when I opened the apartment. Many a night during the previous week, I had simply taken off, unable to stay there, roaming in my car till the wee hours. I sat down now, on the floor, by the door, miserable. As precisely as a song heard on the car radio could transport me to a specific period in time, the rain sounds returned me to childhood and the uncertainties of those monsoon days. I could see my mother sitting by the fire, stirring the ashes, peering into it for hours, unresponsive to human voices, my father as invisible and silent as ever.

My friendship with David, during its inception, and during the heady period when our lives revolved so much around each other, had held out the promise of leading somewhere, to something extraordinary, some vital epiphany—what, precisely, I couldn't be sure of. Still, that was how it *felt*—magical, special. And that was enough; that was reason to keep going.

Playing tennis seemed to express this, as if it were a beautiful experiment we two had created out of thin air. The uniforms were simple, the equipment rudimentary, but in our rat-a-tat volleying at the net, in our mastery of spin, in the rallies, in the way the rackets functioned as extensions of our bodies, in the way we came to know each other's tics and idiosyncrasies, in the way we controlled the movement of a yellow ball in space, we were imposing *order* on a world that was fickle and capricious. Each ball that we put into play, for as long as it went back and forth between us, felt like a charm to be added to a necklace full of spells, talismans, and fetishes, which would one day add up to an Aaron's rod, an Aladdin's lamp, a magic carpet. Each time we played, this feeling of restoring order, of mastery, was awakened. It would linger for a few days but then wane. The urge to meet and play would build again. I had no solitary ambition with the tennis itself—I wasn't trying to raise my game in order to enter a tournament, collect trophies, and yet it was terribly important to keep playing with David, to play beautifully, to play exquisitely, and with great care, as if the universe rested on the flight of a ball.

People we knew and saw in the hospital led lives that to us seemed complex, unnecessarily encumbered, frivolous even: family reunions, office parties, the ski vacation, the big boat, the small plane . . . while the two of us stood apart from all that, as if we knew there was something more—we didn't know what—that we sought, but by God, we were heading there. We led our solitary but parallel lives, on the border, looking in, waiting for the event that would transform us completely.

Of course, it never came. The world ticked on without much of a hitch—Warren Beatty married Annette Bening, Mike Tyson went to jail, Johnny Carson signed off on the *Tonight* show, Arthur Ashe died . . . David relapsed . . .

Now it seemed to be a delusion of ours—of mine. What had manifested itself was David's gradual unraveling, and my increasing despair that whatever it was we were aspiring to became less and less attainable with every passing week.

O

Now that David was gone, I felt a curtain had been drawn back to show me the apartment the way it really was. What I saw was a small space overrun with books, not a single thing on the walls, none of the creature comforts—a sofa, a microwave, a bed—that it seemed stupid to do without. I felt guilty for subjecting the boys to this, even though they thought it was charming just the way it was, a tree house.

I resolved to buy a condo, or perhaps a cottage. Someplace to lay down a doormat, etch my name in curlicue letters on a wooden plaque, and put an end to this exile, this transiency that now felt like quarantine. I pictured a bedroom for me, and one more for the boys. Books aplenty, but this time in bookcases. What it must have, what I could see most clearly, was a kitchen with blue tiles, a zinc sink, a zinc refrigerator, gleaming pots and pans hanging from the ceiling, and a giant oven that I would fire up, keep aglow, my hearth from which I would not be uprooted. I was ready to stake my claim to this edge of the world.

42

"Did you hear?" I said, setting my tray down in front of Gloria and taking off my coat. I didn't know her well enough to justify this familiarity, but as far as I was concerned, in these few weeks after David's departure, all the old rules and civilities had been suspended.

She paused in midbite. Her body tensed. Her pupils dilated, perhaps imagining he had robbed a bank, or worse.

"He relapsed. They sent him to a place in Atlanta for doctors with drug problems."

"I'm not surprised," she said finally, after swallowing what was in her mouth.

"I was," I said.

She studied me. At any other time I might have been self-conscious, embarrassed.

"I'm sorry . . . sorry for you," she said.

I shrugged, as if it were no big deal. But she had diagnosed me.

"He cared for you—" she said.

"Didn't care for himself too well—"

"—cared for you, but he's destined to disappoint."

We paused. These were more words than we had ever exchanged before. She smiled now.

"I've written him out of my life. *I've* stopped feeling responsible for him," she said, looking at me meaningfully. Perhaps she was amused at how *serious* I was about all this, the gravity with which I had delivered my news.

"Welcome to the club," she said. "You're in a long line of people who had faith in David."

"I guess you're still angry with him?"

She shook her head. "I'd have been furious with *myself* if I were still with him and he relapsed. No, I don't have time to be angry with him, or to give him much thought."

I proceeded to unload the dishes from my tray, busy myself arranging the food in front of me, pushing the tray off to the side, trying not to look at her. Except for a trace of eye shadow, she seemed to dispense with makeup. The dark green pharmacist's uniform which, in the haute-couture, dress-shop milieu of the workplace, might have robbed another woman of individuality seemed to bring out hers. Her hooded eyes flitted from her food to me, and then away. If other women I observed in the cafeteria lived life at the surface, in the top layer of clothing and face powder, Gloria seemed to reside somewhere deeper. I remembered my impulse the second time I'd seen her with David to whisk her away. To sit with her like this was the next best thing. She had finished eating, but felt compelled to stay.

"Did you know about the drugs," I asked, dropping my voice, ". . . when you met him?"

She sighed. She could have told me to push off. She could have said this was the past and she didn't want to reopen it. She put her hands on the table, examined the backs of her nails.

"I was too busy 'falling in love.' I remember thinking a couple of times that the way I was feeling—'the love'—was almost too good to be true . . ."

We all had such clarity of thought when it came to bygone loves.

"But needles? Cocaine? When did you find out?"

"In 1989," she said after some thought. "One day, Dr. Binder called me to ask if I knew where David was. I didn't even realize that people knew David and I were seeing each other. Hospitals are such incestuous places—"

We both glanced around to see who was watching us.

"I said to Dr. Binder, 'David can't be gone. I've been speaking to him—or rather, he calls.' I assumed he was calling me from his apartment. But Binder said David's roommate hadn't seen him for days. Then Binder told me . . . the *history* . . ." She waved her hand, the gesture meant to stand in for David's past drug use, the amphetamine factory as a graduate student, the relapse in Lubbock, every sordid event that had preceded her meeting him.

"The story doesn't gel with the man, does it?" I said. "I mean, the David—"

"But I *should* have known," Gloria said, making a motion of striking her forehead with her palm. "It explained the Jekyll and Hyde changes, the long sleeves. In fact," here she paused, in awe of this memory, "I saw tracks on his arm. I *still* didn't want to believe . . ."

She had drifted off, lost her train of thought.

I told her how I had not turned him in when he had confessed to me. She smiled knowingly.

"Maybe *you* should go to Al-Anon," she said, teasing. "They'd call you codependent."

She gathered her tray. Perhaps she felt she had said too much, opened up her old wounds for my sake. She stood next to me, calm, composed, only her eyes fiery from the memories, the anger that had been stirred up. I thought she looked at me with something like tenderness.

"Abraham, David is like a sponge . . . Always *taking*. Relationships come easily to him and then he doesn't know how to maintain them, only how to destroy them, how to let people down. Which is why you feel the way you do."

She took a step, and stopped. "Tell her not to waste her time, to pull away now. She'll thank you in the end."

I knew she meant Emily.

She walked away. When David was around, I had insisted on seeing her as someone who held power over him; I had resented her. It was astounding how differently I saw her now that he was gone.

○

I saw Gato almost every day, sometimes with students, sometimes alone. It had been difficult to find veins in his arms for his intravenous antibiotics, and so we'd put a catheter in his subclavian vein, under the collarbone. He became a familiar sight pushing his IVAC pump ahead of him, going down in the elevator to smoke outdoors, or sitting in the visitors' lounge, looking professorial with his bifocals. He knew the nurses by their first names, and learned the hospital routine better than people who worked there.

At the completion of his four weeks of treatment, we made arrangements for him to go to a halfway house. Before he left, I saw him in his own clothes: a short-sleeved shirt worn over a white undershirt, gray polyester pants, and black shoes. He had a pen and a little notebook in his vest pocket. He looked dapper, handsome, but with a faint air of menace about him—a lady-killer, and I told him so.

"Maybe I'll get lucky, Doc. It's been a while. When you're doing the needle, nothing else is as important."

We shook hands. "Good luck," I said.

"Come and check me out sometime, Doc. I'll give you the guided tour."

"Of the halfway house?"

"Naw—nothing to see there. Same old AA bullshit, 'attitude of gratitude.' No, I'll show you El Paso, the places your buddy hung out."

I nodded.

"Don't worry, Doc. I'm going to beat this thing." He smiled as he said this, a winning smile.

He and I knew that he said this for my sake, a parting gift, to keep up appearances. To make me feel better.

43

In June, alone in the apartment, I watched the French Open final between Jim Courier and Sergi Bruguera on television—without baguettes or Brie.

Many Grand Slam finals were anticlimactic, bloodless after the passion of the semis. But this final was a jewel, a four-hour epic, one for the archives, well worth my having set the alarm and woken up early for.

Bruguera, a tall, handsome Spaniard, with dreamy eyes and thick, sensuous lips, looked like a hero from a Márquez novel come to life. He had the modern strokes—a crisp, compact, two-handed backhand hit close to the body, as precise as a bullet from a marksman's rifle, and a windmill Western forehand. But often, on the return of serve, and whenever he was pulled wide, he had a habit of slicing under the forehand—a forehand equivalent of David's elegant backhand slice. I had displayed that shot for David one time, sticking my arm out, my wrist and racket laid back, the face slightly open, blocking his serve with little backswing and a firm follow-through. I had been pleased with myself and the trajectory of the ball. "What possessed you to slice the forehand when you have a perfectly decent topspin forehand?" David had called from across the net. It was a lazy, antique stroke, and I had put it away forever, keeping only its cousin, the forehand-slice approach, as a means of taking the net.

Time after time, after pulling Bruguera wide on the backhand, Courier would follow it up with a crosscourt to Bruguera's forehand. Bruguera, his stance open, almost in a split, slid on the loose clay, stretched his long arm to his side, and scooped at the ball, drifting it back with underspin. It was a defensive shot that floated low over the net. And each time, as Courier pounced and hit the forehand

again, back to the exact same spot, I felt my anxiety rise—it had sim-
ilarities with the pivotal set-point rally I had had with David. Yet,
strangely, in its consistency, Bruguera's forehand put the burden
squarely on Courier, tempting him to go for too much or to change
direction. I realized that Bruguera was a born clay-courter, willing to
stay out there for days, getting the ball back one more time, throwing it back, drifting it back, coaxing it back, until it triggered
Courier's desire to end the point. The shot was defensive in nature, a
relic of a bygone tennis gentility, but in his hands, it was not only
timeless, it was also a winning strategy. Big Bill Tilden, who thought
tennis should be played "as a defensive game with an offensive
mental attitude," would have approved. Bruguera won.

It was the end of a brief era: Courier had been the dominant male
player, the clear number one in the world in '91 and '92, but now, as
he graciously accepted the runner-up trophy, it was clear to me that
the other players had caught up with him, that his attack had
become tautology: big serve, run around the backhand, inside-out
forehand from midcourt. Bruguera had come up with an effective
counter.

○

It felt as if David had rolled up the court and taken it with him. I
had not played in weeks. That morning, after watching the final, I
went to the club, knowing that I would probably run into Emily. On
weekends, Ross Walker and his assistant pros held a "men's development": four courts that you cycled through—four stations—each
pro working on various drills. At the end of an hour, you were
paired off for a doubles match. It was an activity I had noticed
before when I'd gone to the club with David.

○

I had not spoken to Emily since the day of David's sudden departure. She had gone to California, I knew, to visit friends, get away
from El Paso. We had left messages on each other's phone machines,
long, chatty messages, as if we hoped these would stand in for a
meeting—seeing each other would have been too much.

I spotted Emily through the window of the pro shop, gaunt, with-
drawn, bent over a textbook, a highlighter poised over the pages.

Immediately, I felt guilty for not having sought her out.

She came around the desk and hugged me, and I her, as if, after some natural disaster, we were relieved to find the other alive, safe.

She closed the shop for a few minutes and came out to the lounge area with me. We sat at a table, across from each other.

"Fine!" she said when I asked her how she was. Hearing the false bravado in her own voice, she laughed.

"Shitty, actually. He left—just left everything. I had to get all the furniture out, gather his stuff up, vacate the house. By the time I got to his car at the hospital, it wouldn't start. Had to have it towed. There were bills to be paid. And the bad checks he's written are still coming . . ."

"I should have helped you," I said, ashamed that I had given no thought to the logistics of his sudden departure, only what it had meant to me.

"I had help. That wasn't the problem. It was just this sense of . . . *he* screws up and walks away! And here I am cleaning up after him, tidying the mess he left behind. I had to sell the engagement ring to cover his bad checks. Pawn the jewelry my grandmother gave me. That really killed me . . . ," she said, her eyes tearing.

"He hasn't called me," I said.

She looked directly at me. "I was up there a week ago." She seemed embarrassed to admit this.

"To Atlanta?"

She nodded. "Spent money I didn't have. I really hated to go. I had to break away from school on a weekday . . . I felt sorry for him, to tell you the truth, that's why I went. Think about it: He doesn't have a soul in this country, no one other than me and you. And he'd write letters every day begging me, just *begging* me to go up there . . . 'I love you, I'm sorry; I screwed up, forgive me; I love you . . .'"

From her expression it didn't appear that those phrases meant very much to her.

"'Family Day' they call it," she said, as if still unsure why she had gone up and needed to justify it. "I thought, If it helps . . ."

"Did it?"

"It helped him, I suppose. It's an unbelievable place. To see all those doctors there . . . It beats anything David has been to before, anything I've seen. They cut right through his bullshit, you can see it in his face."

"I should write to him," I said. But what would I say?

"He's embarrassed to talk to you. He knows he let you down."

There was no joy for either of us in this talk of David. Emily's eyes gave away her conflict, her ambivalence. She was, I realized, in the very same position Gloria had been in: A relationship that had begun full of promise had been turned on its head by David's relapse. And now, to all appearances, she was in deep, but in her heart she was uncertain. Or else she was certain, but did not yet have the gumption to make the break.

"Are you having second thoughts . . . ?"

She didn't answer directly. She drew imaginary circles with her finger on the Formica table.

"The session with the therapist was brutal. She went over what she is working on with David. His fantasizing about other women, the stuff in his journals, the magazines that titillate him . . . *sexual* issues that she thinks are part and parcel of his drug use. That precede his drug use. I had no idea. But I know she's right.

"The therapist is telling me this, and all the while David is sitting there, sincere, trying hard, you know? *Earnest*, the blond poster boy of recovery. But he's looking at me kind of worried . . . can I handle what I'm hearing? Then we move on to Gloria and the way he began to fantasize about her, withdraw from me . . ."

Her features were stiff with anger.

"Can you imagine his living with me and fantasizing about her?"

It was more than that, Emily, I said to myself. She didn't seem to know about his approaching Gloria in the cafeteria, declaring his love and saying he'd go back in a heartbeat. He had held that back from Emily and from the therapist.

"Can you imagine how it made me feel to hear all this? I sat there thinking, What am I doing here? Later, when I had a session alone with the therapist, she says to me, 'Be prepared, he might have more relapses with you. You're going to have to be careful. Sexual compulsion is part of his problem. He's easily titillated. You can't leave a Victoria's Secret catalog lying around. You can't do this, you can't do that' . . . And I'm looking at her, thinking, Can I live like this? Can I see twenty years from now trying to screen what's on TV, what comes in the mail?"

Everything I was hearing suggested she wanted out. Why not just end it?

"But he's so needy, so pathetic, so penitent, Abe," she said, anticipating my thought. "Clinging to me, literally clinging—a hand on my sleeve the whole time I was there. Waiting for my letters. Terrified that I'll leave him for another man—even though that kind of betrayal is his specialty."

She reached for a napkin to dry her eyes, and her lips were quivering.

"I couldn't bring myself to say . . . to even express the anger that's building up inside, because it would be . . . like kicking a dog. It's like the time he hit himself: Suddenly his pain is greater than mine so I have to shut up. I wanted to scream at him when I was hearing all the sexual stuff, 'DEAL WITH IT, OKAY?'"

"So, you haven't given up on him, you—"

"We were *engaged*, Abraham," she said, rubbing the place on her finger where the ring had sat. "We were planning a family together. If the timing had been a little different . . . I might already have been married to him . . ."

That was a scary thought.

"I can't just disappear now. He obviously needs me. I . . . I need him too."

She touched the napkin to her nose.

"Meanwhile, every worldly possession of his is in my father's garage. Including a boxful of his journals."

"Did you read them?"

"No. Believe me, what little I saw while moving them made me not want to read them. They are from some dark, hellish place. I knew they would only bother me more."

○

There were about sixteen of us who showed up for men's development. On the first court, Ross stood at the net feeding balls from a grocery cart. He had me hit ten forehands, and then ten backhands, then it was the next person's turn. When you tired of this, you moved to the next court where an assistant pro carried out other drills: overheads, volleys, a three-ball drill.

"Abraham," Ross said when I came back to his court, "try standing a little farther away from the ball on your forehand."

I could feel the difference at once. I was transferring power more crisply to the ball, seeing it zing across the net and come off the ground with greater pace. He let me hit a slew of forehands. As I jogged off, he nodded, pleased with the result of his intervention. At each station, I picked up something new, some hitch that had crept into my game and that fresh eyes spotted. But the tip on the forehand was priceless. I would be sure to enter it into my notebooks when I got home.

○

In the doubles that followed, I was paired with three others whose games were much weaker than mine. Afterward, I sat in the shade and watched Ross and another pro who had paired up with two of the better students. Their doubles was entertaining, and I was envious. The fluidity, the composure, the contained power of Ross's game was so refreshing to watch; his fellow pro had the same quality to a slightly lesser degree. It was rare that they looked awkward.

Ross and his partner won. As I gathered my things to leave, Ross came up behind me.

"Keep coming. Don't stop playing. We'll get you some matches," he said, tapping me on the shoulder. I knew then that he knew about David.

I watched him walk away. It struck me that in all the time I had been coming to the club, watching Ross coach juniors or give a private lesson, I had never heard him raise his voice, never seen him with an expression other than that of equanimity, never seen him without that gentle smile. There was to Ross (and to Pancho Segura) an abiding quality, a steadfastness that David did not have.

It reminded me of my childhood belief about tennis, a belief that David had almost shattered: If you mastered the art of tennis, the art of hitting a ball that was never in one place, it brought about a parallel and salutary effect on the psyche.

○

It took me three months from the time I decided to move to find a condo that I thought was perfect for me. It was two miles from where the boys lived, in a development on the slopes of the Franklins. In place of a view, it had a secluded patio off the living room, a patch of lawn beyond that with a willow tree in its center, and behind that steeply terraced plant beds leading up to a tall rock wall. Ivy, juniper, and pyracantha with bright red berries all but hid the rock wall. It made me think of a Florentine garden, and from my bedroom window, I could look down on to this. It had a one-car garage, two bedrooms, and two and a half baths.

In an orderly way, I got a mortgage approved and went to the closing. The boys loved this new space in the same way, I now understood, that they would love any place they could claim as their own. We went to a furniture store to pick out bunk beds. Their only dispute was who would sleep on top.

I called Manuel the mover. He came to the apartment promptly, this time with a new assistant, "Tiny."

"Very nice place," Manny pronounced when we arrived at the condo and once he had inspected it. "You look happier already. Didn't I tell you last time it would be all right?"

"You did."

"Now you need some furniture, Doc."

"It's on its way."

"There you go!"

The bunk beds and a queen-sized bed for myself arrived that afternoon. Lying on my bed I could see the shimmering leaves of the willow tree through the picture window. From across the border, I purchased a circular, rough-hewn dining table with four matching chairs. The old dining table—the taped-up U-Haul box—I brought with me in my car, reluctant for Manuel to see it. I stored it away carefully in the garage.

44

Most afternoons when I left work I picked up something new—a wind chime, a southwestern-style mirror framed in beaten tin, a jasmine plant—as if I wanted to weigh down my new home, anchor it with objects that were mine, keep it from flying away.

I could hear the phone ringing as I fumbled with my key with one hand, the other hand encumbered with yet another jasmine plant.

"Abraham!" David said, his voice unaffected, and so cheerful. I realized suddenly how much I had missed him. If I had imagined that this might be an awkward moment, he proved me wrong.

"David!" I said, matching his tone. "God! How *are* you?"

He had arrived in El Paso the previous day and was staying with Emily, at her father's home.

He wanted to play tennis right away, that very minute.

"Of course!" I said, and set out for our secret court, all but singing to myself on the way, "David is back!"

When I got there, I saw Emily's car by the court. David stood some distance away, looking out to Cristo Rey. He came running over, tanned and more muscular than I had ever seen him. The wrinkles around his eyes were deeper, as if his smile had found a permanent place on his face. He was animated, like a boy let out of school for the summer.

"God, yes!" he said, spitting on his palm, bringing the racket handle—my racket, which had been stored at Emily's place—back to life after its long layaway. I turned the lights on and unlocked the gate and he all but ran on the court. "Great to be back." He peered up at the sky, licked his finger and tested the wind, slapped the net cord, seemed delighted that it was so taut, and looked around the court as if he had missed it.

He seemed beyond his shame, his manner that of someone who had no more secrets, someone who was no longer pretending to be anything other than what he was.

Being in his presence, seeing the faded yellow El Paso Tennis Club T-shirt, the once white shorts, the right sneaker worn down at the big toe, I felt strangely nostalgic. The September sun hung very low in the sky and, despite the lights, sent long shadows across the court, adding to this feeling that five years, not five months, had gone by. I felt jubilant. David had weathered his troubles and was back on track. Regardless of what had happened (I pushed the memory of it away quickly), the important thing was that it was behind him.

"I feel like I never went through rehab before. Like this was the first time. All those months I spent in other places were such a waste. Talbott was the best . . ."

He was talkative, authoritative about his condition, as if he had not just gone through rehab but had graduated from it.

"How are Steven and Jacob? Have they been playing more tennis? And the pneumonia study? You moved?"

"Whoa! David! Let me catch my breath! Hold up! First things first, let me look at you . . . ," and I put my hand on his shoulder and spun him around. He twirled like a marionette, and our laughter echoed in the canyon, collapsing time, as if only yesterday we had been on the court and had laughed like this.

But he could not be restrained about the Talbott-Marsh clinic. He had so many insights that he wanted to validate by sharing them with me, so many friendships he had forged with others who had made similar voyages. He had heard incredible stories of compulsion and dependence. He had a firm sense of emerging from a dark tunnel.

When we began to rally, the echo of the ball, the scamper of our feet sounded like a continuation of this conversation. I had played sporadic matches at the club, attended "men's development" frequently, and in the process I had forgotten how much I enjoyed this extended baseline exchange, how much I relished playing with someone whose strokes I knew so well—even the spin of his ball, the arc of its flight, was familiar.

When he had been gone, sometimes I'd wondered if there had ever been anything special about our tennis, if a trick of memory had made something prosaic appear extraordinary. But it was real, and it was at the root of my connection with David.

We tried out every skill in our repertoire, lingering on the dink'em, horsing around hitting soft but severe angles almost parallel to the net, laughing as one ball danced twice on the net cord, then dribbled down the side of the net. We did down-the-line and crosscourt drills to the point where I could feel a blister forming on my right toe. When the moon crested the mountaintop and seemed to hover right above us, it gave us new energy, and we played a few service points.

"I see you've been practicing your half volley," he said.

"There was never anything wrong with it," I said.

When we were done, David crab-walked to the bench, groaning and loosening his laces. I was completely exhausted.

"You know what my real problem is?" David said. His face was open, a window to his soul, his eyes holding my gaze, inviting me to peer in—the opposite of when I had last seen him on the court. I wondered if this was common to all doctors who came out of the Talbott-Marsh clinic—did they develop an institutional countenance? "My problem was not cocaine, but sexual addiction." He pronounced the word self-consciously, as if he were still getting accustomed to its sound on his tongue.

"You too?" I said, teasing him.

"I know, I know . . . sex is wholesome, all-American, right?"

"If you're getting any."

"But it wasn't all A-OK for me. I might have been sober, but my sexual addiction was untreated. It led me into situations, generated guilt that undermined my recovery. Then," he said, making a vulgar stabbing motion with his hand, "when I shot up, *that* got everyone's attention."

This sounded a bit facile. "What are you saying? That your horniness is different from mine?"

"You see?" he said, irritated. "As a society we can't take sex seriously—"

"I take it seriously."

"—such mixed messages on TV. And in advertising. I couldn't put it all into perspective. Perhaps you can? But I couldn't."

"I'm sorry . . . I wasn't making fun of you—"

"It's tough for people to understand. My sexual activity had the same compulsive quality of my cocaine use. I'd get preoccupied with it, get into a trancelike state, feel powerful, good, take risks, then feel shitty, then go back for more to feel better—a vicious cycle. It was also progressive, just like drugs . . ."

I wanted to accept this for his sake. But even though Emily had mentioned it, it now felt as if it had been sketched out on a blackboard, and therefore it came off his lips sounding a tad hollow. It begged the question, Why didn't you just stop it? Where were the brakes?

"I thought you were having difficulty taking responsibility for your actions," I said. "Being loyal and fair to Gloria. And Emily. But acting out sexually . . . ?"

I was startled to see the old twitch come back to his face, a sobering sight, a reminder of the dark period before he'd gone to Atlanta. Perhaps sexual addiction *was* his problem, maybe this wasn't just a cute recovery label.

"Those are our darkest, deepest secrets, aren't they? No one knows about them. But it's not just . . . fucking"—he spat out the word, as if its sound was loathsome—"it's toying with people's emotions in the process. Using them. There was one nurse . . ."

I tried to imagine which one.

"I'd say and do anything, and later forget what I had said. She bought me an expensive tennis bag. She didn't have that kind of money. I told my sponsor about it—he made me give it back."

"That hardly justifies the label 'addiction.'"

"Abe, I'm telling you. There were so many others, the most unlikely people you can imagine. Old, young, ugly, pretty, strangers—many strangers. Anonymous sex, and afterward the race to get clear, to get the hell out of there . . ."

I wondered if David was bisexual. Did "unlikely people" include men? I couldn't bring myself to ask this. I felt much like Emily had: I didn't really want to hear this.

"But the next day, I'd be back at it. To have a woman open her body to me was a great affirmation. If you don't have self-esteem to begin with, it becomes a drug."

Yes, but we all feel strong sexual urges, I wanted to say; we all struggle to control them or at least to not allow them to get us into trouble. What allowed him to label his struggle an addiction?

"When Emily came up to Atlanta, I could see how much my behavior had hurt her. Not the cocaine, but all the stuff that preceded it. Obsessing over Gloria, the stuff she uncovered in my journals . . . She only knew a small fraction of what I had been up to."

My mood had become subdued, different from when we started. We sat in the dark, the spectacle of the night lights of the twin cities before us. What he was revealing was unsettling, difficult to match with his sunny disposition, his cheery affect, which had not diminished at all.

"Thank God for you and Emily intervening," he said, standing up, "thank God you called Jim. Because if I hadn't gone to Talbott, I'd never have dealt with this. I've been through the cocaine business so many times. No startling insight to be had there. But the SA business was a revelation."

Before we parted, he said, "I have only one disappointment. Dr. Talbott felt I shouldn't go into the emergency medicine residency. That it was the worst thing for me." He laughed, catching himself. "It's a moot point 'cause I doubt the EM people would take me now, anyway. Dr. Binder said I could finish my transitional internship, get credit for that. After that, with my record . . . God knows what I'll do," he said, smiling genuinely, looking up at the sky again. "I can't worry about that, though. I'm grateful to be here. To be around."

○

I drove home slowly, my exhilaration about his return, about our game, dampened by the turn our conversation had taken. If sexual addiction—and I hated that term—was at the root of his drug addiction—if it was, in fact, true, true and related—it didn't bode well. He would have to be celibate, or else risk relapsing into cocaine. Was he capable of exhibiting the same restraint Emily showed toward food? It was all very confusing, yet David spoke as if he had insight. I hoped he did.

I was glad Dr. Talbott had vetoed emergency medicine. EM was an adrenaline-driven field—the difference between cocaine and adrenaline a matter of a few carbon atoms. Perhaps I had been right: Internal medicine might suit him best. Perhaps I could talk to my chairman about David's situation.

○

Dr. Binder came by my office a few days after David's return.

"The Talbott-Marsh folks want David's first two months back to be really light. No night call, no disruption of his sleep cycle. I thought perhaps he could be with you in November and December?"

Hesitantly, I told Lou how I had become caught up in David's relapse, had shielded him, albeit for only one night, how I had felt torn between my institutional role and my role as his friend.

He smiled, indulgently. "Don't feel bad about it. As far as I'm concerned, it showed you cared. You know he plotted that relapse for months?"

I must have looked puzzled.

"Yeah, he figured out when the pathologist was going to be on vacation. Figured out that it was unlikely that anyone else there would take the initiative to call him in for testing. He plotted it for months."

I was flabbergasted.

"Perhaps at that time you didn't appreciate how bad his disease was?"

When I didn't respond, Lou went on. "You know the disease concept? Thousands of American soldiers in Vietnam used heroin, but only a small percentage continued to use when they came back? Some genetic disorder in the forebrain made the ones who continued using vulnerable."

I remembered having read this, but I had glossed over it. My focus with patients who were addicted was much more clinical.

"It's why we've given him so many chances," he said simply.

"But, Lou, *he* knew what steps he needed to take to keep the disease in remission. That's where he was at fault—surely he is responsible for that?"

"Oh, absolutely! We're not letting him off the hook for that. He has a physician compliance contract that's more rigorous than before—four meetings a week, reports from his sponsor, more frequent urine tests, visits with a therapist here in town. It's not going to be easy at all. He'll have very little free time."

Lou smiled.

"Of course, he doesn't *have* to comply. But if he wants to complete his internship, if he is ever to get a license, then this is the route he must follow."

○

I called Emily's place on a Friday night to speak to David.

"He's at a meeting, Abraham," she said. "It'll be a while before he gets back. He has to take the bus, unless someone there gives him a ride."

"Doesn't he look great?" I said to Emily.

"He's okay," she said.

"And you?"

There was a long pause.

"I'm struggling. I'm up to my ears with schoolwork. To be quite honest, he's driving me nuts."

"What—"

"I'm happy he's better and gung ho about his recovery. I just don't have much time for him." Her tone was aggrieved.

"He's being a nuisance?"

"No, worse," she said, and laughed for the first time. "He couldn't be more accommodating. He can't figure out why I'm not the way I used to be . . . Things have changed. My priority is school. He's just so needy. It's, like, suddenly our roles are reversed: I'm taking care of him, and he's clinging."

"Maybe he should move out. Maybe he can stay with me. I have enough—"

"He *is* moving out," she said, adding under her breath, "thank God." Both the Talbott-Marsh people and his sponsor thought it unwise for him to be staying with her. His sponsor wanted him to go to a halfway house in the old Sunset Heights neighborhood where David and Emily had lived. There, he would be part of a rigorous recovery experience, not unlike the one at Talbott-Marsh: meetings with his housemates every night, household chores to fulfill.

Emily's voice dropped to a whisper. "To be honest, Abe, I kind of cringe when he touches me. The other night he says, 'You won't touch me.' And I said, 'I have no desire to.' I'm just not ready for that, not after everything he has told me. He has to accept that." There was a long silence and then she said, "I don't know, Abe. He's assuming it's all okay. I know it's not. But I don't want to precipitate anything. I don't have the time."

○

"How do you define FUO, or fever of unknown origin?" I asked.

I had two medical students, a corpulent internal medicine resident, and David, in tow. We were heading up the stairs, only David relishing the physical effort.

"FUO is . . . fever for at least three weeks where no cause is evident . . . despite a week of intense . . . investigation," the resident said breathlessly.

"Right. And when they are admitted to a teaching hospital, they are the special purview of the infectious-disease specialist. She's our baby, in other words."

We had taken the stairs because the elevators were slow, and I was anxious to see this consultation. Sorting out an FUO was, to me, the quintessence of the skill we practiced.

One of the students found the chart.

"She's in six-eleven," he said, and we proceeded down the hallway, all of us flushed and panting a little.

The patient was nineteen years old. According to the chart, her fever had gone on for three weeks. A week into her illness, she had gone to Juárez for a shot of penicillin administered by a pharmacist. When that had not helped, she had seen a doctor in El Paso who put her on another course of antibiotics, ran some tests. Still the fever persisted, and soon she was too weak to get out of bed.

I was attentive to the aura of the room, vigilant for her icons—a doll, rabbit-ear slippers, a prayer card, her own nightgown. I inhaled discreetly so that her scents, all the eructations and effluvia that were hers, the redolence that might spell the name of the disease lurking below, could land on the free nerve endings of my olfactory nerve. Smells registered in a primitive part of the brain, the ancient limbic system. I liked to think that from there they echoed and led me to think "typhoid" or "rheumatic fever" without ever being able to explain why.

I taught students to avoid the *Augenblick* diagnosis, the "blink-of-an-eye" label, the snap judgment. But secretly, I trusted my primitive brain, trusted the animal snout; I listened when it spoke.

Already, in that first sight of this awkward, fearful young woman with the skin of a baby, eyes as wide as those of her doll, I could picture myself returning many times, as if to revisit the crime scene. Perhaps my patience would be rewarded with a spleen that one morning became palpable. Or the appearance of a soft, blowing, heart murmur. Each new finding would lead us down a narrower diagnostic pathway, help nail the diagnosis.

If the diagnosis eluded us in the first few days, her chart would thicken as pages of computer printouts bearing witness to the blood urea, the serum creatinine, the liver enzymes, and other soundings accumulated. But no computer could make the mind-pictures I could form if given the right clues: a liver hobnailed from cirrhosis and weeping yellow ascitic fluid; a spleen swollen like a giant and angry thumb from mononucleosis; a smooth-walled cavity in the lung apex within which a fungus ball clatters like a bead in a baby's rattle.

○

I introduced myself to the patient, explained our purpose. I asked if she minded if I put drops in one eye before we began. I then quizzed her in great detail about the onset of this illness (gradual), her past health (excellent), her recent travel (the one crossing to Juárez), her diet (no goat cheese, no poorly cooked pork, no herbal products), her pets (a cat and an outdoor dog), her home (out in the lower valley, well water, an outhouse with a septic tank), medications (oral contraceptives), occupation (community college student), family history (a brother in Ohio with a "kidney disease" at age twenty-five), social history (occasional pot, hated beer, no needles), and sexual history (active with her first and only boyfriend who she swore was not into needles or men).

I felt her pulses. I looked into her eyes, the right pupil now fully dilated so that in that darkened room the students got their first good look at a retina through my ophthalmoscope. I used a tongue depressor to sweep every nook and cranny of her oral cavity. I felt for glands in her neck, armpit, and groin. I listened to her heart while she lay recumbent, and then while she rolled to her left side, I switched from the diaphragm to the bell of my stethoscope, the better to hear low-pitched murmurs. I felt for the spleen three different ways and then percussed for it. I examined all her joints, and then her nervous system, testing muscle power, coordination, reflexes, sensation, and the cranial nerves.

By now the bed was cluttered with the instruments I had pulled out of my pocket and not resheathed. One last search for rheumatic nodules in the places most easily overlooked: behind her ears, at the back of her neck, behind her elbows. And another once-over from scalp to sole to make sure I hadn't missed petechiae or a rash, or the cigarette-burn lesion of disseminated gonococcal disease.

I summed up what I had found for the patient and the students: tenderness and perhaps synovial swelling over a few larger joints. An oral ulcer. A spleen that I thought was palpable. Enough clues here to support my first suspicion—that this was either lupus, or an unusual presentation of rheumatoid arthritis. But there were many other possibilities.

I talked to her at length about what tests I would order. She was to have her mother call Ohio and get more details on her brother's kidney disease—he could have lupus-related renal failure. Her mother was to call me when she came to visit.

Outside the room, my entourage seemed as excited as I was, caught up in the diagnostic puzzle.

"Jennifer, I want you to make a brief presentation to us on the major causes of FUO. Vincent, I want you to compile a list of the causes of splenomegaly."

We split up now, the students and the resident heading to the library to read on FUO, David coming back with me to the office. This was his first day back, and we needed to resurrect his pneumonia study.

"Awesome," David said. "What happens if the tests come back negative?" David said.

"We dig deeper. Go over the history again. Pursue other leads."

"And if there's still no answer?"

"We'll have an answer on her—"

"But what if . . . ?"

"One famous professor would discharge and then readmit the patient to another medical team at the same hospital. But he'd withhold the chart and the results of all the tests. What he wanted was a fresh, unbiased eye, a fresh taking of the history, a thorough physical by a new group of doctors. The old team had perhaps become too entangled in a web of assumptions, too biased to see the patient objectively. And after a few days, he'd give them the results of the previous tests."

As I said this, I thought it could also be a metaphor for David's return to the hospital. I had given him a clean slate, dismissed the confusion of the months before he relapsed, the cyclothymic moods, the shilly-shallying of his commitments to Emily and Gloria. He had been readmitted and I wanted to look at him without bias.

○

In my office, I saw David's eyes go to my desk, looking for the stack of papers from the pneumonia study.

"I put them back there on the shelf, behind you," I said.

He took the folder down and set it on the table.

"I put in an article there on hantavirus. You heard about that outbreak in New Mexico?"

"It was in the news, wasn't it?"

"A fulminant pneumonia. Related to rodent exposure. Made me think of Mr. Rocha. If you can dig out his serum that you saved, we could send it for testing. Maybe that's what he had."

David said, "Cool!" but when he looked up, there was sadness in his face.

"You okay?" I asked.

"Just being back. People looking at me. I had to go to the lab for a urine screen. Dr. Boman, the pathologist who does the testing . . . I apologized to him for something I had done. He was angry and had every right to be."

It was on my lips to say, I know what you did, but I let it pass.

"Then I saw the residency director for emergency medicine before I met up with you. I could see that he was disappointed in me. There wasn't much to say."

"You expected all that. Just shrug it off."

"Yeah," he said, sitting up in the chair, remembering his new-found spirit. "By the way, the FUO was fascinating."

"The *patient* with FUO."

"It was like watching you build something over the patient's bed. Kind of like an operation, but all in the head—"

"Maybe that's why they call it *internal* medicine."

"—and I could see how you were doing it, I understood the process better than before."

"Could you see yourself doing it?"

"What? Internal medicine? . . . Yeah, yeah, I could. That's what I was thinking about when we were in her room. It's a different kind of skill, but just as intricate as . . .

"Surgery?"

"Doing something with my hands. Do it with the head instead—"

"What if I could get you into internal medicine? Here."

A flush came to his cheeks.

"I'd resigned myself to finishing the internship and then going to work in a . . . prison," he said, bursting into laughter.

"You're not serious?"

"I really didn't think anyone anywhere else would take a chance on me!"

"The question is, would you *want* to be in an internal medicine residency? Not just because you might be able to get a slot. You can't later say—"

"God, yes. It would be a bloody miracle!"

"You could then go on to do cardiology—"

"Or critical care, or gastroenterology."

"Stuff with the hands and the head."

"Yes!"

"Go over and talk to Dr. Casner," I said. "He's expecting you."

"What? . . . You spoke to him? . . . You think he really might . . . ?" He was on the edge of his chair, as if I had handed him a new lease on life.

"It's in the bag, mate," I said. "If it's what you want."

He stood up now. "I definitely want it."

"You sure, now?" I said, turning deadly serious. "'Cause he's going out on a limb for you. Mostly because I asked him to."

45

David moved from Emily's place after living there for just a few weeks. He accomplished the move alone, borrowing Emily's car. She had been busy with school.

"I would have helped you," I said to him when I saw him at work, thinking back to when he had offered to help me move.

"Couldn't take much. I left most everything at Emily's. The room I'm moving into is tiny."

We were together at work every day, but with all his meetings, and not having a car, it proved difficult for us to play tennis. His weeknights were tied up, my weekends revolved around the kids and fixing up the condo. After a month with me, he had picked up the routine of the consultation service, and he was of great help. In his free time he was analyzing the data from the pneumonia study and he was poised to write a first draft of what I knew would be a publishable paper.

On a Saturday afternoon, I went by his place in Sunset Heights. I followed his directions to a grand old house. It had two floors, an attic, and a basement, but it faced the freeway. Broad stairs led to a wraparound porch. A black man in his forties in a flannel shirt opened the door. I introduced myself and he shook my hand, mumbled his name from behind a beard that hid his lips. David appeared behind him.

The living and dining room were clean but cluttered, the furniture mismatched. There was a grayness to this common area, as if every one who had trafficked through it over the years had peeled off a shade so that it no longer had a color of its own.

We took the stairs up to David's room, a narrow room above the front of the house. It had a cot along one wall and a small study table by the window; the view was of Juárez. He shared a bathroom down the hall and there was a communal telephone on a chair in the hallway.

David was apologetic about his room. There were, David said, seven or eight of them in the house, all with varying periods of sobriety, all working or going to school. David grabbed his tennis racket and was ready to go.

I felt sorry to see him in that tiny, stuffy room.

"Has Emily been here?"

He shook his head. I imagined it was difficult for him to endure living this way, not because it was spartan, or strict, but because just up the road sat the house he and Emily had lived in. That house had been airy, uplifting, a home, while this place was dark, gloomy, weighing on me like an old Salvation Army coat that carried in its sweaty seams the despair of lonely, abandoned men. Mickie's place would have been preferable, more like a home.

"My sponsor insisted," David said, looking at his room with distaste, eager to leave. "Ah, well, I was allergic to Emily's cat. I'm breathing better here."

We went down the stairs and then climbed into my car. Once we were out of the house I felt as if I had shed a weight.

"It's bloody intense," David said, looking back at the house. "Four meetings a week here. Two more NA meetings in town. But I'm getting to know my housemates. They're okay."

I took that to mean that he had nothing in common with them other than the addiction. This was no Talbott-Marsh Recovery Campus.

"Yesterday's house meeting surprised me—powerful testimony. Solid AA stuff."

At least he was able to look at the bright side.

○

It was cold and blowing on the court. I found it difficult to loosen up. I was hitting into the wind, swinging hard but still struggling to get the ball deep. David merely tapped the ball and the wind did the rest. Perhaps it had been a bad idea to play, but when he'd called, I had felt obliged to come get him, sensing his need for a break from his routine, hearing loneliness in his voice.

He was solicitous, hitting to my backhand repeatedly when he saw me making adjustments on my slice, trying to make it flatter with just a hint of underspin—more like his stroke.

"Don't consciously think of coming *under* it," he called out. "Just take your backswing high, and hit *through* it. The high-to-low swing gives you just enough slice."

I was reminded of the very first time we had played. His focus then and now was entirely on the game. He was relaxed, laughing at his errors, not bothered by the wind, while my head was somehow not quite there.

"Did you see the French Open this year?" I asked.

"Read about it."

I described the match to him and the forehand slice that Bruguera had hit that day.

When I hit to his forehand, he tried it. "You mean, like that?"

"Exactly."

"I can see why he'd use that on clay," David said, "especially when you are stretched wide. I'm surprised Courier didn't make him pay for it."

"He tried. Bruguera had faith in that stroke—you could tell *he* didn't think of it as defensive."

We were now both trying the stroke, laughing when it floated off too high.

The tennis felt lifeless for me that day. Perhaps after the first blush of excitement when he had returned, I had come to see how difficult it was to carry on just as before. It was like trying to step into the same river twice.

"Eyes on the ball," David called out, because my attention had wandered.

"I'm trying."

O

At Dolce Vita, without Emily, it should have felt just like old times. David was happy to be there, garrulous after the tennis and away from that house. He was still full of recovery-speak—the "pink cloud" Emily had called it. I was listening, but found myself restless.

"Whoa! Check this out," I said, spotting the gorgeous brunette who had served us so many moons ago, tall and fetchingly uncoordinated.

He looked at her, and then deliberately looked away. This irritated me. Like a dipsomaniac proudly making a show of refusing a drink at a party, it rang hollow. David picked up the thread of his conversation, resumed the drugalogue.

○

We drove back to his house in silence. Across the street, a father and son were stringing up Christmas lights. David stayed in the car, looking at them, then up to the window of his room.

"I'm here for a good reason. I'm just grateful to be here, to have this chance. Ah, well . . . What are you doing tomorrow?"

"Soccer in the morning. Kids in the afternoon—"

"Soccer?"

"Had to do something when you were gone. And you?"

"Church in the morning. I have to take the bus over to the SA meeting in the afternoon. Then I'll probably be back here. Emily is busy—she has a test on Monday. You want to play again?"

"I should probably pass. After the soccer, my knees would complain. I'll probably stay home and read."

"If you change your mind . . . ," he said, and opened the car door. "I've been trying to read my *Harrison's*, the chapter on lupus," he said, shaking his head. Our young patient with FUO had turned out to have lupus, as did her brother in Ohio. The fever subsided promptly when she was begun on corticosteroids. "I tell you, for so long I've had my mind set on emergency medicine, it's tough to switch gears. It's sad to have to give up that dream." His voice had turned high-pitched, whiny. "Really tough to picture myself in internal medicine. That book . . . there's *so* much in it."

I didn't reply. Just a few weeks before, he had considered it a miracle if internal medicine would have him. And now that my chairman had decided to take him, David was moaning about it. I waited for the positive spin he would give to this.

"Thanks, mate," he said. He went up the stairs and disappeared into the house.

○

Our last consult of the day. I had kept David busy for the two months he was with me, given him charge of the students taking the elective. He led rounds with them on the old patients, and he helped the students gather data on the new consultations and polish their presentations to me.

In her room, the patient was irritable, and shuffling around, fiddling with her IVAC pump. She had an intravenous line that had been placed in her neck, and taped there with a bulky dressing. Her hair was disheveled and had fallen in front of her face, hiding her eyes. Her lower lip was bruised and swollen. She turned her back to us.

"Why don't you come back later?" she said, as if we were door-to-door salesmen who had intruded on the privacy of her home. "I have to go to the bathroom."

"Oh my God," David said, under his breath.

"We'll be back," I said.

"Did you recognize her?" David asked when we were outside.

"I recognized the legs."

It was Angelina Cortez. Her hair was now blond. Without makeup, her face looked completely different.

For the benefit of the others, David explained that we had seen her on the ward service and had treated her for heart-valve infection, and from there she had gone to a rehabilitation facility. It had been almost a year since her last hospital visit, and she looked ancient now, ravaged by her habit.

"She's been using," I said.

"She's about to use right now," David said gently.

We waited a long while outside her room, until we heard the bathroom door open. She was in bed, calm, with her eyes closed. Her legs were weepy tree trunks, perhaps bigger than they had been before. The lower half of the left leg was the color of raw beef. She roused when I put my gloved hands on her leg. She opened her eyes, smiled, muttered, and then nodded off. She was quite arousable, not in any danger.

"Dr. Kumar," I said to the intern as he was about to read from his case notes, "I think she needs an urgent X ray of her leg."

"I already have one, sir; it's normal, there's no air in the soft tissue."

"Let's get another one, stat. I'll explain why later."

He looked puzzled, but went off to write the order. We waited till

the orderly came and wheeled her away. She was still nodding off;
David looked at her with an expression of utter disgust.

"Shall we give her some Narcan?" he said.

Narcan would reverse the effect of the heroin, bringing her back
to normal.

From her face, from the ecstatic expression on it, I thought I
understood her state perfectly: Heroin was magical, sacred, orgas-
mic, and it took her to another world. She tolerated the track marks,
the pockmarked feet, the swollen flesh, the fever, because they were
symptoms from this world, a world Angelina chose not to occupy.
Who was to say which world was better?

"No, let her be," I said.

In her bedside drawer, wrapped up in tissue paper and then
placed in a plastic bag, was a diabetic syringe and a bottle cap.

"Did she shoot her legs again?" a student asked.

"No," David said, "she used her IV. Probably the first time she has
mainlined in a while."

"Cocaine?"

"No, heroin," David said. "See where the bottle cap is burnt at the
bottom? She cooked it with a lighter. Cocaine dissolves at room
temperature. Her sedation, the nodding off—that's heroin. With
cocaine she'd be super alert, paranoid, seeing shadow people, hearing conversations taking place in the next room."

"Or imagining them," I said.

○

"I see he's back."

I recognized the voice before I turned. The students and David
had rotated off service, and I had no students assigned until the holidays were over. I was on the sixth floor, following up on Angelina,
writing a note in her chart.

Gloria had her hair gathered behind her, revealing her ears.
She was wearing a pharmacist's smock, carrying a clipboard, and
appeared to be in a hurry.

"Yes, he's back, I hope this time—"

She didn't let me continue.

"He had the nerve to send me a letter from Atlanta. To tell me he
was over me!" She laughed, and shook her head. "He said he was

writing to put closure on this relationship once and for all."

"Part of his therapy—"

"He doesn't get it, does he?"

Before I could reply, she said, "Didn't mean to interrupt you. Got to run. Did you have a good Christmas?"

I nodded.

She smiled, touched me on the shoulder, as if to make it clear that she had no beef with me.

46

On New Year's Day of 1994, David telephoned. From my bedroom, where I was half asleep, I heard his voice on the answering machine downstairs. I rolled over and went back to sleep.

I came downstairs about noon when Rajani brought the boys over. She appeared dressed to go out. The boys ran in, happy, bustling with energy, hugging me, then one heading upstairs, one out to the porch, too busy to converse, as if the condo were an extension of their play space.

Rajani brought mail that had arrived at her place for me. I gave her a package I had set aside for her: an asthma inhaler with a letter that she wanted to take to the school nurse for Steven's occasional wheezing.

"Happy New Year, by the way," I said as she hurried out.

"You too," she called over her back. We were, I noticed, exceedingly, almost sarcastically, polite with each other. That we should get along well, and be so functional and practical now that we were apart was vaguely embarrassing. It had been so difficult to do so when we were together.

At Christmas, Jacob had said to me, "We're lucky. We get to open presents twice!" I was thrilled to hear him say that. My life and Rajani's were on different tracks, the boys crossing back and forth freely. They seemed to have completely accepted this state of affairs as normal. There were even advantages—I allowed video games and had cable TV while she did not; I had no room for a dog, but she had one at her home.

My guilt had diminished. It helped to see my sons thriving, blooming as vigorously as her roses. If we did not bring up the discussion of divorce just yet, it was perhaps out of fear that our facade of politeness would collapse, it would bring acrimony, it would disrupt this shared parenting that was clearly working and that showed in the faces of my sons.

○

It was warm enough to take my coffee to the porch, pull my chair into the sun. Steven took down the hummingbird feeder and refilled it. We watered the jasmine plants, which were doing famously. I weaved some of their shoots through the trellis that sat between my neighbors' property and mine. I hoped one day to have a wall of jasmine here, its scent filling the air and calling up the memory of evenings in Madras, strolling on the freshly swept and watered pavement, past the glittering sari shops in Mambalam. Every few yards, women with nimble fingers had sat stringing together jasmine flowers, selling them by the foot, jasmine to be taken home and given to the wife, jasmine that I would buy and take to my hostel even though I had no woman to give it to.

I put off calling David. If he wanted to play tennis, I'd have to pick him up, drive to the court, then later, Dolce Vita, then back to his house—it would shoot the rest of the day. As much as I loved tennis, it felt like too much effort for New Year's Day.

○

Much later that night I listened to David's message, and felt guilty because I heard loneliness. All he'd said was, "Abraham. Just seeing what you're up to. Bye." As I went to bed, I told myself that I cared for David, we had a bond, but the headlong plunge I had taken into the friendship early on had been unfruitful. The enforced hiatus in Atlanta had imposed the requisite distance, one that allowed the tie to remain strong and yet flexible, allowed it to weather whatever changes were ahead in both our lives.

I resolved to check on him at work in the morning. He was about to begin a month's cardiology elective, and then, in March, he would begin his internal medicine residency.

○

When I got to work the next day, I saw David at the table in the small conference room around the corner from my office where, early each morning, Dr. Jorge Martinez-Lopez pored over the electrocardiograms (EKGs) done in the previous twenty-four hours at Thomason, each one with a story to tell. I liked walking by and seeing Jorge, white-haired, white-coated, and never ruffled, surrounded by his students, a pile of EKGs before him, taking the morning pulse of the hospital.

In my office, I called the microbiology lab to check another sort of pulse: All over the hospital, patients with fever had their blood sent for culture. Some of these cultures were now turbid, growing bacteria, and the lab would read me the list of culprits, each organism telling a story. That morning a *Salmonella arizonae* had turned up in a blood culture. It meant someone had either eaten poorly cooked rattlesnake meat, or else had swallowed rattlesnake pills prescribed as an all-purpose tonic and aphrodisiac by a *curandera* in Juárez. I jotted down the patient's name and room number.

Half an hour later, when David poked his head in, there was a story in his face too, the letters displayed so clearly in the lines around his eyes and at the corners of his lips that I already knew what he would say.

"Emily broke up with me . . ."

He remained in the doorway. He had to rejoin his cardiology team, which was heading to the ICU to meet the patients whose EKGs they had just read.

"Said she couldn't go on."

He had to leave then, as Dr. Martinez-Lopez appeared behind him, waved at me, and clapped David on the shoulder.

○

I called Emily and heard the rest.

She had driven over to David's place. It was her first visit there in all that time. He had come down the stairs to the curb, to her car, smiling, excited, certain that her surprise visit augured well for '94.

"I just couldn't go on with it anymore, Abe. I'd been pushing him away, not making time for him, focusing on my studies. I was so afraid to tell him."

"Did he know it was coming?"

"No . . . he'd call and I'd make excuses not to drive out there, not to go to a movie. 'Why are you doing this to me?' he'd ask."

"I thought since he was with you at Christmas . . ."

"I didn't have the heart to tell him at Christmas. I'd made up my mind then. *Before* then, actually. But I wanted the semester to be over."

I was glad for her. If her heart wasn't there, it was better that they both moved on.

"He took it hard. He had no idea. He cried. I felt so bad. He said he had come back to El Paso just for me. Is that true?"

"If he wanted to finish his internship, be a doctor, he had to come back."

"He said, 'Now I've lost everything. I've lost you. I've lost my residency in emergency medicine. I'm stuck in internal medicine, which I hate.'"

"What? He said that?" Suddenly it felt as if the conversation was about me. Blood rushed to my face. I felt betrayed.

"Just crying his eyes out. But I had to do it, Abe. It was dishonest to go on."

"But what he said about internal medicine—"

"All he has is the two of us, you and me. Other than meetings, he doesn't do anything with anyone but you or me. I was scared to pull away, scared because—" I was hardly listening. I felt as if I had just overheard a good friend make an uncharitable remark about me. "—he came back too soon from Talbott."

That stopped me. I waited.

"He's not whole," she said. "That whole 'attitude of gratitude' is slipping away. He's getting on his pity pot. The pink cloud is gone."

"You mean, since you broke up?"

"No. Before. Long before. I could tell."

○

When David managed to sit down with me at the end of the day, I felt awkward. I wanted to confront him with what I had heard, but I restrained myself. His version of the breakup was, surprisingly, the same as hers. Unlike the breakup with Gloria so many months before, a breakup precipitated by his seeing Emily, this time there was no external force to blame. This time, as he sat quietly, dejected, he was not in denial, he was not trying to recast it to suit himself— he saw it for exactly what it was.

"She just doesn't want it anymore. She said she doesn't love me, doesn't feel what she once felt." He shrugged. "What could I say to that?"

"Well . . ."

"She said I was too needy. That she couldn't be my whole world."

"I'm sorry, man," I said, but my mind was still on what I saw as his betrayal of me. I realized now he had called my house minutes after the breakup.

"You've got to go on. You've come so far. You'll meet others."

His face twitched and I realized there were already others in the wings.

"I loved her so much."

○

I stewed with anger, frustrated by the fact that his pain over Emily's leaving made it impossible for me to bring up my beef with him.

"How," I wanted to ask, "did an internal medicine residency at Tech go from being a miracle to pissing you off? Where did you think you'd find another residency? And you sure as hell aren't getting into an emergency medicine residency—even if they'd take you, the Talbott-Marsh people would veto it."

The Texas Tech system, and then too, only our department, had once again stuck its neck out to clear a path for him. He would be the only American medical graduate in the internal medicine residency. Even though we provided excellent training, residency programs like ours were stigmatized by the fact that we hired foreign medical graduates. It was a catch-22: The specialty was not in great demand, there was a glut of positions, and so you filled your slots with foreign medical graduates. Once you did that, when it came to selecting internships, your own medical students shunned your program because it was all foreigners.

If the residency training system in America was caste ridden, hypocritical, unable to conceal its inherent bigotry, I had assumed all along that David, as a foreigner himself, was beyond this. When I had first introduced myself to him in the parking lot, I had sensed a commonality partly based on that belief. Now it felt as if he had renounced me.

I was certain that if he were offered an internal medicine residency at an Ivy League university hospital, he would have none of these qualms. What he did not realize was that in a system where foreign graduates were pariahs, he was even farther down the ladder. He had no other options.

Perhaps when my anger subsided, when he was over Emily, I'd sit him down, talk to him about his attitude—how he needed to see the glass as half full, see his situation as not half bad. *Yes, David, it truly is a miracle.* He could excel at Tech, show his mettle, study hard, take great care of his patients, publish papers, become the chief resident, perhaps inspire future Tech students to give something back to the program. Temperament, adrenaline, or his preferring to work with his hands was no excuse: He could go on to become an interventional cardiologist, spend all his days in a cath lab, using his hands to probe people's hearts—plenty of adrenaline there.

But there was no point in telling him that the problem did not lie in the merits of one specialty over another, and that *he* was the problem. There was no point in saying any of this because I had already heard the gates slam shut; I had seen the pessimism in his face and in his attitude. In tennis terms, he was tanking the match.

47

On the last day in February, I called David before he left for work. Officially, he would start his residency in internal medicine on March the first. I felt guilty for not seeking him out more. Perhaps this would be our last chance to play for a while.

We had seen each other at work regularly. I knew he had bought a white Hyundai for a couple of hundred dollars. When we chatted, it was about this car, a safe and familiar theme. But he never voiced to me the rumblings I heard from others: that he was pissed off at Emily, pissed off at the fact that he would be in internal medicine, pissed off that he couldn't do emergency medicine—somehow, we were to blame. It was the reason I had not pushed very hard to play tennis.

He picked up the phone on the first ring.

"David!"

"Yes?" His voice was wary, suspicious, as though he had expected someone else. Or, he thought I was calling for a reason other than the one I voiced. I told him to bring his racket, perhaps we could leave for the court after work.

"All right," he said, but again the voice was distant, suspicious.

When I arrived at work an hour later, I found out why.

David had submitted a handwritten letter of resignation.

I walked down the hall to find Lou Binder.

"You heard?" I said.

"I'm sure he's relapsed," Lou said.

"How do you know?"

"I don't, but I will in a few minutes," he said. "There were two urines tested last week—David, and one other person. I just called the lab; one of the urines is positive. I asked them to tell me if it's opiates or cocaine—if it's cocaine, it's David. The other guy never used anything but opiates."

The phone rang.

"Yup, yup, okay, thanks," Lou said and hung up. "Cocaine. It's David. Do you know where he lives?"

○

We got off at the downtown exit, and made our way to Sunset Heights.

"What are we going to do if we find him? I mean, if he's resigned, that's it, right?"

"He's *relapsed*. That's the issue," Lou said. "His disease is very bad. His use escalates quickly. We get him into detox and then back to treatment."

I was in shock, unprepared for all this, while Lou was matter-of-fact, knew exactly what to do.

I was angry with myself. Angry that I hadn't sat him down and read him the riot act when I should have. Somehow I had let it happen again: I had forgotten about the cocaine, focused instead on his self-pity, on his pessimism. It was all so predictable in hindsight. I felt as if I had been sucker-punched.

"I *am* very upset with him," Lou said, though he didn't look upset. "It's a pity. David has a very bad disease. Perhaps the worst of all the people I've dealt with."

I had knots in my stomach and, as the house came into view, I felt my chest tighten. My anger had given way to fear.

The street was deserted except for David's Hyundai. We parked behind it. I put my hand on the hood. It was warm.

The house loomed over us, sinister, offering no clues. I pointed out David's bedroom window.

I followed Lou up the stairs from the curb and onto the porch, our steps resounding on the wooden boards. He rang the bell repeatedly but there was no answer.

The hair on the back of my neck stood up, and with every passing second, I was getting more anxious, hearing my heart pound in my ears, physically fearful, but not sure why. I had the eerie sense we were being stalked.

The house was enveloped in a cloak of silence, the freeway sounds held at bay. Every nerve in my body was alert, as if waiting for the signal to flee. The sound of the doorbell echoed deep in the bowels of the house. David's roommates were surely all at work.

"Maybe he's not there, Lou," I said. "Maybe it's just his car . . . and he's gone."

Lou, a stout man with a loud voice, now shouted through the closed door, "DAVID. OPEN THE DOOR. WE KNOW YOU'RE IN THERE."

"I think we should go, Lou." I was halfway down the stairs.

Lou followed, but as it turned out, only so he could look up at the window to David's room and shout, "DAVID!"

There was still no answer. Now he used his cell phone to dial David's number. No one picked up, though I could faintly hear the phone ring in the house.

"Lou, let's go."

But Lou wanted us to go around the house and try the back door. I followed him down the steps, up the rough driveway to the side of the house, the windows of the dining room and living room too high for us to peek through.

We rounded the corner, and I ran into Lou because he had stopped suddenly.

There, coming toward us, its eyes lowered, not having seen us yet, was a creature I knew but did not recognize. It muttered under its breath, and the sight chilled me, froze me to one spot. It resembled David in its general appearance, but the face was hollowed out, and the facial planes peaked at the nose. I recognized the warm-up suit as a present from Emily. A large tennis duffel bag was clutched in one hand, the ends bulging.

When he saw us, he snarled, and swerved and walked away from us, to the side fence.

"David!" Lou said.

"David?" I said.

"Get away from me!" The words came out in a low growl, an octave below David's voice. The appearance of this beast was terrifying, the face fixed in a scowl, the pupils so wide that they appeared unfocused, the ears splayed back, the head retracted into the muscles of the shoulder and neck, which were tensed like a rottweiler about to pounce. He paused, as if he were cornered. But like a sewer rat, he knew every exit, every back door, every hole, every tunnel, every canal, every escape but the front door.

"David," Lou said, taking a few steps forward, but even he seemed to hesitate for the first time that day. "Where are you going?"

I put my hand on Lou to pull him back, to stop him from going forward.

From the first moment we spotted him, he had not stopped moving, pacing with small steps, as if in a frenzy, first this way, then that.

"Leave me alone," he said, a louder snarl. Then he found the opening he had been looking for behind the garbage cans, and swiftly, muscling aside a plank, he clambered through and made his way into the alley, ran between two houses, and was gone.

○

Once we were in the car, Lou got on the phone. He spoke to one of the psychiatrists at Texas Tech.

"We've got to get him into detox," Lou said.

We went from there to the courthouse downtown, and took out a protective custody order to pick David up.

While Lou filled out the forms, a woman in her late forties came up to me.

"*¿Señor? ¿Por favor, me puede ayudar?*" she said, holding out the clipboard and pen.

That was when I noticed that my hands were trembling.

She had orange hair, but skin that was my color. Her face was lined from smoking and worry. She tapped a nail that was a dark purple to show me how far she had gotten and where she needed help. The person she was taking the PCO out on was her son.

"*Mi hijo . . . me destruyó la casa . . . me pegó.*"

Under "Reason" I put down: Son has assaulted mother, destroyed property at the house.

"*¿Por qué lo hizo?*"

"*Las drogas,*" she said simply. "*Cocaina.*"

48

When I spoke to Emily that night, told her what had happened, she was distraught.

Even though there was no reason for it, we felt responsible.

"I was spooked, Emily. It wasn't David I saw. It was someone else."

"What do we do, Abe?"

"Nothing," I said, remembering the advice of David's sponsor the last time this had happened. "David is responsible for David. There's nothing to do."

"No, we have to find him, get him into detox. He could have a seizure, he could . . ."

"You can't take him against his will, Emily. Only the cops can do that."

"We must try and find him, get him help."

○

I could not concentrate on work the next day. Twice I checked in with Binder and once with Emily, but there was no word.

That evening I drove slowly down Alameda Street, a likely place for David to get his cocaine.

I hoped perhaps to spot his car, if he hadn't sold it already. Used-car lots were cheek by jowl on both sides of Alameda for several miles. A pickup truck or a four-wheeler—the he-man car—was given center stage, its back end raised rakishly on a ramp. But on either side, a monotony of hoods made it impossible to focus. Banners screamed: SE VENDE BARRATO!; SI SE PUEDE!; AUTOLIABILITY BY THE MONTH!; NO DOWN PAYMENT! I gave up looking at cars and instead looked at faces.

O

On my second pass, just a mile from the hospital, I saw an older man sitting on a stoop, smoking a cigarette, his attitude jaunty, as if he owned that space.

It was Gato. I had not seen him since he'd left the hospital weeks before. I circled back and stopped in front of him. He looked at me with suspicion, then his brow relaxed. He glanced up and down the street, and sauntered over.

He was freshly shaven. When he leaned into the car, I could see the pack of Marlboros in the pocket of his safari shirt, and I caught the scent of tobacco mingled with aftershave.

Doing well, he said. Still at the halfway house. No, he didn't have a job yet, but he was looking. Not too many people wanted to fool with an ex-con.

"Say, Doc," he said, "let me take you to a place where you get the best *caldo* in town. Good for your strength," he said, holding up a stiff forearm like a *lingam* and grinning lewdly.

"I'm fine," I said. "But you probably need it . . . I'll come."

O

"*Es mi* doctor," Gato said proudly to the shapely but very pregnant proprietress of the tiny cafe. The kitchen was separated by a counter from the rest of the room. We sat down at one of the three tables.

I told him about David.

"That cocaine shit is bad," he said. "Once they start hearing the train, those fuckers are crazy. The train? It's like a *wheeoou-wheeoou.*"

"And you? Have you shot up since you left the hospital?" I asked once the proprietress had taken our order.

"Hell, I won't lie to you, Doc," he said, showing me his square teeth. "I came down here two days after I left the hospital. I split a dime bag with somebody. It didn't do shit for me. The stuff around these days, it's pathetic. Used to be, if you got arrested or went into the hospital, you'd be all shaky and sniffling. Now they bust guys in jail and they don't even sweat. They don't puke. It's no good, the stuff they're selling."

I didn't ask if he had shared needles. In the hospital, he was HIV negative, and surprisingly showed no exposure to hepatitis B or C.

The food arrived, spilling over the bowls.

"You like spicy food, eh?"

"Love it."

"They have some chilies here. Stronger than jalapeño. *Pequin*. Pure dynamite. Watch yourself with it, okay?"

He gave instructions and the pregnant lady returned with a fiery red liquid in a tiny bowl. I cautiously put some in my *caldo*.

"I grew up right here. Ran a bar just around the corner."

"Is that when you started?"

"Hell no! I looked down on the hypes . . . fucking junkies nodding off. No. I was crazy about women and dancing. I would never be a hype."

He ate his *caldo* with relish, spooning out a few pieces of meat and putting it into a tortilla, holding this self-rolled burrito in his left hand as he spooned the soup up with his right.

"I got into a fight out there. Self-defense. Killed a guy. I was sixteen. Reform school for two years. I came back, and still you couldn't get me to use dope. When I ran the bar, I'd make good money selling to the junkies. My dealer kept after me, 'You need to try it, you must try it.' I tried it and puked like crazy. He kept after me and I tried it two more times, and by the third time I was into it. I was a big-time dealer. Ask anybody, Doc. I was the man here. Had my *gente firme* around me wherever I went. Broads. Cars. Even God had nothing on me."

It was stuffy in the cafe, and the clients coming in were mostly older men, looking not too different from Gato.

"I always carried my shit in my hand, slept with it in my cheek so I could just swallow it if the narcs busted in. One time I swallowed a packet this big," he said, making a fist. "Choked on that son of a bitch. I made bail and brought it out as soon as I got home."

I paid, and he stood up.

"Come on, Doc. You want I give you the quick tour? We'll look for your buddy?" He smiled mischievously.

Men like Gato made you feel that your manhood was being tested. There was nothing about his life—the hard time he did, the drug use, the manslaughter—that you envied, and yet when he flashed that arrogant grin, it was as if he dismissed everything you had done in your life as being sissy, *joto*. It tempted you to take some foolish risk just to prove him wrong, to show him you were one of the boys.

"Let's go," I said. "You think he's been around here? He mentioned under the bridge . . . the canal."

"I doubt it. I know most of the hypes around here. A guy like him would be pretty noticeable."

In the car, Gato kept up a commentary. "See that guy? He just got out of the pen after eight years and he's back in that shit . . . She's an old *puta* and I can't believe anyone pays her—she'd have to pay me and blindfold me to fuck her . . . God, will you look at that—" he said, eyeing two very young teens hitching a ride"—let's stop and get us some of that. Pussy in a gift box."

"No thanks," I said. "I like mine well-done."

He had me turn off Alameda. One block away, we came to a little bridge that spanned an irrigation canal, a canal that ran from the Upper Valley all the way to Socorro.

"Park here. The car is fine."

Gato calmly walked down an alley between two houses to a back fence. He squeezed through an opening that I had not seen.

"Come on, Doc! Don't worry."

"Gato, what about the people whose yard we just walked through?"

"Aw shit! Everyone knows me here." His swagger was more exaggerated. If the stoop where I had found him was his pied-à-terre, this was his manor.

The moon was out. Lights shone down from the windows and backyards of houses that adjoined the canal. The muddy water in the canal shimmered and ran swiftly with a pleasant whirring sound. On both banks, weeds and trees had overgrown, creating little grottos. "See down there?" he said, pointing in the direction of the water flow, "Under the bridge we just drove over? That's where we used to shoot up a lot. Especially when it was hot. You can always find some hypes there, using. Water's up now because of the rains."

So much for the tour. I was ready to turn back. But Gato was marching ahead, along a little path that ran parallel to the canal, behind houses and backyards, ducking branches as he went and pushing back weeds.

We rounded one clump of bushes and heard voices. I saw three pairs of legs. I felt a surge of adrenaline. I was ready to run.

"Hey!" I heard Gato say and walk into the clearing. When I followed, I saw three chocolate-skinned men in scruffy laborers' clothes, sitting on the ground and looking at us, swimmy-eyed. If I was scared of them, they seemed more scared of us. They sat there as if they had come to admire the view. *"¿Qué pasó?"* Gato said. *"Nada,"* one of the men replied, and said in Spanish that they were just resting. Gato took slow steps past them, fearless, studying them as if deciding whether to allow them to stay. Then they were behind us as we continued along the narrow path.

"Who were they, Gato?"

"Ah, fucking wetbacks. Said they were just resting. Maybe so, maybe they just came over the border." He was scanning the ground ahead of him, a bloodhound following a scent.

No more than twenty yards along the path, behind a clump of bushes, another three men. They must have heard us coming but they didn't stop what they were doing. A man in a purple shirt and orange aviator shades was kneeling on one leg, shooting into his forearm with an orange syringe. Another man, also kneeling, his back to us, was similarly engaged. The third simply stood there, as if shielding them.

"Hey," Gato called out, "how you guys doing?" When he got closer, he realized he knew all three. He shook hands with the man who was standing, peered over at the two shooters. *"Oye! Chingado!* Come here, see this? Don't worry, Doc, I know these guys," he said, beckoning me forward to watch the shooting, while he himself looked at the scene lovingly, the way women will bend to coo over a baby.

It was an eerie spectacle, almost a ballet set piece: two men kneeling, one standing, forearms bared, fists clenched, veins bulging, moonlight and a naked backyard bulb washing over them, glinting off the needles. They were younger than Gato, in their twenties. The man in the purple shirt tossed his head, throwing his carefully styled hair out of his eyes. He looked familiar, as if during the day I had seen him behind the counter of a fancy store or sitting in an expensive restaurant. I couldn't take my eyes off him. He stood up, animated, sniffing, looking me up and down, and then engaging in a rapid-fire exchange in Spanish with Gato. He had almost certainly injected cocaine, not heroin.

Unlike his clipped, staccato English, when Gato spoke Spanish, it was smooth and musical, but still full of *chingolés*—fuck words. He looked ready to spend the evening.

Gato looked my way and I pointed in the direction we had come from. I wanted a tour, but if the cops or the people against whose back fences we were congregating took a notion to chase us, how would I explain my presence? If we didn't leave soon, Gato would probably shoot up. This world, so normal to him, was terrifying to me. I wondered for a second if they were planning to rob me, or worse.

To his credit, Gato recognized my discomfort, and didn't mock it or turn on me.

"Hey, we'll catch you guys later," he said, and we headed back. As we passed the first group of men, who were still sitting there, the man in the purple shirt, who was following us, called out to Gato. I didn't hear quite what he said, but Gato said over his shoulder, "No, I got to go. Can't."

Just as we were about to slip back through the fence, Gato said, "Let's check out this one spot."

We were off in the other direction now. "See here," he said, pointing to a clearing in the weeds the size of a tiny pantry where a soggy mattress lay, bottle caps, needles, and empty water bottles all around. "Someone slept here." He grinned. "I probably slept here, except I don't remember."

We walked on another ten yards and saw a pair of legs sticking out from the underbrush. Gato strode confidently forward. "What have we here? Let's see, let's see . . ."

A chubby man in his twenties was seated against a wall, his legs stretched out in front of him. His sweatshirt said HARVARD in white letters on a background that might once have been crimson. He wore a filthy ball cap. Only when we got closer could I tell that he was a white man. His face was puffy and lethargic and he barely looked up.

"Hey!" Gato said, moving in briskly. "Hands up, man!" The kid made as if to rise and obey. "Just kidding, kidding, man. Do I look like fucking police, *pendejo*?" Now he was striding over the boy's outstretched legs. "See here, Doc," he said, picking up a bottle cap and handing it to me. "Peel out the rubber and make you a great cooker."

I put it in my pocket.

He bent down, sniffing out new evidence, as if the boy were not there. Three unsmoked cigarettes lay in the dirt next to the boy's legs, and Gato fingered one of these. "These yours?" The boy mumbled unintelligibly. Gato dropped the cigarette and picked up a syringe, caked in mud. And then he wrinkled his nose.

"Smells of shit," he said. He spat and looked at the boy. "How can you sit here in this shit? *Chingado!*" He spat again, took a step back. "Stupid fucker. Sitting in his own shit."

I thought the boy was a schizophrenic because he was so disconnected and mute. He sat rooted in the dirt. "There's a little something here, if you want . . ."

Gato peered, his sight not very good. All I could see was mud in the boy's hand.

"No," Gato called. "You go ahead. You have it." He laughed to himself. "Stupid fucker."

We slipped back out through the fence. Gato was pleased. He had promised to show me his world and he had found it intact, just the way he had left it.

○

Alone now, I drove into downtown proper, studying faces, faces that were so obviously *not* David, but my eyes lingering nevertheless, as if a face might transform into his. I turned onto Ochoa, then San Antonio, where a number of gay bars clustered together, the patrons spilling into the street, the flashing strobe lights visible under the windowsills, the deep bass thumping through the walls. A transvestite looked at me inquiringly and then, on St. Vrain, a hooker took my examination to be an invitation. She showed me the finger when I shook my head.

In the late 1800s, when Sun City was better known as Sin City, this part of town had boasted the grand mansions run by Gypsy Davenport, Tillie Howard, and Alice Abbott—El Paso's best-known madams. In the parlors of these houses on what was then Utah Street, a small orchestra played, and a staff of servants waited on the visitor. For the less wealthy, women could be found at the Monte Carlo and the Jim Burns Red Light Dance Hall. For a dollar, you could go to their crib on Utah Street. Or, if she were a colored girl, to Overland Street.

I passed Café Central, which had the best cuisine in El Paso. I was a block from where John Wesley Hardin was gunned down. At the stoplight, a group of brown-skinned, tubby Brahmins in tuxedos crossed over to the Camino Real Hotel, going to a black-tie reception, I imagined. I read worry in their faces, the strain of keeping uneasy tabs on their younger wives—maybe their daughters?—who glittered ahead of them.

I left downtown, took the freeway, and instead of going home, decided to drive up Transmountain Road, something I had never done at night. It would take me to the side of town where David had lived with Mickie. Cattle rustlers years before had found a path—Smugglers Gap—that cut through the Franklins from the east side to the *bosques* of the Rio Grande on the west side, where a man and a good-sized herd of cattle could hide in the tangled jungle of cottonwood and mesquite. Transmountain Road commemorated the smugglers' route. The long straightaway, on which there were no other cars, rose several thousand feet. Then came a series of white-knuckle curves that were carved in a canyon. I sped through, shadow and moonlight alternating on my windshield. I came out to a long downhill straightaway, the lights of northeast El Paso displayed for me.

On Dyer Street, I thought of Angelina; this had been her beat. There were many motels, bars, strip joints, and nightclubs here. But now I was fed up, tired, my heart no longer in this search. My back was sore from sitting in the car. I parked and entered a dance hall to use the rest room, and then I sat at a dark corner table. The music was happy, polkas and *corrida*s alternating with Texas blues and even rockabilly.

I wanted to forget about David for a while, push him out of my mind, something I had been unable to do since the morning he had resigned.

I studied the animated expressions of the dancers. I saw the faces differently now, saw them as if I were an anatomist or an anthropologist cataloguing the compilation of noses and eyes, of lips and brows, of teeth and jaws, and the infinite variations possible as you mixed and matched. I could see clearly the traces of the Indians, colonists, conquerors, friars, trappers, traders, forty-niners, gunmen, gamblers, fancy women, hucksters and hookers, *Villista*s and *Porfirista*s, pimps and madams, lawmen and railwaymen who had made this town, a town in which David had successfully disappeared.

49

*I dash out of the hospital into the bright sunlight. It is two in the after-*noon and windy. Other than the police, at this moment, as I cut between cars in the parking lot, I am the only one who knows that David is dead. For the people who haven't heard, David's death is yet to happen. For them, he is still alive.

I run into an intern, a big, affable El Salvadoran sporting a bright green tie.

"Dr. Verghese, about Mrs. Escobedo—"

"Not now." I grip his arm. "I have to go to the morgue."

Then I say it: "David Smith is dead."

His face goes slack and his head lolls back as if I have hit him. He stumbles, reaches to support himself against a car that is not there. I grab him. I have a moment of perverse pleasure in seeing how he reels and totters, imagining how his day is now unhinged. I picture how the shock waves will spread through the rest of the staff— David's fellow interns in particular—and leave them frozen in door-ways. They will rack their brains for the memory of the last time they saw him, the last thing he said to them. They will play the before-and-after game that I am now playing.

○

On Alameda Street, leading away from the hospital, there is a pro-cession of hopeful signs: LUCKY CAFE, GOOD LUCK BAR, LUCKY TAVERN. Between the hospital and these neighbors only the cemetery inter-venes, claiming four city blocks. From the hospital's upper floors, patients look out through their windows over a sea of crosses.

The morgue, which I have never visited before, seems to sit *in* the cemetery even though it is not of the cemetery. With its mirrored glass front, stepped skylights, and large panels of marble and stone, it resembles a giant mausoleum.

Inside, it is cold. The orange carpeting, the modular furniture, and the ficus plants of the atrium have been imported directly from a Scandinavian furniture showroom. No echo here. No green tile. I sniff like a bloodhound, but not a whiff of formalin escapes.

The coroner's secretary is pretty, solicitous, experienced in these matters. She offers me coffee and a chair, but with her eyes she takes my pulse. I thank her and decline both. Yes, his next of kin are in Australia and are unlikely to come for at least a few days. A few code words into an intercom and then she weaves down a baffle of short corridors. I follow into the labyrinth, my eyes on her shoulder-length black hair that bounces with every step. Suddenly we are in another room. She positions me in front of a large glass partition and then she disappears.

I bring my hand up to shield my eyes from the glare of my own reflection. I see into a spotless, darkened chamber. My eyes fix first on the tiled floors—at last something morguelike here—and then, almost hidden in shadows, swinging double doors to the right. David will come through them. No, David's *body* will come through those doors.

I try to picture how it will look. The police have asked me to identify David's body. They need me to be certain it is he. They are pretty sure . . . I am pretty sure . . . still—

O

Wait, wait, I want to say when I hear voices and sense movement on the other side of the glass partition . . .

Overhead lights click on and chase away all shadows. The tiles become lustrous. The swinging doors bulge open and disgorge onto this stage-lit scene the backside of an attendant, then a stainless-steel gurney, then another attendant.

I have seen both the attendants around Thomason. One of them is a ringer we sneaked on to our internal medicine soccer team, a left-footed, fluid striker. They are surprised to see me. I raise a hand and then am embarrassed by this gesture. They are wearing thick rubber gloves, the kind you use to attend a mare in labor.

The attendants jockey the stretcher back and forth until it is right below me. I push against the glass and look down at the body on the gurney.

○

David's face is intact.

I feel a huge relief. I worried that I would carry away a horrible and lingering vision of him, of a face blown away, a grotesque *after* picture, a gaping hole of a death mask that would terrorize me at night, distort and supplant the memory of the real face of my friend. A stored-up breath leaves my body in a long exhale.

Still, the bony scaffold behind David's face is shattered, causing it to sag back as if it were a deflated football. The right eyeball has popped neatly out of the orbit and dangles by the optic nerve, staring at the toes of the corpse. It is, strangely, not repulsive to me: A splendid anatomical specimen has been delivered from its housing by a careful dissector. The eyeball is undamaged, a perfect sphere, shiny still, with a tinge of blue to the sclera and turgid from the vitreous fluid within. From the back of the eyeball, the optic nerve gathers its fibers together like a carefully combed ponytail and slips back between the closed eyelids.

There is a bloody pool at the back of David's head where it meets the metal of the gurney, a pottage of hair, sero-sanguinous fluid, brain. David put the muzzle of the shotgun in his mouth, pointed it up and back against the soft palate, perhaps shading to the right just a hair. The eyeball must have been forced out by the explosion that went off within the confines of the skull. This same dangling eye witnessed the shape and form of the treason about to unfold. And then he pulled the trigger.

A memory from when I was a medical student, a fragment of text from a forensic book, appears in my head. Criminologists of the late nineteenth century tried to dissect out eyeballs of murder victims, hoping to find the image of the killer preserved on the retinae. Now, in the presence of this body, I can see how that silly thought was formed.

○

I pull my gaze away from that eye and start again, clinically, through the glass, to examine this face. My hands reflexively reach for the instruments in my coat pocket. Their touch against my fingers is reassuring even though they are completely useless in this building. I see the blond hair, the small jaw that is so much like Rod Laver's . . .

The body looks smaller than how I remember it, perhaps because the oversized gurney dwarfs him. He wears boxer shorts and an El Paso Tennis Club T-shirt.

This looks like the T-shirt Emily gave him two days before he died. Yes. I had seen it in her car. She had been carrying that T-shirt and a tracksuit and a Bible for him in the backseat, just in case she spotted him a third time walking on the street. Each evening I had driven up and down Mesa Street looking for him, but it was Emily, on her way to and from school, who had run into him three different times. The last time he again told her to get away. He didn't want to talk. And he wouldn't tell her where he was staying.

But he accepted the change of clothes and the Bible and the fifteen dollars she put in the Bible, weeping suddenly, she told me, at this act of thoughtfulness and concern on her part.

"Why are you doing this for me?"

"Why are *you* doing this, David?"

He trotted out his worn excuse: She had left him, he couldn't do emergency medicine, he hated internal medicine.

"I wish you'd get your crap together and quit this," she said.

"I want you to know, I never, ever cheated on you." It seemed terribly important for him to tell her this, even though by now I knew that this was not true.

"You're going to be fine one day," he said. "You're going to have a husband and you'll be happy." He pushed away all her other offers of help. "Tell everyone thank you," he said.

Off he went, heading in a different direction each time, never toward the motel he was staying in.

○

One moment I was eating the lunch special, dipping into a bowl of *caldo de res* rendered fiery by home-canned serrano chilies being passed around the cafeteria table. The next moment, sweating slightly, my mouth on fire, I answered a page and was told David was dead. When I could speak, though not make my words come out straight, I had confused the sergeant with my questions.

Now, as I stare at the body, I reconstruct David's last moments: He was in bed. The Bible was on the nightstand. The TV was silent on its pedestal. Perhaps he was asleep. Or staring at the exposed rock wall that ran the length of his room, a feature of this motel that, when it first opened, must have seemed as radical as the wood-patterned Formica on the nightstands, or the bright yellow vinyl on the chairs. The tennis bag I had seen him disappear with, and which had surely held his shotgun, sat on the shaggy green carpet along with seven bottles of unused Vaseline Intensive Care hand lotion, each representing a bad check, a trip to Furr's where he would buy lotion and pay for it with a twenty-dollar check, pocketing the difference.

The cops knocked at the door of his motel room, ignoring the PRIVACY PLEASE sign. There was no peephole. David got up and cracked open the door.

Are you Dr. David Smith?

Yes.

We have a warrant for your arrest.

What for?

Bad checks.

That was our doing, we the friends-of-David. After checking at every motel on Mesa, we had tracked him to this one. He was registered in his own name. We sent the cops after him. To catch him and take him straight to the El Paso County detox, bypass jail, get him off the street.

David closed the door, as if to slip the chain off. But instead, he turned the dead bolt.

One cop ran to the back of the motel, thinking he might be diving out the window. The other cop banged on the front door. David made a phone call. "Mickie? MICKIE!" Mickie, his former landlady, was out and only her answering machine recorded the despair in his voice, the pounding in the background . . .

And then came the boom of a shotgun, a deafening blast that reverberated down the corridors.

The cops took cover.

Motel guests were flushed from their rooms.

The SWAT team arrived and with them the press and every other scanner hound nearby.

It was a while before they stormed into David's room and found his body.

○

The coroner's assistant materializes beside me. I am petulant. Where was she all this time? I am resentful of her tidy appearance, her perfume, her professionalism, her matter-of-factness, the way she wears the reserve and severity of this building. There is a process here that she is comfortable with but that hasn't been explained to me sufficiently.

"I can't be sure it is him," I say finally. "Can I go in there?"

She goes out to ask the coroner.

I wait.

The two attendants stand deferentially on the other side of the glass, their hands resting on the gurney. I know how they feel: This is just another body to them, and yet they have to act a certain way in the presence of the living. Once I'm gone they can resume their chatter, the Tex-Mex Spanglish patois that I caught from behind the closed door before the stretcher came through.

The assistant returns. "You can go in."

She escorts me out and around and through the double doors and then she leaves.

○

Suddenly, I am on the other side of the looking glass, under the theatrical lights, in the tiled room, beside what is left of my student, my intern, my tennis partner, my friend.

There is a visceral smell now, the miasma of a freshly opened cadaver, not unpleasant but leaving me feeling as if I had stumbled on to someone's most intimate scent, the kind left on their bath towel or that wafts up from their laundry hamper. There are so many odors in medicine; if I had students next to me now, the pedant in me would recite the list that I have memorized: the moldy-hay smell of typhoid, the mousy odor of liver failure, the sweetish acetone odor of diabetic coma . . .

But this odor is not in my canon of odors.

I move closer and lean over the body. My hands come out of my coat pockets, restless again, an instinctive response when you put me close to a recumbent figure. David's face is as I saw it from behind the glass. The skin is dry and flaking, there is three or four days of stubble around his chin, the fine wrinkles at the corners of his eyes are exaggerated by the light. But, as a face, it yields no more clues. My fingers want to reseat that eyeball in its socket.

Instead, I lift up his T-shirt. The scaphoid belly and the thin, hairless chest look like David's. A loss of at least fifteen pounds in the last two weeks. I run my fingers down his arms. There is a salmoncolored bruise and a pale puncture mark in the crook of his left elbow. Before I am aware of it, my fingers are rooting reflexively on the inner side of his biceps tendon. A cold, pulseless, brachial artery submits to my touch.

His hands are ensconced in brown paper bags. I reach to remove them.

"Don't!" one of the attendants says. "Sorry, Doc. *Es que*, they need to do the gunpowder test."

"Like there's some doubt as to who pulled the trigger?"

He shrugs and smiles.

I leave the paper bags alone. I inspect the lower torso, the thighs, the knees.

○

I turn at last to the feet.

And then I know for sure it is David.

His feet are pointed down and turned out at the heels to make a V. I see the toes with the prehensile curl in them, toes I recognize from the locker room, and from when he padded around my apartment barefooted. I see the pearl-like calluses over the joints of his second and third toes, and the knobby excrescence of hardened skin on the side of the big toe of the right foot. The toe cap of his right sneaker would wear out long before the left, from his dragging that foot to the line as he launched into his serve.

○

His battered toes carry the stigma of his past life, before he was a doctor, when he was a professional tennis player. Those toes were shaped by scuffing on ant-dirt courts in Australia, sliding on clay and skidding on grass in Europe, pounding on American cement and Har-Tru. They are surprisingly coarse when contrasted with the grace of his movements on the court.

I laugh. The attendants have been watching me with concern and now they are positively alarmed. I want to tell them how he said when he was playing college tennis his feet ached so much that he would limp off the court after a match, then limp around all week, limp during practice, eventually limp back onto the court for his next big match where he would leap and pivot and scramble brilliantly only to limp off again . . . it was a running joke among his teammates. And I remember the way he told me this, laughing at himself, his smile so broad that his eyes were buried in the crinkles that formed around them.

I straighten up. I don't say any of these things.

I adjust his T-shirt, pull it back into place, tug it down so it covers his boxers.

This is undoubtedly David. But I am reluctant to leave. This is the picture I have been left with: a deflated face, a wasted body . . . the familiar curl of his toes.

50

The plane gathers speed. Steven and Jacob clutch the armrests, and are pushed back into their seats. Their faces are anxious but their eyes are bright with excitement. We are heading to Florida for Thanksgiving with my parents and my brothers. For days now, the boys have had their backpacks ready, their swimsuits packed, and they have talked of nothing but this journey.

Steven was born not far from Plymouth Rock, and for both my sons, Thanksgiving is simple, uncomplicated, genuinely their celebration. For me, this holiday is more involved, still an acquired ritual, one that I learned in my twenties. There is the complication of the *other* Thanksgiving: Oñate's arrival at the Rio Grande, celebrated in April in El Paso. And, I wonder, should there be a day to balance Thanksgiving, a day to ponder sorrow and remorse?

After all the anticipation of this trip, my sons found the waiting at the airport intolerable, the process of boarding painfully slow, the push back from the gate sluggish, and the taxi to the runway felt like a long tease.

But now, as the plane hurtles down the runway, all is forgiven, speed erases all the aggravation and Steven lets out a "Yes!" as ever so gently the plane lifts its nose, then breaks our connection with the ground.

I love takeoffs, love the steady climb that makes my limbs feel heavy and makes sleep seem so easy. I am looking forward to my mother's cooking, to seeing my father, to taking the boys to the beach—

And suddenly I think of David.

I see his face so clearly. Not the death mask, but instead David laughing, David trying to catch his breath after a rally that was more slapstick than tennis.

When David died, I told my sons he had died in a car accident. His memorial service was not the first they had attended in their young lives. They had seen some of my patients who, later, were not just patients but my friends struggle valiantly with AIDS, fight to live, but ultimately wither and then die. My sons had made home visits with me, come to know and love Uncle Jim, Uncle James . . . I never had qualms about their seeing death: Perhaps it would lend urgency and poignancy to their lives.

But when David died, I could not bring myself to tell them that he took his own life, that such a thing was possible. I invoked a car accident in which he was blameless—the equivalent of a tornado or a flood. But a few months after he died, they found out, overhearing me on the telephone when I thought they were fast asleep in their bunk beds. They came down and confronted me.

"Suicide means he killed himself, right?"

I nodded.

"How did he do it?"

"With a gun," I said, holding my breath, stupidly hoping they would stop there.

"Why?" On their faces I saw uncertainty, fear, disappointment that I had lied to them. A death had occurred a certain way, they had come to terms with it, and now they had found out that it had, in fact, happened in another way, had completely different implications.

I have come to think of this as the metastasis of suicide, this transformation of a brutal act into a "Why?" in the minds of the living.

O

Perhaps I think of him now because we fly over the Franklins, and the boys point excitedly to the Queen of Peace Church and other landmarks near their house and mine.

Emily and I climbed high up a trail off Transmountain Road to scatter his cremains, the duality of this new term appealing to me. It amazed me that David's body could be reduced to fill a plastic-lined carton that fit into a backpack. What we poured out—powdery and dry, black with flecks of white gristle—disappeared without a trace into the rock and sand and creosote. I saved a handful, feeling most of it escape between my fingers even as I tried to stuff it in my pocket. After our trek, we drove to the court he and I had loved and I emptied my pocket. The wind was gusting and perhaps none of it stayed on the court, blowing straight out of my hands into thin air.

I have found myself telling our story to strangers: how I still feel betrayed by David, by his death. How I was his teacher and his mentor, and how, on the tennis courts, he fulfilled those roles for me. How we had found a third arena outside the defined boundaries of hospital and tennis court, found it at a time in both our lives when friendship was an important way to reclaim that which had been lost. We had built it up, carefully, the way two boys fashion a sand castle with spades and buckets, ignoring the rising tide. But it was not the tide that washed it away. David knocked down his half; it lay sightless and bloody in a cold mortuary.

○

I have come to a sacrilegious belief: The living, vibrant essence of David—his psyche—pulled the trigger. But even as it did that, at some unfathomable level his psyche must have thought itself immortal. Why take your life unless you believe death is a transformation to a more agreeable state? And how can you even think "agreeable state" unless you also imagine some particle of yourself surviving to witness the change? David shoved aside the hands that reached to help him, and instead with his shotgun blasted through the brick wall he had come up against. In so doing he made his final assertion: I walk alone.

I have talked to the experts, read all the theories that apply to David. "David just fucking loved cocaine," was the opinion of one therapist, an astute man who knew David well. "He killed himself because he had blown it as far as being a physician, had no more stomach for rehab, and didn't want to do anything else with his life. One last, great coke run, one bad-check spree to beat the band, and then the shotgun to make his escape."

I have formed my own opinion. David's illness was far removed from the mere act of sticking a needle in a vein. I can only imagine that his disease began in childhood, and that it was a disease of the soul. I know almost nothing about his childhood, but I know that what he felt was universal. A child will always feel insufficient and powerless in a world of adults.

We grew up, and on the surface, we left our childish ways, overcame these feelings. Then, in the middle of the journey of our lives, we found ourselves, like Dante, on a dark path. It was there my road diverged from David's. My dark path, no matter how many times I relive it, would never have led to suicide. There was too much I believed in, too many things I held sacred. My escape from the dark path came from reaching out, primarily to him, but also to my parents, my brothers, my friends, a network of human connections. It was *David's* hand more than any other that pulled me free, set me back on my feet, made me feel I was not alone. Gratitude for that is at the root of my love for him.

Sadly, I could not do the same for him. His dark path, his pain, created an isolation, and pretty soon he became an island unto himself, a prisoner in a solitary cell of his own construction. Drugs were a way to at once further the isolation and yet ease its pain, to keep the world and its people at bay. Such a pity that the drug effects lasted only a few minutes, that they never effected a permanent change, and in the end, even the drugs failed him. Chasing success—first in tennis and then in medicine—was another way he sought to cure his pain, his dysphoria. Like so many of us, perhaps he was drawn to doctoring because he subconsciously thought that if he attended to the pain of others, it would take care of his own.

○

I have come to believe that AA and NA worked for David (albeit temporarily) by leading him out of his isolation, showing him he was part of a community, he did not walk alone. Recovery forced him to repopulate his world again, bring down the walls of his prison. It introduced him to extraordinary people like Emily and Mickie; it brought him the wise counsel of Dr. Doug Talbott, the advice of Jim, his sponsor. I have seen the same phenomenon in my HIV clinic: A newly diagnosed man feels his world has ended. Reluctantly, he joins a support group, all of whose members have the same diagnosis. It is at first reassuring, then uplifting, and enables him to shed his secrets, to be honest and open with himself and his family. And two years later, despite falling CD4 counts and the virus gaining ground, he tells me with some amazement that he has never felt more whole, more alive, never felt happier. As if it were his pre-HIV world that had been the fatal illness, now cured.

"Within your secrets lies your sickness," Dr. Talbott had said to me when I talked to him long after David's death. If David never sustained a lasting recovery, it was because he never let go of his secret, there were some bars that never came down. His secret is still with him. He still walks alone.

O

I cannot help but believe that David's aloneness, his addiction, was worse for being in the medical profession—and not just because of ease of access, or stress, or long hours, but because of the way our profession fosters loneliness.

Despite all our grand societies, memberships, fellowships, specialty colleges, each with its annual dues and certificates and ceremonials, we are horribly alone. The doctor's world is one where our own feelings—particularly those of pain, and hurt—are not easily expressed, even though *patients* are encouraged to express them. We trust our colleagues, we show propriety and reciprocity, we have the scientific knowledge, we learn empathy, but we rarely expose our own emotions.

There is a silent but terrible collusion to cover up pain, to cover up depression; there is a fear of blushing, a machismo that destroys us. The Citadel quality to medical training, where only the fittest survive, creates the paradox of the humane, empathetic physician, like David, who shows little humanity to himself. The profession is full of "dry drunks," physicians who use titles, power, prestige, and money just as David used drugs; physicians who are more comfortable with their work identity than with real intimacy. And so it is, when one of our colleagues is whisked away, to treatment, and the particulars emerge, the first response is "I had no idea."

It is not individual physicians who are at fault as much as it is the system we have created. So many doctors and medical students came to my office after David's death, cried with me, expressed concern for me as if I were the grieving widow. Over a hundred people showed up at the funeral home for David's memorial service, all of them deeply affected by his death, sitting as one body behind his sisters and his father, behind Emily. Gloria was there too, in the back pew, weeping.

Mine was the only eulogy at the service. I blush to remember how nakedly in that eulogy I expressed my sorrow, my shame. But I am proud too that I celebrated his life, consecrated our friendship. It would have amazed David, but perhaps not have saved him, to know that at the end, even as I stumbled through my last words, my voice breaking, that so many others wept for him.

○

We are at thirty thousand feet, slowly but surely leaving West Texas, the gray-brown of the desert, the colors of my adopted home, now giving way to greener, undulating land. On the right side of the plane, the sun is setting on a curved horizon, while on the left, night has come and the stars are visible. My sons, after all the excitement, after dinner, fall asleep, their necks lolling on their shoulders, their faces in sleep revealing an innocence that is, I think, still at the core of every one of us. I adjust their bodies so they are wedged against me.

I close my eyes and still see David. I hear the squeak of his sneakers, and watch him plant his front foot at just the right distance from the oncoming ball. I see the grace of that pose, just before he leans into the ball, the racket held high and laid back, his arm straight, his lips slightly parted, his left hand gently cupping the throat of the racket . . .

I recall that moment when we turned off the lights at our secret court, throwing it into pitch darkness, groping our way like blind men to the bench. Then, as our pupils adjusted to the night, and as we looked heavenward, it was as if one by one, then by the tens and hundreds, the stars appeared, a private showing for just the two of us. It was an illusion of course; they had been there all along. That panoply of stars dwarfed us, rendered us insignificant, made the ritual of the yellow ball and its flight seem absurd.

But soon, another thought followed, the converse of the first: that at this moment, nothing was as important as the two of us keeping that ball in play. The universe and our very lives depended on this one thing: Get the ball back over the net just one more time.

Acknowledgments

Many people gave me their time and were patient with my questions. I particularly thank Kristen Kelley, Gloria Esparza, Mickie Canciennce, Raj Masih, Lou and Nancy Binder, Joe Kasberg, "Duke" at El Paso County detox, Trey Carter, Sonny and Pat Farr, Pamela Lynch, Bruce Berman, Luis Jimenez, Brian Nelson, Darius Boman, James and Barbara Farnum, Barbara Allen, Jack and Adri Peacock, Max Ponce, Chevo Quiroga, Karen Marasco, Pedro Blandón, Armando Meza, Karen Davis, Stuart Levitz, Jo Seibel, Earl and Janice Greene, Helen Cherry, Pete Duarte, Delia Gallo, Olga Ortega, Belia Parra, Tommy Holmes, Martha Cornog, Coco Balew, Timothy Perper, Joe Old, Keith Wilson, Ken Wiant, Art Anderson, David Kruzich, and the staff of the Texas Tech Medical Library.

Doug Talbott welcomed me, gave me housing, and despite his hectic schedule, took great pains to educate me, even finding time for a squash lesson. To him and to the staff of the Talbott-Marsh Recovery Campus, as well as to the residents undergoing treatment who shared their stories with me—particularly Al—I am eternally grateful.

Several books were of great help:

For the Southwest: *El Paso: A Borderlands History*, by W. H. Timmons; *Pass of the North: Four Centuries on the Rio Grande*, volume 1, by C. L. Sonnicksen; *Border: The U.S.–Mexico Line*, by Leon C. Metz; *Great River: The Rio Grande in North American History*, by Paul Horgan; *The Texas Monthly Guidebooks: El Paso*, by Eric O'Keefe; *Legends of the American Desert: Sojourns in the Greater Southwest*, by Alex Shoumatoff; *The Franklin Mountains: Beginning of the Rockies*, by Michael Moses and Alex Apostolides; *La Frontera: The United States Border with Mexico*, by Alan Weisman.

For tennis: *The Courts of Babylon,* by Peter Bodo; *Big Bill Tilden: The Triumphs and the Tragedy,* by Frank Deford; *Match Play and the Spin of the Ball,* by William T. Tilden, II; *Pancho Segura's Championship Strategy,* by Pancho Segura with Gladys Heldman; *Bud Collins' Modern Encyclopedia of Tennis,* by Bud Collins and Zander Hollander; *Winning Ugly: Mental Warfare in Tennis Lessons from a Master,* by Brad Gilbert and Steve Jamison; *Hard Courts: Real Life on the Professional Tennis Tours,* by John Feinstein; *Love Match: My Life with Bjorn,* by Mariana Borg; *Golf Dreams: Writings on Golf,* by John Updike; *Arthur Ashe: On Tennis,* by Arthur Ashe with Alexander McNab; *Top Spin: Ups and Downs in Big-Time Tennis,* by Eliot Berry; *Ivan Lendl's Power Tennis,* by Eugene L. Scott.

For medicine: *The Pathology of Drug Abuse,* second edition, by Steven B. Karch; *Suicide and the Soul,* by James Hillman; *Should You Leave?,* by Peter Kramer; *Zebra Cards: An Aid to Obscure Diagnosis,* by John G. Sotos, M.D.; *Smell: The Secret Seducer,* by Piet Vroon.

The lesson with Pancho Segura appeared in a different form in *Sports Illustrated.* A portion of chapter 17 appeared in a different form in *The New Yorker.*

The names and identities of patients who appear in this book have been changed in order to protect their anonymity. The name "Emily" is also a pseudonym.

Melanie Whiley provided valuable secretarial assistance for well over two years, for which I am deeply grateful. Ross Walker went over the tennis elements in the book, and Leon Metz read all references to El Paso, but I am responsible for any errors.

I am deeply grateful to Mary Evans, my agent and friend, for her hard work and her constant encouragement, which began in Iowa in 1991 and continues to this day. Jonathan Burnham and Alison Samuel of Chatto & Windus offered valuable advice, as did Abner Stein in London. Joëlle Delbourgo and Tim Duggan of Harper-Collins shepherded the manuscript through its final stages.

This book would not have been possible without the extraordinary efforts of Eric Steel, out of whose vision this project emerged. He served as my editor, first at Simon & Schuster, then at HarperCollins and, when he moved to Scott Rudin Productions, somehow found the time to continue putting in many hours on the manuscript. His clarity of thought, his discerning eye, and his judgment at every stage made this book what it is and I am deeply grateful to him.

To David's sisters, Phillipa and Paula, who supported this project, gave me their time, shared photographs and memories, painful as it must have been, I hope this will help to heal the wounds.

To the two women who were most significant in David's life, and who shared their stories, their understanding, held back nothing, and trusted me to tell this story, you have my undying admiration and gratitude.

Finally my wife, Sylvia, her mother, the rest of her family, and my sons put up with me through the long gestation period of this manuscript, allowing me the luxury of writing. Sylvia gave birth to a true masterpiece while I labored on this book: our son Tristan. To all of them, all my love.

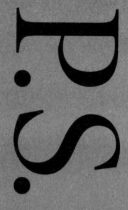

Insights,
Interviews
& More . . .

Meet Abraham Verghese

ABRAHAM VERGHESE is known for his acclaimed nonfiction work, including *My Own Country*, which was based on his experiences as an AIDS physician in Johnson City, Tennessee, and became a finalist for the National Book Critics Circle award. His second book, *The Tennis Partner*, was a *New York Times* notable book and a national bestseller. His third book, *Cutting for Stone*, published by Knopf, is a *New York Times* bestseller. He has published extensively in medical literature, and his work has appeared in *The New Yorker*, *The Atlantic*, the *New York Times*, and the *Wall Street Journal*.

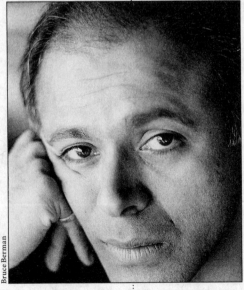

Board-certified in internal medicine and in pulmonary and infectious diseases, Verghese attended the Iowa Writers Workshop at the University of Iowa, where he earned his MFA. He is currently on the faculty at Stanford University as senior associate chair and professor of the theory and practice of medicine in the Department of Medicine. ❧

Bruce Berman

Match Point
A friendship that developed across the net turns into a matter of life and death for one of the players.

By Caroline Knapp

This review appeared in the New York Times, *August 30, 1998. Used by permission of the Doe Coover Agency.*

Abraham Verghese—fervent tennis player, physician, and author—is mesmerized by the sound of the human heart. As a boy growing up in Africa, he first heard echoes of it in the steady "thunk-a-thup" of a tennis ball against a racquet, a profoundly soothing sound that served as a balm against the claustrophobic unhappiness of his parents' home. As a medical student in Madras, India, he was "carried . . . to the exact same state of mind," transported and calmed, by the "lub-de-uh, lub-de-uh" of the real thing. Tennis and medicine have remained Verghese's primary passions, and they have turned him into an astute observer, a man who not only listens to heartbeats but also recognizes their darker and more mysterious workings. *The Tennis Partner: A Doctor's Story of Friendship and Loss* is Verghese's account of his friendship with David Smith, a young Australian intern Verghese met shortly ▶

3

after joining the department of internal
medicine at the Texas Tech School of
Medicine in El Paso. It is, as the subtitle
suggests, a story about many things—
medicine and relationships and grief—
but it is above all a story about human
nature, about the heart's baffling capacity
to lead us either toward one another or
astray, to generate either healing or pain.

When Verghese first meets Smith,
his own life is in a bit of a shambles:
a full professor at thirty-seven, he
is doing well professionally, but his
marriage is falling apart and he's
lonely, an outsider both as a foreign
medical graduate and a newcomer to
Texas. He feels an immediate kinship
with Smith, who not only shares
his outsider status and its attendant
edge of self-consciousness but also his
fanaticism about tennis: Smith came
to Texas on a tennis scholarship and
played on the pro tour before enrolling
in medical school. The two begin playing
together twice weekly; a ritual—and a
friendship—is established.

Verghese is a fine writer, lyrical
and controlled, and he captures the
attachment between the two men—its
motives, its allure—with both precision
and charm. He is refreshingly honest
about his own vulnerability in the
early stages of friendship—its promise
evokes in him almost childlike feelings
of longing and excitement, making him
feel at times "like a boy eager to turn
a first date into a romance"—and he is
eloquent about their growing need for

each other. Both men, it turns out, are rather lost souls: increasingly estranged from his wife, Verghese moves out and takes up residence in a barely furnished apartment; Smith, who rents a spare room in a boardinghouse and is virtually friendless when they meet, leads a similarly Spartan personal life. Over time, tennis becomes both a vehicle and a metaphor for connection, placing them on common ground, allowing them to come "to know each other's tics and idiosyncrasies," helping them to fill some of their shared emptiness. "It pleased me," Verghese writes, "to think of his life and mine being parallel, overlapping, as if the sum of our two lives created a safer shelter than what we could construct alone."

That there is—or will be—trouble ahead is obvious from the outset: the book opens as a mortified and panic-stricken Smith is hauled off to the Talbott-Marsh clinic in Atlanta, a drug and alcohol rehab program specifically designed for physicians. But from there Verghese loops back to their first meeting, and the narrative takes on the feel of a mystery novel. Between rounds of tennis and postmatch chats at a cafe, there are glimmers of trouble, clues that something is deeply awry: an involuntary twitch occasionally flashes across Smith's face, "fleetingly bringing to the surface something darker, something wrenching and painful"; other staff members at the hospital seem oddly mistrustful of him; his ▶

Match Point *(continued)*

relationships with women have a frantic, tortured quality; the confidence and poise he exhibits on the court is strangely lacking off it. Smith finally reveals to Verghese that he's a recovering cocaine addict and that he's suffered several nasty relapses, the most recent one eighteen months earlier, during his fourth year at Texas Tech. The confession cements their friendship: one newly sober, one newly separated, both men are struggling to put their lives back together.

The Tennis Partner tackles complex, emotionally loaded subjects—addiction and recovery, sexual compulsion, friendship and intimacy, the elusive nature of change—and it would be easy to be heavy-handed with any one of them. But Verghese's style is understated and admirably free of psychobabble, and the narrative is as laudable for what it leaves out as for what it covers. Verghese doesn't pretend to understand the roots of his friend's troubles, describing his addiction simply as "a disease of the soul," and although he is quite self-aware and candid about his own emotions, he neither presses Smith for details about his inner life nor attempts to explain it himself. Instead, he relies on the tools he employs as an internist—careful observation, painstaking attention to detail—and simply tells the story: what it's like to find and love and need a friend, what it's like to watch that friend self-destruct.

This deliberate, restrained approach

gives a vivid sense of what addiction feels like to the nonaddict, the bystander left on the sidelines, helpless and confused. As Smith's life begins to spiral out of control, he grows more distant and unpredictable; his love life grows more chaotic; he reports that his A.A. and N.A. meetings "are getting to be a pain"; his earlier humility is replaced by an alarming edge of arrogance. There is horror in the transformation; there is also a wrenching sense of betrayal. The two men, Verghese writes, had built up a friendship "carefully, the way two boys fashion a sand castle with spades and buckets, ignoring the rising tide. But it was not the tide that washed it away. David knocked down his half."

The Tennis Partner is in some respects about a physician's particular vulnerability to addiction: Verghese describes quite poignantly the way the medical profession fosters loneliness, discourages the expression of emotion, leaves individuals to battle their demons alone. But in his search to understand what happened to his friend Verghese also touches upon more universal truths. Wise and compassionate, *The Tennis Partner* is about how we all cope with feelings of insufficiency and powerlessness in the world, how some of us manage to transcend fear and loneliness by connecting with others, and how some of us—no matter how well loved—fail. ⮑

A Reading Group Guide to *The Tennis Partner*

Topics for Discussion

1. Do you think David might have been a happier and healthier person had he chosen a different profession instead of medicine? Is there something about medicine that attracts addiction-prone individuals or that causes people to turn to drugs?

2. After returning from the Talbott-Marsh clinic, David proudly tells Verghese he has at last found "true recovery." A short time later he is back on drugs and more desperate than ever. What happened? Why does he relapse so quickly and tragically?

3. In a sense, this is a book about foreigners adjusting to a new country. How does Verghese use foreignness and alienation to heighten the intensity of his narrative? Talk about David's story as a kind of dark underside of the American dream of renewal.

4. "Tennis was so much more than a game," Verghese writes at one point—and yet, as he acknowledges at the end, it is also just a game: a simple, even slightly absurd ritual "of the yellow ball." How does Verghese manage to tie together so many of the book's complex strands through tennis?

5. Do you think Verghese is being honest—with himself and with us—about the sexual element in

his attraction to David? Do you think this is basically a healthy relationship? Or do you feel Verghese is unaware of how deeply involved and dependent he is on David?

6. David stands at a juncture between two opposite paths: an orderly middle-class existence in medicine with a wife and a "dream house"; and a hell of drug addiction, shame, poverty, disease, and death. Does David choose hell in part because the respectable middle-class existence is so hollow, so spiritually vacant? What other alternative could there be for someone like David? What about for Verghese himself?

7. Do you really believe that drug addiction is a "disease" comparable to diabetes or cancer, or do you think that talking about it in this way is harmful because it somehow absolves the addict of responsibility? Which view does Verghese endorse?

8. Talk about the statement that "David is responsible for David" and how it plays out in the two men's relationship in the final pages of the book. How can a true friend deny responsibility for his friend in crisis? Did Verghese act responsibly in calling the police or did he betray his friend's trust? ❧

Recommended Reading

Cutting for Stone by Abraham Verghese
(Knopf, 2009)

My Own Country by Abraham Verghese
(Vintage, 1995; Simon & Schuster, 1994)

Don't miss the next book by your favorite author. Sign up now for AuthorTracker by visiting www.AuthorTracker.com.